Removable Partial Prosthodontics

This Book is Dedicated to My Wife
Mary Louise without whose Encouragement
and Infinite Patience this Book Would Still
Be a Dream in the Mind of a Teacher

Removable Partial Prosthodontics

Ernest L. Miller, D.D.S., M.S., F.A.C.D.

Professor of Dentistry,
Department of Prosthetic Dentistry
The University of Alabama, School of Dentistry
Birmingham, Alabama

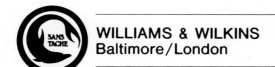

WILLIAMS & WILKINS
Baltimore/London

Made in the United States of America

Reprinted 1976
Reprinted 1978
Reprinted 1979
Library of Congress Catalog Card Number 72-75363
SBN 683-05989-0

Composed and printed at the
Waverly Press, Inc.
Mt. Royal and Guilford Aves.
Baltimore, Md. 21202, U.S.A.

PREFACE

It is often said that the mandibular complete denture that has failed might have been a successful removable partial denture, had the dentist who prescribed the prosthodontic service been endowed with better clinical judgment. This is more apt to be true today than at any other period in history as a result of advances in the fields of periodontics, endodontics, and preventive dentistry. While the need for full mouth extractions has certainly not been eliminated, an ever increasing number of partially edentulous, as opposed to completely edentulous mouths, are being seen in our offices and treatment facilities. One consequence of this phenomenon is that a sound understanding of this phase of prosthodontics is becoming more and more a *sine qua non* of successful dental practice. The purpose of this textbook is to provide the student as well as the practicing dentist with a straightforward approach to the basic principles of the subject so that he can conduct this phase of his practice with the sure knowledge and understanding that begets success.

For far too long it has been customary to begin the planning of the removable partial denture after all of the other needed dental treatment has been completed. Diseased teeth are removed and inlays and amalgams are placed in the teeth before any serious thought whatever is given to the design and construction of the prosthesis. A more error-prone, less efficient method of operation would be difficult to imagine. Planning for the prosthesis logically begins at the time of the examination or better yet at the time that the patient proffers his hand for the introductory handshake. And by all means before any treatment has been rendered, other than to allay pain. At this juncture, all options are open and amenable to intelligent exploitation in order to create conditions that favor a prosthesis of the most ideal design. This is the time when all relevant factors either favorable or unfavorable to the success of the prosthesis should be recognized and assessed. Armed with this knowledge, the designer can incorporate into the treatment plan the proper clinical procedures to fully exploit the former and most expeditiously compensate for the latter. Nothing serves better to illustrate the futility and wastefullness of piece-meal planning than the abutment tooth that has been restored with an MOD inlay, which reveals upon analysis on the surveyor that it has no usable retentive undercut. Or the discovery that insufficient interocclusal space has been provided to accommodate an occlusal rest in a gold crown that has been cemented to place on the abutment tooth. Accordingly one of the dominant themes of this book is to stress the critical importance of proper planning procedures.

Emphasis has been placed on clinical procedures as distinguished from laboratory techniques in the belief that the trend in dentistry is unmistakably in the direction of the delegation of ever more subprofessional tasks to auxillary personnel, thus making it possible for the dentist to concentrate his talents on the phases of patient treatment that he alone is qualified to accomplish. Moreover, there are excellent manuals available that describe laboratory techniques with commendable clarity and in beautifully illustrated detail.

In similar vein, the handling characteristics of chromium-cobalt alloy, as opposed to gold alloy, are stressed throughout the text since relatively few large castings are being made of gold today, largely as a result of economic imperatives. Indeed, it seems altogether logical to train the dental student in the techniques of handling the chromium-cobalt types of alloy since the odds so greatly favor his working with the "white" metal following his graduation.

In the final analysis, the merit of any textbook must rest on its capability of imparting knowledge to the reader. A dental text should be designed to accomplish this by either of two methods: first, as assigned reading for the student during his preclinical and clinical years and secondly as a reference source for either the student or the practitioner to look up a specific bit of information which temporarily eludes recall. Accordingly this text has been fashioned with a two-fold objective: (1) to explain basic concepts and principles of removable partial denture prosthetics as they relate to management of the clinical patient and (2) to provide a source of current authoritative information on all phases of partial denture planning and construction. To the extent that it presents a lucid explanation of basic concepts and provides an abundant storehouse of pertinent facts it will have attained its objective.

ACKNOWLEDGEMENTS

Successful publication of a textbook is often due less to any inate talent of the writer than to fact that he has been fortunate in the individuals with whom he has associated. I have been singularly blessed in this regard. I owe much to Dean Charles McCallum who provides for his teaching staff the sort of academic environment that stimulates and encourages creative effort. My deepest intellectual debt is to Dr. John Sharry who encouraged me to undertake the writing of a text in the beginning and who stood steadfastly by with scholarly counsel when it was needed. I am indebted to Dr. Frank Adams for his artistic talent in interpreting the crude drawings of the author with extraordinary insight and transforming them into technically accurate, meaningful illustrations. I should like also to acknowledge the guidance of Williams & Wilkins Editor, Mr. G. James Gallagher, who was enormously helpful in plotting a course around the shoals and reefs of the world of publishing. And finally I would be remiss were I to fail to mention the invaluable assistance of my wife who transcribed the countless drafts into beautifully typed manuscript with speed and accuracy.

CONTENTS

Chapter 1

EXAMINATION OF THE PATIENT

This chapter describes the procedures which are followed in examining the patient who is a candidate for a removable partial prosthesis. It is organized according to the following subject areas:

Introduction
The Preliminary Examination
Obtaining the History
The Visual-Digital Inspection
The Radiographic Survey
The Planning Cast
The Definitive Examination

Introduction

In no other phase of dentistry is the need for knowledgeable planning and forethought so vital to a successful outcome as it is in the practice of removable partial prosthodontics. The multitude of procedural and clinical details that must be coordinated into an orderly sequence makes it imperative that all factors bearing on the treatment be carefully evaluated so that each phase of therapy can be coordinated with the overall plan. Nothing serves better to illustrate the futility of piecemeal planning than the removable partial denture that cannot be worn comfortably because adequate space has not been provided for an occlusal or cingulum rest, or for some other essential part of the prosthesis. Or, of the discovery, following the cementation of a gold crown, that a vitally needed retentive undercut has not been incorporated into the wax pattern because at the time that the pattern was contoured the overall design of the prosthesis had not been considered. It cannot be overstressed that a comprehensive overall plan must be formulated well before any definitive treatment is begun.

The planning process for convenience of discussion may be divided into three major phases: (1) the examination, which includes the history, the visual-digital inspection, the radiographic survey, and the study cast analysis, (2) the selection of the prosthetic service to be prescribed, and (3) the formulation of the treatment plan. The interrelationship of these three steps in the overall planning of partial denture construction is depicted in Figure 1.1. Enumerating the types of clinical treatment that will be required cannot be done until the type of prosthesis or combination of prostheses is decided upon, while similarly the prosthodontic service cannot be prescribed until a thorough examination has been accomplished. The inseparable interrelationship and mutual dependence of these three phases of the planning process for a removable partial denture is thus illustrated. This chapter will be confined to a discussion of the procedures for conducting the examination. The succeeding two chapters will deal with the factors which are involved in prescribing the prosthetic service and in formulating the treatment plan.

The Preliminary Examination

Essential to the selection of the most appropriate prosthetic service and to the formulation of a thorough treatment plan is a comprehensive understanding of the individual who is to wear the prosthesis, so that the many judgments that must be made can be based on a thorough insight into his systemic health and emotional makeup, as well as on a detailed knowledge of his dental condition. The only

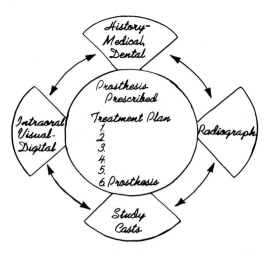

Fig. 1.1. The planning process involved in the design and construction of a removable partial denture consists of three major phases: (1) the examination which includes the visual-digital inspection, obtaining the history, the radiographic survey, and an analysis of the diagnostic casts (shown in the outer circle), (2) the selection of the prosthetic service to be prescribed (at the top of the inner circle), and (3) the formulation of the treatment plan (inner circle).

possible source of this information is by means of a thorough, orderly workup of the patient. The examination is customarily divided into a preliminary examination conducted at one appointment and a definitive examination which is accomplished at a subsequent one. A minimum of two appointments is needed because of the fact that radiographs and study casts are integral parts of the examination, thus requiring that time be programmed for processing of the radiographs and pouring and mounting of the study casts. The interval between appointments might well contain a period of time purposely set aside during which the clinical findings can be reviewed and the pros and cons can be weighed concerning the various types of prosthodontic service that may best serve the patient's interests.

Every dentist should develop his own routine of conducting the examination so that all relevant diagnostic procedures are accomplished in an orderly sequence. A methodical routine will minimize the pos-

sibility of inadvertently omitting an essential portion of the examination, thus setting the stage for subsequent faulty judgments.

The Covert Examination. Over and above the information that can be elicited from the history, the intraoral inspection, and the various other phases of the examination, the astute clinician can glean much additional knowledge of value from a discerning observation of the patient's behavior during his series of personal contacts with him. This is referred to as the "covert examination" and it begins when the patient is first greeted in the waiting room or the operatory. The unconscious deportment of an individual reveals much information to a trained observer and oftentimes these "personality clues" are invaluable in establishing a soundly based doctor-patient rapport in addition to being an aid in prescribing the most suitable type of prosthetic service.

The patient discloses by his appearance whether he is delicate, robust, or obese; by his gait whether he is well or poorly coordinated, vigorous or phlegmatic. The type of handshake which he proffers is meaningful. A moist, limp hand denotes nervousness and uncertainty; a firm handshake with a dry hand, confidence. A grossly untidy person of slovenly demeanor portends a very low quality of oral hygiene which will auger poorly for his success with an oral prosthesis, unless he can be persuaded to change deeply ingrained habits. Personal habits may be noted, such as nail biting, clenching, grimacing, and the like, any one of which might add to the difficulty of fitting the patient with a successful prosthesis. For example, a clencher would place additional stress on an oral prosthesis that would tend to overload the supporting tissues. A chain smoker or a nail biter may denote a hypertensive individual with a lower than average "discomfort threshold." The face may reveal calmness and composure which may be interpreted as favorable to the prognosis, or tension and irritability, as evidenced by a flushed frowning demeanor, which would be less favorable. Paleness traditionally denotes delicacy and fragility and very likely a lower than normal tolerance to inconvenience or annoyance. The voice, by its tone and volume, reveals confidence, fear, or hostility. The patient who is confident and eager to face the world is usually considered a promising candidate for an oral prosthesis, all else being favorable. A well modulated voice and a clear speech pattern indicates an above average level of intelligence. Such an individual ordinarily is well equipped to deal effectively with the relatively minor vexations which may be anticipated in adapting to a prosthesis. A weak tremolo is more indicative of a person who lacks confidence in himself and who will probably have a less than average capacity to adapt to a new situation. The eyes are well known as a source of clues to the inner person; dilated pupils betoken a sense of well being, contracted pupils signify uncertainty, fear, or an unfavorable reaction. The astute clinician will be armed with a wealth of pertinent information concerning his patient very early in their relationship as a result of having trained himself to be alert and perceptive.

Obtaining The History

Obtaining a good history is perhaps the most frequently neglected phase of the dental examination although it is a productive source of information that may directly affect the success of the treatment. The information revealed by a good history will often provide the supplementary bits of information which illuminate the way to a wise decision as to the type of prosthesis that the patient can wear with serenity, comfort, and health. For convenience it may be divided into a medical history and a dental history.

The Medical History

The medical history may be obtained either by what has been termed the "vending machine method," by a direct interview with the patient, or by a combination of the two methods. The vending machine method consists in handing the patient a printed questionnaire and in-

structing him to fill in the blanks. The second method is a structured interview in which key questions are posed to the patient regarding his health and the information is noted on an appropriate record. A combination of the two methods is perhaps most effective from all viewpoints. Certainly the dentist who takes the time to sit down and converse with the patient at eye level is making the most of an unmatched opportunity to establish a congenial rapport early in the doctor-patient relationship.

Obtaining the medical history will probably be more successful if it is prefaced by a simple explanation to the patient of its purpose. Most individuals are unaware of any connection between the state of their general health and the wearing of a prosthesis but they are quick to appreciate the significance when it is explained to them.

Areas to be Investigated. The prime purpose of the medical history is to establish the status of the patient's systemic health. Questions used to elicit this information should be structured so as to obtain a maximum amount of pertinent information with a minimum number of questions. The patient's age is significant because it provides a frame of reference for his physiologic status. Such things as puberty, menopause, pregnancy, and senility are age-related and each could have a bearing on the type of prosthesis that the patient will best tolerate. As age increases the individual's neuromuscular skills decrease and it is generally conceded that older people do not adapt to new situations as readily as do members of the younger age groups. Moreover, the oral epithelium of the aged patient tends to become dehydrated and lose elasticity; there is a diminution of salivary gland activity and the soft tissue in general loses its resistance to traumatic insult. Recording the age will identify the postmenopausal female who may have osteoporosis. This is typically associated with hormonal imbalance in which there is a decrease in estrogen output which in turn exerts an atrophic effect on the oral epithelium.

Systemic Health. The history should

reveal whether or not there is or has been any systemic illness, or if the patient is taking any drug that might affect the prognosis for an oral prosthesis. It should reveal any illness of which the patient is aware, and it is not unusual for a good history, as a part of a thorough dental examination, to reveal evidence of an incipient illness of which he has no knowledge. When some systemic disorder is suspected of which the patient is ostensibly unaware he should be referred to his physician for consultation. The utmost in tact should be exercised so as not to provoke needless anxiety.

Systemic Illnesses of Significance. Several systemic diseases can directly affect the patient's ability to wear a prosthesis comfortably, and the existence of such a disorder should become a part of the dentist's knowledge of the patient as a product of the examination. In addition to the ailments that are brought to light as a result of the medical history other disorders may be discovered by an alert examiner by a recognition of the oral symptoms. Some of the more common illnesses which may have oral manifestations and that can affect the patient's ability to wear a prosthesis comfortably follow.

Anemia. One of the most commonly encountered systemic disorders of significance to the prosthodontist is anemia. The anemic patient may have a pale mucosa, reduced salivary output, a sore, red tongue, and not infrequently gingival bleeding. He is much more prone to experience difficulty wearing a prosthesis comfortably than is the normal patient.

Diabetes. The prevalence of diabetes is quite high in the general population and the busy prosthodontist will encounter it frequently. Although the controlled diabetic (one in whom the blood sugar level and the glycosuria are controlled by diet or drugs or both) may as a rule wear a prosthesis without undue difficulty, the uncontrolled individual is a very poor risk for prosthodontic therapy. The diabetic is usually dehydrated, as manifested by a diminution in salivary flow. There may be macroglossia, and the tongue is sometimes red and sore. The teeth frequently loosen due to alveolar breakdown and there may be a generalized osteoporosis. The uncontrolled diabetic bruises easily and heals slowly, and represents a classic pitfall awaiting the unwary dentist who fails to avail himself of this information.

Hyperparathyroidism. The patient with hyperparathyroidism is prone to suffer rapid destruction of the alveolar bone as well as generalized osteoporosis. The dental radiographs typically show a complete or partial loss of lamina dura. Such a patient is a very poor risk for partial denture therapy.

Hyperthyroidism. The individual with hyperthyroidism may show no oral symptoms other than early loss of the deciduous teeth followed by an accelerated eruption of the permanent teeth. However, these are usually hypertensive individuals who are prone to be hypercritical and who typically possess a very low discomfort threshold. By and large they are poor risks for prosthodontic therapy.

Epilepsy. The patient with epilepsy may be taking Dilantin sodium, a drug which frequently produces hypertrophy of the oral mucosa, to control the disorder. Gingival surgery is usually indicated for such a patient prior to construction of a prosthesis. Following removal of the hyperplastic tissue, the patient who has demonstrated a tendency toward hypertrophy as a result of medication with Dilantin sodium may be switched, by his physician, to another drug which does not produce this side effect.

Arthritis. Treating patients with any type of arthritis raises the question of whether the disease may have affected the temporomandibular joints and this possibility should not be overlooked. If any of the usual temporomandibular joint symptoms are present, a careful assessment of the condition is recommended before constructing a prosthesis.

The Dental History

The valuable contribution made to the examination by a thorough dental history can scarcely be overstated. It is important, for example, to ascertain how the patient arrived at his present state of semiedentulousness. If the teeth were lost as a result of periodontal disease, the prognosis for the remaining teeth and the bone will not be as favorable as it would be if the loss were attributable primarily to dental caries. If the teeth were lost as a result of caries, this knowledge can be applied both in selecting the most suitable type of prosthesis to be prescribed and in formulating the treatment plan.

Patient Attitude. Many an oral prosthesis falls short of complete success because too much emphasis is placed on the purely mechanical aspects of construction while too little attention is paid to the fact that the patient is an individual with a unique psyche, with likes, dislikes, hopes, and fears peculiarly his own. Obtaining the dental history affords an unparalleled opportunity to learn exactly what the patient expects of the treatment he is seeking. A candidate for an oral prosthesis may reveal to a perceptive examiner, often inadvertently, expectations which no man-made prosthesis could possibly deliver and any treatment for such an individual should be prefaced by some preprosthetic conditioning. The fact that treatment with an oral prosthesis is a mutual effort of dentist and patient must be established early in the relationship. Failure to do so is to court defeat.

The Patient's Prosthetic Experience. An effective approach to gaining an understanding of the patient's attitude toward the contemplated treatment is to investigate his past experience with dental treatment in general and with prosthetic treatment in particular. The objective is to determine his attitude toward any oral prosthesis that he has worn or is wearing, or even more important, that he has been unable to wear. Does the present one fit? How many previous ones has he had? Is it comfortable? Is it acceptable in appearance? In short, what is right and what is wrong about it? When the fact is revealed that he was unable to wear a previous prosthesis it is important to establish the reason that he was not able to tolerate it and if possible the prosthesis should be inspected if it can be made available. The patient may complain that it "covered the roof of the mouth and I couldn't tolerate it" or that "I couldn't stand the bar under my tongue," for example. Some preprosthetic conditioning is obviously called for in such an instance before the treatment goes forward, or the new prosthesis may be foredoomed to end up beside the first one entombed in a dresser drawer. The experienced clinician will encourage the patient to ventilate on this subject knowing that the answers to these questions will provide valuable clues to his mental attitude as it may effect the wearing of a prosthesis and will augur well or poorly for success of the planned treatment. Interestingly enough it is not unusual to encounter an individual who, although having had a very limited personal experience with dentistry of any kind, has experienced vicariously some dental episode, perhaps through a close member of his family, which has served to color his opinions and attitude strongly. A spouse who has had an unusually unsatisfactory experience with a prosthesis is not an uncommon example. Any bit of information (or misinformation) which has influenced the patient's attitude towards dental treatment is germane to the dental history and could bear importantly on the type of prosthetic service which will best serve his needs.

Although the dental history is treated separately for convenience of discussion, it may be most expeditiously accomplished during the intraoral phase of the examination. If questions are carefully thought out and adroitly phrased the amount of time required to acquire this essential psychological insight will be inconsequential. If obtaining the dental history establishes a clear line of communication and a mutual understanding between patient and dentist so that the former knows what he can reasonably expect and the latter what is expected, it will have served an extremely useful purpose indeed.

The Visual-Digital Inspection

A meticulously thorough visual-digital inspection of the oral cavity is the very heart of the dental examination. It should be carried out under good lighting with a mouth mirror, explorer, and periodontal probe. An air syringe should be available to dry off certain areas as they are scrutinized since saliva is notorious for its ability to camouflage some oral structures. Indeed some areas can be so effectively obscured by droplets of moisture that important diagnostic signs are completely overlooked; calculus in the gingival crevice being a classic example. Either a printed form or a mental check list should be employed from which each phase of the inspection can literally or figuratively be checked off as it is accomplished. This will minimize the possibility of overlooking an important detail. For example, the teeth can be inspected for caries in one step, the periodontal inspection made in another, and the occlusion examined in a third. By concentrating attention on one phase of the examination at a time the chances for an oversight are greatly reduced.

Caries and Defective Restorations: The Caries Index

This part of the examination consists of a tooth by tooth inspection in which carious lesions are probed and the quality and condition of existing restorations are noted and charted. This information will be corroborated and may be supplemented when the radiographs are available for viewing at the second appointment. Not to be overlooked are the so-called "root caries" frequently found in the mouths of the partial denture candidate. These lesions are sometimes found on areas of the tooth where gingival recession has occurred and they are at times virtually impossible to restore properly because of inaccessibility. When such a lesion occurs on a tooth which is of strategic importance to the design of the prosthesis the decision to attempt a restoration or to sacrifice the tooth may be an especially difficult one. Marginal ridges on adjacent teeth which are of unequal height (Fig. 1.2), or not well aligned, are frequent causes of fibrous food impaction. The condition may be amenable to im-

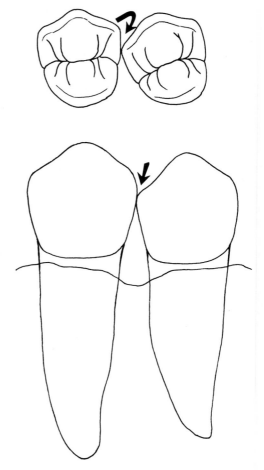

Fig. 1.2. Marginal ridges on adjacent teeth which are not well aligned (*top*), or of unequal height (*bottom*), are a frequent cause of food impaction between the teeth and should be corrected prior to construction of the prosthesis.

provement by inserting a properly contoured restoration.

The Caries Index. This is a logical juncture at which to make an assessment of the patient's inherent susceptibility to caries. It is worth noting, however, that a high caries index is not necessarily to be inferred from the fact that the patient has multiple restorations. He may have passed through a period of very high caries activity and have then arrived at a plateau of relative immunity. On the other hand, when the index is unmistakably high this fact must be given due weight not only in the type of prosthesis to be prescribed but in the overall treatment. For example, a complete denture might be prescribed in preference to a removable partial denture for the patient who is obviously caries-susceptible. If a removable partial denture is prescribed for such a patient, full gold crowns might be placed on abutment teeth which would not normally require full coverage.

Determining the Vitality of Questionable Teeth

It is important to identify any tooth for which there is evidence of degenerative change that might eventuate in loss of vitality at some future date, thus jeopardizing the useful life of the prosthesis. Certainly the possibility should not be overlooked that placing a clasp on a tooth with a pulp of uncertain status might activate a quiescent infection. Discolored teeth which elicit a history of traumatic injury or which exhibit abnormal symptoms should be tested for vitality. The radiographs may serve to disclose further evidence of viability or pathology when they are available for interpretation, although it is well known that a tooth can contain an unhealthy pulp while being completely asymptomatic clinically and disclosing no sign of abnormality in the radiograph.

A healthy pulpless tooth can be as useful as an abutment for a removable partial denture as can a tooth with a vital pulp, provided it meets the other criteria customarily applied to abutment teeth, and provided also that it has received proper endodontic therapy. An infected tooth, on the other hand, is a menace to the health of the individual and like any focal sepsis should either be returned to a state of health or removed. Several misconceptions once prevalent in regard to the pulpless tooth have been convincingly dispelled over the past few decades as a result of both clinical trial and reliable investigative work. For one thing it has been well established that the pulpless tooth is not a "devital" tooth as long as it is suspended in its alveolus by a healthy periodontal membrane which is attached to healthy vital bone. The apical nerves and vessels give off branches before they enter the apex of the tooth which innervate and nourish the periodontal ligament. The ligament is also nourished and innervated by nerves and vessels which reach it by means of small foramina in the bony walls of the alveolus. Although pulpless, such a tooth retains its proprioceptive mechanism, is vulnerable to attack by dental caries, and must be anesthetized to be painlessly extracted; in fact, the only sensation that is not retained by the tooth is pain of pulpal origin. While the concept of focal infection has long been recognized, the present concensus holds that a properly treated pulpless tooth is not a logical suspect as a focus of infection. Such a tooth should virtually never be extracted in the vain hope that this procedure may bring about a cure or meliorate some systemic illness.

The Periodontal Evaluation

The prevalence of periodontal disease in the general population is so high as to be considered epidemic. This has profound significance in partial denture construction since it is a basic tenet that an oral prosthesis inserted in the presence of periodontal disease is foredoomed to failure, and as a rule it will be early failure. By the same token, a properly designed prosthesis is an essential link in the treatment chain for the partially edentulous mouth that has been periodontally treated. Clinical observation bears out the fact that the candidate for a removable partial denture typically has periodontal disease and that the patient with periodontal disease is very apt to need a removable partial denture as a part of his total treatment. A properly designed prosthesis will prevent drifting and extrusion of the remaining teeth, help to prevent food impaction, assist in stabilizing the remaining teeth, and by restoring normal function forestall the process of deterioration which so often follows the loss of natural teeth.

The periodontal examination should begin with an inspection of the marginal gingiva and the interdental papillae for evidence of inflammation or infection and

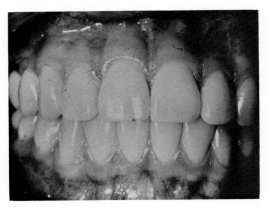

FIG 1.3. The gingival tissue illustrated in the photograph is in a state of health. The mucosa is firm, stippled, and coral pink. The gingival margin is smooth in texture and knife-like in form as it tightly envelopes the tooth. It extends occlusalward in the interproximal embrasure to the contact points to form the interproximal papilla.

the presence of materia alba, bacterial plaque, or calculus. The assessment of the health status of the periodontium should be based on the extent of deviation from normal. A healthy mucosa (Fig. 1.3) is firm, although slightly resilient, and coral pink. The gingival margin is smooth in texture and knife-like in form as it tightly envelopes the tooth. It extends occlusalward in the interproximal embrasures to the contact points to form the interdental papilla. The free margin is protected from the full impact of the bolus by the contour of the crown of the tooth while still being exposed to the gentle, physiologic stimulation from the flow of food during mastication. Immediately adjacent to the free margin is the attached gingiva. Its surface is stippled in appearance and as the name implies, it is tightly bound down to the underlying bone.

The use of a gentle stream of air directed into the gingival crevice should be routine when inspecting the gingival attachment. Evidence of mobility and pocket formation is significant, and the depth of any pocketing between the gingiva and the tooth or between the bone and the tooth should be carefully measured with the probe. Areas of food impaction should be noted since these are often

due to faulty interproximal contacts which are usually correctable. When inspecting tooth contacts for food impaction one should be on the alert for the contact which is ostensibly intact when the occlusal surfaces of the teeth are viewed with the mouth open but which separate slightly when the teeth are occluded under pressure. Many a periodontal pocket has been allowed to worsen because the clinician failed to make this observation. Gingival recession is especially significant in the mouth of a candidate for a removable partial denture because exposed cementum is particularly vulnerable to decay, and for this reason should not be covered with a clasp.

The Tooth with a Doubtful Prognosis

Tooth mobility and crater formation, as well as bifurcation and trifurcation involvement, are profoundly serious problems for the patient who is to wear a partial prosthesis, and when present their probable influence on the contemplated prosthesis should be carefully assessed. Arriving at a decision as to whether to extract or retain the periodontally involved tooth for the partial denture candidate requires a high order of clinical judgment. However, in the cold light of logic one must conclude that the tooth which has a doubtful or unfavorable prognosis should, with rare exceptions, be extracted in the best interests of all concerned. The practice of retaining a tooth with a doubtful prognosis, in the hope that it might respond favorably after the prosthesis is made, is ill-founded and all too often an exercise in futility. Sometimes a so-called "contingency design" is recommended so that in the event the questionable tooth is subsequently lost a replacement can be conveniently added on to the prosthesis. If a thorough examination is made and sound clinical judgment brought to bear this should rarely if ever be necessary.

The Quality of the Oral Hygiene

The patient's oral hygiene should be evaluated early in the examination procedure because this factor figures promi-

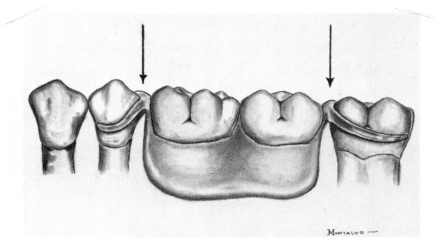

Fig. 1.4. The very important role that the terminal abutment plays in supporting the partial denture base is illustrated in the above sketch. When the prosthesis can be entirely tooth-supported, stress is directed along the long axis of the abutment teeth, which is the type of stress that they best withstand.

nently in the decision as to the type of prosthetic service that is to be prescribed. The patient whose oral hygiene habits are lax and who cannot be prevalied on to improve is not a promising candidate for a removable partial prosthesis, and in many instances the interests of such a patient are better served with a complete denture. In order to identify such an individual at the earliest possible juncture a regimen of home care should be instituted as soon as circumstances permit so that the result of his efforts to improve his oral hygiene can be observed throughout a long enough time frame to have validity. If the results of an effort to motivate such an individual to practice good home care are disappointing the prognosis for a removable prosthesis must be correspondingly downgraded. Anything less than assiduous home care augurs poorly for the success of a removable partial denture.

The Residual Ridges

Examination of the residual ridges focuses attention on the extremely important contribution that can be made to the stability of the removable partial denture by a terminal abutment tooth (Fig. 1.4). When the partial denture is supported entirely by natural teeth, all stresses are directed along the long axis of the abut-

ments, which is the type of stress that they best withstand. When no distal abutment tooth is available, horizontal and torsional stresses are transmitted to the abutment which may be damaging to the periodontium (Fig. 1.5).

The residual ridge in each edentulous area should be investigated both visually and by palpation in order to determine its contour and assess its potential load bearing capacity. If palpation is routinely employed the examiner will quickly develop a "feel" that will acquaint him with the structure being explored far better than would a mere visual inspection. The mucosa should be firmly pressed against the underlying bone to assess its thickness and resilience as well as the contour of the bone. If the patient evinces pain as the residual ridge is palpated with moderate pressure, his ability to wear a prosthesis with comfort is open to serious question and an effort to find the cause of the pain should be made so that some remedial treatment may be accomplished prior to beginning fabrication of the prosthesis. If radiographs reveal that the bone is rough and spinous, alveoloplasty may be helpful, although it may be that additional healing time is all that is needed. The same general area on the contralateral side may be palpated for comparison if it is compa-

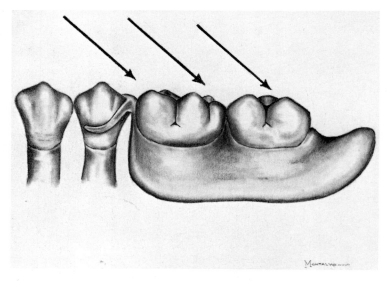

FIG. 1.5. When the denture base is supported at only one end by an abutment tooth and must be partially supported by the residual ridge, the stresses that are transmitted to the abutment tooth have both horizontal and torsional components. This type of stress may be damaging to both the periodontal apparatus of the abutments and to the bone of the residual ridge.

rable in structure. If the edentulous ridge is destined to support a portion of the prosthesis, then the bony contour as well as the thickness and density of the overlying mucosa are of critical importance. If, on the other hand, the prosthesis will be entirely tooth supported then this factor diminishes somewhat in importance. Much variation in both the contour of the bone and the type of density of the overlying mucosa will be found between the maxilla and the mandible, as well as in different regions of each jaw.

Torus Mandibularis. The lingual surface of the mandible in the cuspid and first bicuspid region should be palpated for the presence of bony exostoses. (They occur in approximately 7% of the population.) When present these bony elevations can be a major obstacle to comfortable wear of a prosthesis since the mucosa overlying the torus is invariably thin and easily traumatized (Fig. 1.6). If a lingual bar is positioned so as to avoid contact with the torus it must extend medially farther than normal into the alveolingual space. This places it too far into the domain of the tongue, an intrusion that this curious

organ may not welcome, and a fact of which the wearer of the prosthesis may be made acutely aware. If the lingual bar of a distal extension base partial denture is positioned superior to the torus (Fig. 1.7) in an effort to avoid contact with the edge of the bar, it will descend guillotine-like into contact with the mucosa as the denture bases settle (Fig. 1.8).

At times there may understandably be a temptation to spare the patient the discomfort and inconvenience of a torectomy, particularly when he tends to be resistant to the thought of surgery. It should not go unnoticed, however, that the individual who is thus spared this relatively minor ordeal may well be the one who professes an inability to adapt to the prosthesis because he cannot tolerate the bar under his tongue. It cannot be overstressed that such surgery, when indicated, should be recognized during the examination and programmed into the treatment plan, to be accomplished along with other surgery (gingivectomy, for example) that may be called for.

The Mylohyoid Ridge Region. The area of the mylohyoid ridge should be

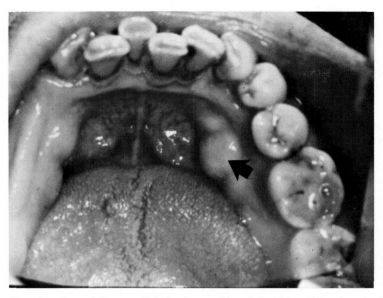

FIG. 1.6. The lingual surface of the mandible in the cuspid and first bicuspid region should be palpated for the presence of bony exostoses (tori mandibularis) which can be a major obstacle to comfortable wear of a prosthesis.

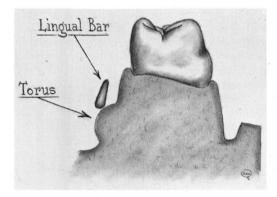

FIG. 1.7. A lingual bar which is positioned superior to a torus mandibularis as shown in the sketch above is a potential source of trouble, particularly in a distal extension base type of partial denture.

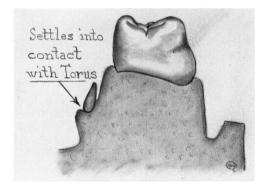

FIG. 1.8. If a bar is placed superior to a torus mandibularis and the denture bases settle even a slight amount, the lingual bar will descend into contact with the thin mucosal covering of the torus and the effect of the edge of the bar against the mucosa will be much like that from a knife.

palpated to determine its contour. The ideal anatomy for this portion of the mandible, from the standpoint of supporting a prosthesis, would be a lingual surface that descended straight downward from the crest of the residual ridge, with both sides of the mouth approximately parallel. The denture flanges could then be extended far enough into the alveolingual sulcus to make light contact with both the lingual surface of the mandible and the floor of the mouth. Flanges so formed would make an important contribution to both the stability and the retention of the denture. Unfortunately, it is much more common for the lingual surface of the mandible to slope laterally as it descends vertically so that a bony overhang is created. Moreover, it is not uncommon for this outcropping to be markedly accentuated by a ledge of bone that juts medially from the lingual surface of the mandible. An analysis of the planning cast in conjunction with intraoral palpation is very helpful in reaching a decision as to whether to alter the contour of the bone by surgery.

The Tuberosities

The tuberosities should be carefully examined if this area of the maxilla is edentulous and destined to support a part of the prosthesis, since this structure can present some vexing problems in denture construction. Difficulties may stem from the fact that one or both tuberosities are: (1) so large in vertical height as to preempt vitally needed interridge space, (2) so undercut as to interfere with comfortable insertion and removal of the prosthesis, or (3) so bulbous as to protrude into the buccal vestibule where it interferes with normal function of the mandible. Articulated study casts are an indispensable adjunct to the intraoral examination in assessing the need for, as well as the extent of, the surgery that is to be performed.

The tuberosity may extend downward so far that it contacts an opposing tooth (Fig. 1.9), or even the opposing ridge if it is edentulous. This fact may be brought to light when the occlusion is evaluated or it may become evident as the tuberosity is palpated. The lateral aspect of the tuberosity may jut into the buccal space to create such a severe undercut that one or both denture flanges scrape forceably against the sides of the tuberosity as the denture is inserted. When this occurs it may be anticipated with near certainity that the patient will return with an abraded mucosa following a brief interval of wear. To avoid this eventuality the clinician is forced to make a value judgment as to precisely how much base material to remove from the tissue side of the denture so that it can be inserted and withdrawn comfortably. If he removes too much base

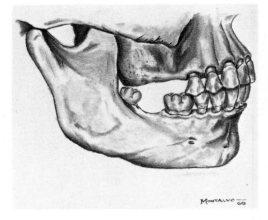

FIG. 1.9. The edentulous tuberosity area should be examined to ascertain its relationship to the mandibular arch. Ideally, there should be ample space for a minimal thickness of denture base and whatever teeth are needed to restore function. The area is sometimes very difficult to visualize in the mouth and the precise amount of space available may not be known for certain until the study casts have been accurately mounted on an articulator.

material from the tissue side, the peripheral seal may be lost. If he removes too little, the patient will probably be unable to wear the denture. If too much of a void is created between the denture and the mucosa the patient may wear the denture in relative comfort but complain of the bothersome space. Removal of only one undercut is often advocated on the premise that this will permit the denture to be inserted over the remaining undercut and then rotated into place on the operated side. This may be satisfactory in the case of the complete denture but is seldom feasible for the partial denture, which must be inserted and removed along a predetermined path of insertion which is seldom parallel to the plane of the undercut.

Much less common is the problem caused by the tuberosity which, although not markedly undercut, nevertheless bulges laterally by an abnormal amount into the buccal vestibule. Since the problem occurs infrequently it may not come to light until the patient reports, following a brief period of wear, that when he opens his mouth the maxillary denture becomes loose or is dislodged. The explanation may be that the denture flange overlying the bulbous tuberosity has preempted so much space in the buccal vestibule that both the denture and the coronoid process of the mandible cannot be accommodated at the same time. Consequently, when the mouth is opened wide and the coronoid process travels forward, it exerts such a strong wedging action against the flange that the denture is forcefully thrust forward and thus dislodged.

The Vestibules. The labial and buccal vestibules in edentulous areas that are to accommodate a flange of the denture should be of sufficient depth to permit extension of the border by a reasonable amount, so that it can contribute support and stability. Scar bands and muscle attachments that interfere with reasonable extension may need to be altered by surgical means.

The Frenula. The labial frenum may interfere with proper extension of the labial flange of a maxillary denture when anterior teeth are being replaced. This structure may be altered surgically to improve the fit and oftentimes the esthetics of the prosthesis as well.

The lingual frenum should be carefully inspected since its position in relation to the alveolar ridge can directly affect the design of the denture. If a lingual bar is to be used it is normally positioned midway in the space bounded by the free gingival margin of the lower anterior teeth superiorly, and the floor of the mouth and the lingual frenum inferiorly. Obviously the breadth of this space is critical. If the lingual frenum is attached at an abnormally high level relative to the crest of the ridge, a lingual plate rather than a lingual bar may have to be employed unless the condition is corrected by surgery.

Tongue Size and Mobility

The size of the tongue, as well as its range of movement and mobility, should be observed even though the tongue per se is rarely an obstacle to successful partial denture wear. When a natural tooth has been lost the tongue normally enlarges slightly, and quickly adopts the habit of occupying the edentulous space during mastication so as to protect the healing mucosa from trauma. Nature has endowed this organ with the capability of protecting the edentulous area from injury by shunting off sharp food particles and absorbing much of the impact of the bolus. When a prosthesis is subsequently fitted into the edentulous space, the tongue finds itself suddenly denied access to an area which had been considered its exclusive domain, and the patient may find the situation bothersome, although fortunately it is only temporary. It may be worthy of mention that tongue interferences with a prosthesis is more apt to be a problem if the natural teeth have been missing for an extended period of time so that habit patterns have become firmly established. A classic example is the patient who has worn a complete maxillary denture with no posterior teeth for an extended period of time and has developed the habit of carrying the tongue high so as to help support the upper denture. This habit may persist after he is fitted with a lower prosthesis, to the detriment of stability. A large tongue may overlie the mandibular edentulous ridge and, indeed, may totally obscure it, particularly if the ridge has undergone extensive resorption. This may complicate impression making, although usually the stock impression tray can be modified sufficiently with either wax or compound to extend the floor of the mouth downward and medially from the residual ridge while the impression is being registered. In extreme instances of alveolar atrophy it may be necessary to construct a custom tray for the mandibular impression. A hypermobile tongue is an inordinately curious organ and the dentist may frequently find it in his field of vision or in a position which denies him access to his work area. However, these minor vexations notwithstanding, the tongue poses no major obstacle to successful removable partial denture wear.

The Saliva

The intraoral inspection must include an appraisal of the character of the saliva, both as to the amount present and its viscosity, since this secretion serves two very important functions in the wear of a prosthesis. A moderate amount of saliva is needed to act as a lubricant buffer between the prosthesis and the mucosa, to help protect this sensitive tissue against scuffing as the prosthesis slides over and against it in function. In addition, a thin film of saliva is indispensable in creating adhesion between the denture base and the mucosa.

Too Much, Too Little Saliva. An overly profuse supply of saliva will not increase the retention and may complicate the impression procedure to a degree. It may be controlled by means of premedication with an antisialagogue. Xerostomia or aptyalism (a lack of saliva) may be symptomatic of a systemic disorder such as diabetes or nephritis. It may also be induced by regular use of certain of the tranquilizing drugs and may be associated with nutritional difficiency, particularly of the B complex vitamins. A mouth which is abnormally dry is a significant finding and should not be ignored without attempting to learn the cause, because the patient with an inadequate supply of saliva will have problems wearing any removable oral prosthesis comfortably. It should be noted, too, that emotional tension is capable of causing a temporarily dry mouth or that the examination procedure itself may cause an increase in salivary flow.

The Thick Viscous Type of Saliva. A thick, viscous type of saliva sometimes reduces retention by interfering with intimate contact between the denture and the mucosa. It may also interfere with obtaining an accurate impression of fine tissue detail, by filling in and bridging over fine grooves and depressions in the mucosa so that they are not registered with complete fidelity in the impression material. This type of saliva can usually be controlled for impression registration with an oral rinse administered just prior to making the impression. It may be of interest to note that this type of saliva is frequently associated with the patient who has a marked tendency to gag, and so may

serve to alert the examiner to this possibility. A very strong, uncontrollable gag reflex might very well influence the choice of prosthesis that is to be prescribed. For example, the confirmed gagger would probably adapt more easily to a partial removable maxillary prosthesis than to a complete denture and it would be far better for the dentist to be forewarned of this fact as a result of a thorough examination than to be suddenly confronted with it following extraction of all of the remaining maxillary teeth.

It is of interest to note that the highly mucinous type of saliva is frequently associated with a diet high in carbohydrates. The implications of such a dietary imbalance should be given weight when a judgment must be made as to the prosthesis to be prescribed. In the opinion of some authorities the character of the thick mucinous type of saliva may be changed to a thinner more watery type by reducing drastically the patient's intake of carbohydrates, particularly refined sugars, and increasing the amounts of fresh fruits and vegetables.

Inspection of the Soft Tissues

An inspection should be made of the lips, cheeks, floor of the mouth, and the palate. Any inflammation, infection, or swelling should be diagnosed and treated before definitive treatment on a prosthesis is begun. The color of the tissue should be appraised and any deviation not within normal limits should be noted. Normal healthy mucosa is usually described as being light coral in color, although a color gradient ranging from light pink to coral pink is typically encountered in a cross section of patients because of racial influences. Pallor is indicative of anemia, which portends a low tissue tolerance to a prosthesis.

The age group from which the majority of candidates for a removable prosthesis comes is one that is cancer prone, and the dentist must be ever on the alert to detect the presence of any neoplasm. Special attention should be paid to the cancer-prone horseshoe in the mandible. According to Ross et al. the horseshoe-shaped area which covers the alveolar ridge and the lateral borders of the tongue extending over the tonsil and onto the buccal shelf is the area in which is found 80% of oral cancer, although it comprises only about 25% of the total oral area.

The Palatal Torus. The maxillary torus is seldom an obstacle in removable partial denture construction since the prosthesis can usually be designed to cover it unless it is massive, lobulated, or undercut, in which case the prosthesis can be designed to circumvent it (the double palatal bar).

The Occlusion

No oral examination is complete without a close scrutiny of the teeth, both anteriors and posteriors in their customary intercuspated position. The lips and cheeks should be retracted, and the operating light properly focused for maximum visibility. A careful inspection of the two arches of teeth in apposition will often divulge relationships between opposing teeth, and between teeth and opposing edentulous ridges, that would never be suspected as a result of simply viewing each arch separately. Accordingly the patient should be instructed to "close on the back teeth" so as to place the jaws into a position of maximum intercuspation, which is by definition centric occlusion. The relationship of the opposing teeth on both sides of the mouth, as well as the anteriors, should be scrutinized. In order to compare centric occlusion with centric relation the mandible should be retracted into its terminal hinge position; a position that may fail to coincide precisely with centric occlusion. If these two relationships do not coincide, an estimate of the extent of the discrepancy between them should be made. A decision will need to be made before definitive treatment is begun whether to accept centric occlusion "as is" or to make the two relationships coincide by means of equilibration procedures. Under some circumstances it may be necessary to mount the study casts on the articulator in centric relationship before this important decision is made. When an equilibration procedure is to be a part of the treatment, it should be carried out before any restorative work is accomplished.

In examining occlusal relationships, the path of closure of the mandible from rest position to centric occlusion should be observed for any sign of deviation to one side or the other as the teeth meet and intercuspate. Any discernible sign of deviation is typically caused by a cusp contacting an opposing incline along which it slides until it reaches a fossa or an embrasure. Cusps in contact with inclined planes powered by the closing muscles exert horizontal stresses against the teeth which are harmful to the periodontium. Ideally occlusal contacts between all of the teeth in centric occlusion should be even and simultaneous. One test of a harmonious occlusion is to have the patient tap the teeth rapidly together. A sharp clear sound denotes even contacts.

Intercuspation in eccentric movements of the mandible should be such that the cusps and inclined planes glide over one another smoothly without tripping or interference. It bears repetition that the equilibration procedure, when it is indicated, should be one of the first steps listed on the treatment plan following palliation of the chief complaint.

The Radiographic Survey

No dental examination can be considered complete without adequate radiographs. The literature is replete with investigative studies which have demonstrated that x-rays of patients who are completely edentulous, in a high percentage of cases routinely divulge the presence of retained roots, unerupted teeth, cysts and foreign bodies, as well as various types of pathology and anomalies, and certainly there is strong presumptive evidence at least, that the mouths of partially edentulous patients harbor a correspondingly high percentage of anomalies (Figs. 1.10–1.12). Construction of a prosthesis without a dental radiographic survey is not only poor practice but it is highly suspect from a legal standpoint. At least 16 exposures, to include two bite wing films, should be employed for rou-

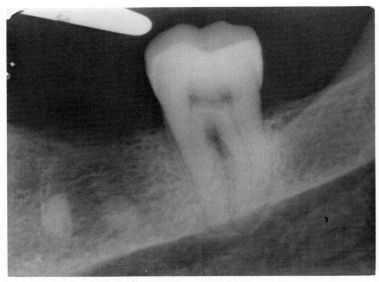

Fig. 1.10. Radiographs of patients who have lost teeth randomly over a period of years will disclose pathology and other anomalies in a high percentage of instances. This photograph shows retained root remnants mesial to the molar.

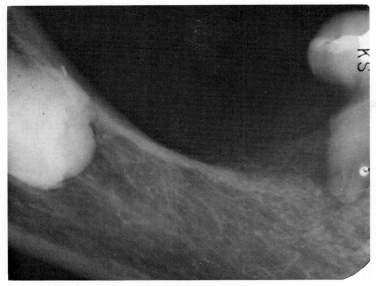

Fig. 1.11. Unerupted teeth, cysts, and other pathology are common findings. This photograph shows an impacted mandibular third molar.

tine diagnostic purposes. Additional films may be needed for special purposes (the occlusal film to locate a root tip in the buccolingual plane, for example).

Radiographic Technique

In viewing radiographs it is well to re-member that a radiograph is a two-di-mensional view of a three-dimensional object. In similar vein one should be aware of the technique employed to expose the films. There are two basic techniques in common use: (1) the long cone or right angle technique, and (2) the short

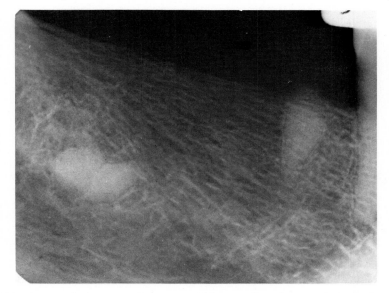

FIG. 1.12. This photograph shows root fragments which were allowed to remain in the bone following extraction of several mandibular teeth.

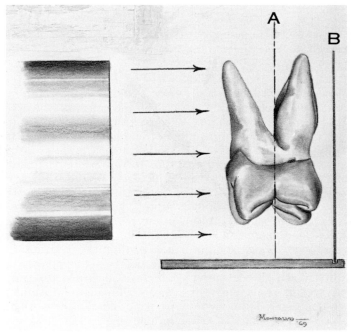

FIG. 1.13. The long cone or right angle technique directs the rays perpendicularly to the long axis of the tooth. *A*, the long axis of the tooth. *B*, the radiograph.

cone or bisected angle technique. The long cone technique directs the central ray perpendicularly to the long axis of the tooth (Fig. 1.13). The bisected angle technique directs the central ray perpendicu- larly to an imaginary line which bisects the angle formed by the long axis of the teeth and the plane of the film (Fig. 1.14). The steep angle of the bisecting or short cone technique introduces some distortion

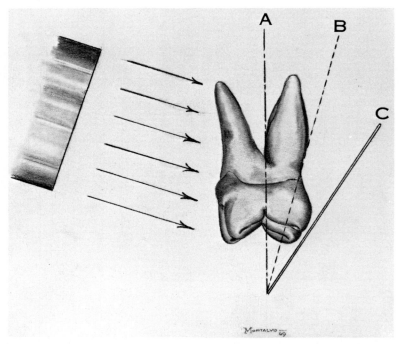

FIG. 1.14. The short cone or "bisect-the-angle" technique directs the central ray perpendicularly to an imaginary line which bisects the angle formed by the long axis of the tooth and the plane of the radiographic film. *A*, the long axis of the tooth. *B*, the line which bisects the angle of film and tooth. *C*, the radiograph.

which if not understood and compensated for can lead to interpretive error. This is especially liable to occur in the maxillary molar region where the bone may appear to vary considerably in height following only a slight change in angulation either vertically or horizontally. Shadows of buccal and lingual plates may be superimposed so that a good level of dense bone on the buccal side of a tooth, for example, is capable of creating the illusion of a similar condition on the lingual side, where it does not exist.

It cannot be overstressed that in order to avoid interpretive error resulting from variations in such factors as film type, exposure time, processing technique, and angulation, a standardized technique combined with rigid quality control should be practiced. Failure to do so will lay the groundwork for mistakes in clinical judgment. A good radiograph will reveal many helpful facts to the knowledgeable clinician; a poor radiograph can lead to grievous error.

Radiographic Interpretation

The information which can be obtained from a knowledgeable interpretation of the dental radiographs is one of the keystones of the dental examination. In addition to disclosing incipient decay, recurrent caries around fillings, inadequate root canal fillings, and the presence of unerupted and impacted teeth, cysts, and other pathology, the radiographs provide the examiner with priceless information concerning the character and probable load-bearing capacity of the undergirding which is destined to support the prosthesis. This is information obtainable from no other source. All radiopacities or radiolucencies not readily identifiable as within the range of normality should be investigated further and fabrication of the prosthesis should not begin until the status of each such area has been either diagnosed and treated or determined to be not significant. A diagrammatic interpretation of the tooth as it appears in the dental radiograph is shown in Figure 1.15.

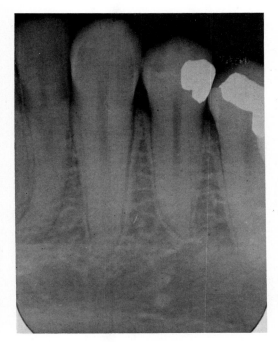
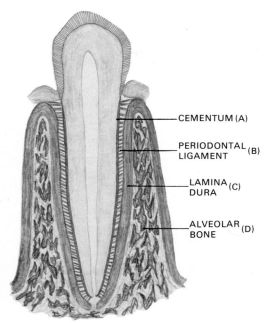

CEMENTUM (A)

PERIODONTAL (B)
LIGAMENT

LAMINA (C)
DURA

ALVEOLAR (D)
BONE

FIG. 1.15. The space occupied by the periodontal ligament (B) is seen as a dark (radiolucent) line immediately surrounding the cementum of the root (A). A thin, reasonably uniform, dark line in the radiograph indicates a normal periodontal ligament and space. When a tooth is out of function, which may occur following the loss of its antagonist, for example, the periodontal ligament and space tend to become thickened, and the dark shadow in the radiograph is usually wider than normal and perhaps more irregular in outline. Such a tooth has usually extruded to some degree and when this is true the periodontal ligament will often appear noticeably thickened at the apex. The periodontal ligament may also appear thickened around a tooth that is being exposed to increased stress, which lends emphasis to the fact that a judgment should not be made on the basis of x-ray evidence alone. A noticeably enlarged periodontal membrane space may also indicate tooth mobility. This, of course, must be verified by clinical test. The lamina dura is the compact bone which lines the alveolus and is seen in the radiograph as a thin white (opaque) line (C). The lamina dura typically thickens in reaction to increased functional demands and tends to become thin if the tooth is taken out of function. The alveolar bone itself (D) is seen in the radiograph as a network of interlaced trabeculae and intertrabecular spaces, the latter being in reality narrow spaces.

In addition to disclosing the presence of pathology and other abnormalities the radiographs will make available information which will be of value in assessing the potential worth of prospective abutment teeth such as: (1) root morphology, (2) bone height, (3) bone quality, and (4) the probable reaction of the bone to increased stress.

Root Morphology. Root configuration is an important criterion in foretelling the probable solidity and durability of a potential abutment tooth. The prognosis may be favorable or unfavorable depending on the length of the root (the

longer, the stronger), the number of roots (multirooted teeth are designed to withstand heavier stress than are single rooted teeth), the shape of the root(s) (irregularly shaped roots are stronger than are straight conical shaped roots), and if multirooted whether fused or spread (spread roots are more stable than are fused roots).

Bone Height. The length of the root per se is not the key factor in forecasting the probable stability and longevity of an abutment tooth but rather the amount of root which is enveloped by bone. This is customarily referred to as the crown/root ratio. The greater the amount of root encased in bone and the shorter the portion of the tooth unsupported by bone, the more favorable the leverage factor. Conversely, the less the amount of bone around the root and the longer the part of the tooth unsupported, the less favorable the leverage factor. A one-to-one ratio for a single rooted tooth is generally considered minimal for a tooth to qualify as a partial denture abutment. A multirooted tooth is sometimes considered usable as an abutment with a crown/root ratio of slightly less than one to one. Like any rule of thumb this one must be applied with judgment since there are numerous qualifying factors which influence the amount of stress to which the tooth would be subjected, thus affecting the crown/root ratio that would be acceptable. Examples are the shape of the roots(s), whether or not there are distal extension bases to control, the total number of abutments to share the burden of the prosthesis, and the structure of the residual ridges, to name a few. Then too, a tooth considered unacceptable as an abutment because of an unfavorable crown/root ratio might be made acceptable by splinting it to an adjacent tooth or teeth.

Bone height can be assessed quite accurately by a study of the radiographs provided the exposure technique is properly controlled. It should be noted that in any comparison of bone height from one period of time to another care must be exercised to maintain constant angulation factors since any alteration in the relationship of the film, the tooth, and the central ray might create a false illusion of height which could result in a misleading comparison. It should be kept in mind, too, that bone level normally decreases with age, a factor that must be given consideration in assessing the potential of a tooth as an abutment.

Bone Quality. Bone which has small, closely grouped trabeculae and small intertrabecular spaces is considered well mineralized, hence strong and healthy. It is portrayed in the radiograph as relatively radiopaque, although a certain amount of variation in size of the trabeculae is normal and to be expected.

Probable Reaction to Increased Stress. When bone responds to increased functional demands by becoming more dense, it is considered an excellent portent for the success of an oral prosthesis. When bone responds poorly to additional stress, the trabeculae become thinner and the intertrabecular spaces larger. The radiograph depicts this type of bone as relatively radiolucent and it is not considered as promising for bearing the additional burden of a prosthesis.

The reaction of the bone around teeth that have been subjected to more than the usual amount of stress, because of having lost the support of adjacent teeth, or having been in hyperocclusion, or having served as abutments for a fixed or removable prosthesis, may be used as a basis for forecasting its probable reaction to future stress.

The Planning Cast

Accurate planning or diagnostic casts contribute information that can be obtained in no other way, and that is invaluable in forming the basis for sound judgments as the type of prosthesis is prescribed and the treatment plan is formulated. Indeed the planning casts serve so many useful purposes that it is difficult to envision a successful partial denture service in which they are not routinely employed. It may be stated without any reservation whatever that it is never too early in the treatment sequence to make use of them.

Major uses of diagnostic casts are:

a. As an aid in planning the design and structuring of the prosthesis to assess the contours of various structures better, as well as their relationship to each other.

b. As a three-dimensional blueprint upon which to note areas of the mouth which require alteration for the purpose of improving the design.

c. As a supplement to the work authorization order (prescription) which is sent to the laboratory technician, the study cast serves to illustrate graphically the prosthesis that is being prescribed and authorized. The design of the prosthesis should be sketched on the study cast and sent to the laboratory along with the *unmarked master cast*. All markings should be made on the study cast, never on the master cast, since drawing on a cast introduces inaccuracies. It then represents a record of the prescribed design which can be referred to in the event of a communication breakdown between dentist and technician. It helps to place responsibility where it should rightfully be: on the dentist for devising and prescribing the design and on the technician for following the prescription with exactitude and precision in his fabrication of the prosthesis.

Additional Uses of the Diagnostic Cast. Study casts constitute a durable, accurate record for future use should the patient decide to postpone treatment temporarily. They can be used to demonstrate a proposed treatment to the patient and are extremely useful in illustrating and clarifying directions to an oral surgeon when a surgical procedure is to be performed as part of the preparatory treatment. The study cast is of value in recognizing and visualizing the need for, as well as the effect of, various proposed clinical and laboratory procedures. For example, anterior teeth can be removed from the cast and artificial ones set in their place in order to visualize better the problems to be anticipated and the cosmetic result attainable, before a decision is finalized to extract anterior teeth for the purpose of improving the patient's appearance. Another use of diagnostic casts is for patient education. The individual who wears a removable partial prosthesis must maintain his mouth in a state of meticulous cleanliness so as to minimize the possibility of erosion under clasps, recurrent decay at the margins of restorations, and of gingival irritations. The diagnostic casts can be very useful in demonstrating proper brushing technique and the use of dental floss, as well as in helping the patient to visualize the problem involved in cleaning tooth sur-

faces that are difficult of access. Finally, the diagnostic cast can be pressed into service as a model upon which to fabricate a special customized tray in the rare instance that the mouth for one reason or another is unusually difficult to register with routine impression techniques.

The planning casts will be studied and analyzed on both the articulator and on the surveyor. This will require that the cast be removed from the articulator and placed on the surveyor and then later returned to the articulator. One of the plasterless type articulators lends itself well to this purpose. If a conventional articulator is employed some type of split remounting device (Split Remounting Plate, Hanau Engineering Co., Buffalo, New York) is recommended.

Cast Analysis—On the Articulator

A study of the casts on the articulator will reveal relationships between opposing teeth and between opposing edentulous ridges that could not be determined by any other method. Special attention should be focused on the following:

The Occlusion. The relationship of the teeth of one arch with those of the other arch can be closely observed (Fig. 1.16). The presence of tipped, rotated, and extruded teeth (Fig. 1.17) can be noted, and the problems in design of the prosthesis which they create can be assessed.

The Occlusal Plane. The status of the occlusal plane is critical in assessing the prognosis for a prosthesis and it may exert a pivotal influence on the type of prosthesis that should be prescribed. A plane that undulates (Fig. 1.18) because of tipped and extruded teeth will make it inordinately difficult to develop a harmonious occlusion. Since a harmonious occlusion is crucial to the success of a removable partial denture the occlusal plane that deviates markedly from normal must be viewed with considerable skepticism. A frequently encountered example which illustrates the difficulties created by a deviant occlusal plane are overerupted maxillary molars (Fig. 1.19) which typically tip bucally to such a degree that the lingual cusps become plunger cusps.

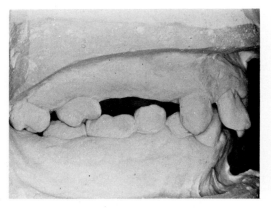

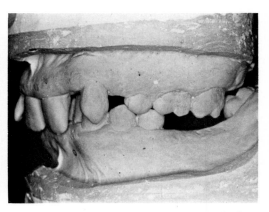

FIG. 1.16. The mounted study casts provide an opportunity to study the relative relationship of the structures of the upper and lower jaws to each other. The problems created by tipped, rotated, and extruded teeth can thus be analyzed.

FIG. 1.18. An irregular, uneven occlusal plane which deviates substantially from the position it once occupied may present an insurmountable problem in terms of articulating the natural teeth with the teeth of a prosthesis.

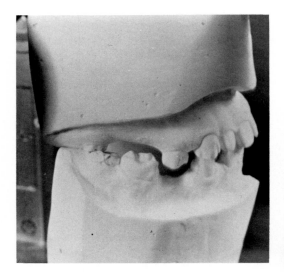

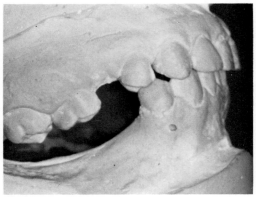

FIG. 1.17. Many times it is apparent at the time of the intraoral examination that the occlusal plane has been lost and that the occlusion has collapsed. Properly articulated planning casts make it possible to make a much more meaningful assessment of the relationship of the extruded teeth to the opposing ridge and to focus attention on the problems that are thus created.

FIG. 1.19. When maxillary molars overerupt they tend to tip buccally so that the lingual cusps become "plunger cusps" which create an exceedingly difficult problem in the establishment of a harmonious occlusion with an opposing prosthesis.

Such teeth inflict considerable damage on the opposing occlusion.

Interridge Space. The amount of space between the edentulous ridges of the maxilla and the mandible should be carefully evaluated. Special attention should be directed to the tuberosity region where bony and fibrous hypertrophy frequently result in contact between the residual ridge and the mandibular teeth, or perhaps between the two edentulous ridges (Fig. 1.20). Interridge space in the incisor region may be nonexistant as a result of extrusion of the mandibular incisors into contact with the palatal mucosa when the teeth are in occlusion.

Interocclusal Space. The space between the occlusal and incisal surfaces of certain key teeth is crucially important. Areas of the abutment teeth that are destined to accommodate occlusal, lingual, or incisal rests should be examined critically so as to assess the amount of space that is available and to estimate the additional space that will need to be provided (Fig. 1.21). When a lingual rest will be required on a maxillary anterior tooth the articulated study casts make it possible to view the lingual surface of the tooth involved with all of the teeth in centric occlusion so that the precise amount of space available for the contemplated rest can be accurately determined.

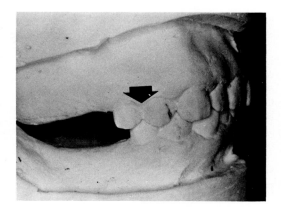

FIG. 1.21. Areas of the abutment teeth that will be expected to accommodate occlusal, incisal, or lingual rests may be closely investigated with the planning casts. For example, an embrasure clasp between the two maxillary bicuspids shown above would obviously not be feasible but it would not be nearly as apparent from a visual inspection of the space in the mouth.

Cast Analysis—On the Surveyor

The path of insertion as well as the design of the prosthesis will be established with the cast on the surveyor, so that all subsequent treatment can be based on this design. The following factors will be noted.

The Distribution of the Remaining Teeth. The number and relative position in the arch of the remaining teeth are important because the design of the prosthesis must perforce relate directly to the location of these potential abutments. From a standpoint of removable partial denture design the ideal would be to have healthy teeth with well contoured crowns and sturdy roots in each quadrant of the arch. Unfortunately this is more often the exception than the rule.

Selection of Abutments. Molars and cuspids make the best abutments from a standpoint of stability and strength with the bicuspids next, although on the basis of claspability the bicuspids are superior to the cuspids. Incisors as a rule make poor abutments because of their poor claspability and weak root structure. Teeth that are grouped together are stronger, all else being equal, than are iso-

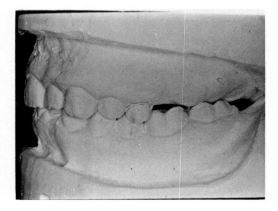

FIG. 1.20. The amount of interridge space in areas that will be expected to accommodate essential elements of the prosthesis can be assessed with articulated planning casts.

lated teeth by virtue of the mesiodistal support which they provide for each other. The claspability of potential abutment teeth can be assessed with the analyzing rod to determine which teeth are most suitable to retain, support, and stabilize the prosthesis. Areas of the abutment teeth that can be modified to bear occlusal, incisal, and lingual rests should be noted.

Interferences. Areas of the mouth or of individual teeth that are potential obstacles to ready insertion and removal of the prosthesis can be identified so that appropriate solutions to the problems which they pose can be devised.

Selection of Guiding Plane Surfaces. Tooth surfaces can be analyzed to determine their suitability as guiding plane surfaces and areas that are to be modified for this purpose can be noted.

Cosmetic Problems and Opportunity. Esthetic problems created by splayed, migrated anterior teeth can be assessed and appropriate solutions planned. The type of prosthetic teeth which will be most suitable from a standpoint of appearance can be tentatively selected.

The Definitive Examination

The definitive examination is carried out at the second appointment when the patient, the radiographs, and the articulated study casts can all be brought together for final study and decision making. At this time all data can be collated and verified. Findings which have been revealed by one diagnostic means can be cross-checked and reappraised within a framework of the overall findings. The mouth may be reexamined for caries and defective restorations, with cross reference to the radiographs. Suspicious areas in the radiographs are verified by reinspection of the mouth with the mirror and explorer. Cross referral may be made between the study casts and the mouth in verifying the amount of interoc-

clusal space, the interridge relationships, and the severity of tipped teeth. Ordinarily there will be little or no change made from the tentative treatment plan which was formulated prior to the appointment. At this appointment the plan of treatment can be presented to the patient and explained with the aid of the study casts.

Bibliography

Applegate, O. C.: Evaluation of support for the removable partial denture. J. Prosth. Dent. *10:* 112–123, 1960.

Bregstein, S. J.: *Interviewing, Counseling and Managing Dental Patients.* Prentice-Hall, Inc., Englewood Cliffs, N.J., 1957.

Burket, L. W.: *Oral Medicine*, Ed. 5. J. B. Lippincott Company, Philadelphia, 1961.

Cheraskin, E., and Langley, L. L.: *Dynamics of Oral Diagnosis*. Year Book Medical Publishers, Inc., Chicago, 1956.

Cinotti, W. R., and Grieder, A.: *Applied Psychology in Dentistry.* The C. V. Mosby Company, St. Louis, 1964.

Collins, L. H., and Crane, M. P.: *Internal Medicine in Dental Practice*, Ed. 6. Lea & Febiger, Philadelphia, 1965.

Glickman, I.: *Clinical Periodontology*, Ed. 2. W. B. Saunders, Company, Philadelphia, 1958.

Kerr, D. A., Ash, M. M., Jr., and Millard, H. D.: *Oral Diagnosis*, Ed. 2. The C. V. Mosby Company, St. Louis, 1965.

Kruger, G. O.: *Textbook of Oral Surgery*, Ed. 2. The C. V. Mosby Company, St. Louis, 1964.

Merck Manual of Diagnosis and Therapy, Ed. 14. Merck & Company, Inc., Rahway, N.J., 1969.

Mills, M. L.: Mouth preparation for the removable partial denture. J. Amer. Dent. Ass. *60:* 154–159, Feb. 1960.

Perry, C. F., and Applegate, S. G.: Study cast. J. Michigan Dent. Soc. *28:* 82–84, 1946.

Presstime Roundup: Dental Times, December 1968.

Ross, W. L., Johnson, R. H., and Hayes, R. L.: Examination of the mouth. G. P. *36:* 78–86, 1967.

Sarnat, B. G., and Schour, I.: Essentials of Oral and Facial Cancer, Ed. 2. Year Book Medical Publishers, Inc., Chicago.

Sharp, G.: Oral manifestations of systemic disease. Oral Surg. *23:* 737–744, 1967.

Sicher, H.: *Oral Anatomy*, Ed. 2. The C. V. Mosby Company, St. Louis, 1952.

Stafne, E. C.: *Oral Roentgenographic Diagnosis*. W. B. Saunders Company, Philadelphia, 1969.

Chapter 2

PRESCRIBING THE PROSTHETIC SERVICE

This chapter is concerned with the judgments that must be made as the prosthetic service best suited to the patient's needs is selected. The numerous factors which must be weighed as the decision making takes place are enumerated and discussed. Subject matter is arranged in the following format:

Introduction

Because of the wide variety of combinations of missing and standing teeth, the numerous types of prosthodontic service available, and the diversity of needs peculiar to individual patients, the selection of the most suitable prosthesis may at times be an inordinately complex process. For purposes of discussion, in establishing guidelines it is helpful to employ as a frame of reference the scale depicted in Figure 2.1.

In making a selection of the most suitable prosthesis or combination of prostheses, the patient with missing teeth may be placed at a point somewhere on this scale, one end of which represents a completely edentulous mouth and the other a full complement of natural teeth. In terms of indicated treatment, the choice for these two extremes would be: (1) complete dentures, and (2) no prosthesis indicated, respectively. In between these two extremes various stages of edentulousness requiring treatment with the fixed partial denture, the removable partial denture, and the complete denture are depicted on the scale. Either one, two, or all three in combination may be indicated in a given instance to reinstate satisfactory oral health and function to an optimum level. The decision as to where on the scale the patient passes from a candidate for a partial denture(s) to candidacy for a complete denture(s) is sometimes a difficult one to make since the choice is often not a bipolar black and white. In making this decision the clinician should weigh the answers to these questions. Assuming an optimum result from whichever prosthesis is selected, which one will best preserve the remaining oral structures while at the same time restoring health and function? If the choice is two or more fixed partial dentures, will the clinical result justify the added expense, time, and effort required for this type of treatment over that needed to construct a removable partial denture? If a removable partial denture is chosen, can it be ex-

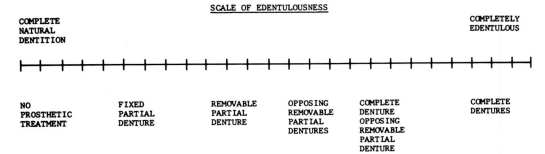

FIG. 2.1. The scale depicts the various degrees of edentulousness and the probable types of prosthodontic care indicated, ranging from no treatment needed for the complete natural dentition (*left side of scale*), to complete dentures needed for the completely edentulous mouth (*right side of scale*).

pected to justify, in superior function and length of service, the additional time and expense required in its fabrication over that needed for a complete denture? What is the status of the patient's systemic health? Does he have the stamina to withstand whatever treatment is deemed ideal or must some compromise be made because of a faulty systemic background? Which restorations will be best for the patient from a psychological standpoint? Will removal of all the remaining teeth be a psychologically traumatic experience for the patient? Which will be the best prosthesis from a cosmetic viewpoint and how much importance should be accorded the esthetic requirement? Is the patient's desire to salvage some of the remaining teeth, in an effort to postpone "old age," so intense as to justify their retention even on a pro tem basis? In short, which prosthetic service is best from all viewpoints?

Extraoral Factors Which Influence the Type of Prosthodontic Service To Be Prescribed

There are a multitude of factors that may influence the decision-making process, some related directly to oral conditions and others more accurately described as extraoral factors. The importance of extraoral factors should not be underestimated; indeed they may at times play a pivotal role in the decision making. Some of the more important of

these are discussed in the following paragraphs.

Age. The age of the patient may influence the choice of prosthodontic service from several standpoints. For one example, the patient under 25 years of age should, as a rule, not be rendered completely edentulous unless there is no feasible alternative. The number of years such a patient can reasonably be expected to live, on a statistical basis, raises the question of whether the bone of the residual ridges can be expected to endure throughout his lifetime for the purpose of supporting his dentures. Certainly the possibility exists that a patient may literally outlive his denture foundation. This fact suggests that every effort be expended to avoid full-scale extractions for patients in the younger age groups.

In similar vein, heroic measures might be justified in salvaging a third molar for an adolescent, even to the extreme of constructing a prosthesis over an unerupted tooth. This approach would be warranted if there were a reasonable expectation that the tooth would erupt beneath (and through) the denture base thus becoming available for use as an abutment at some future date.

In like manner, good clinical judgment might dictate that a maxillary third molar be permitted to erupt beneath the denture base so that as it erupts it will assist in the formation of a normal sized tuberosity. Bone in this region of the mouth is invaluable and can be expected to contribute enormously to the support of a prosthesis in future years.

Generally, teeth are not extracted for the extremely elderly individual except for reasons of discomfort or systemic health, unless there is reason to believe that function will be materially improved. Many oldsters shun any change in routine or environment, and moreover, there is typically a diminution in their ability to adapt to change. One must be reasonably sure that a contemplated treatment will, at the very least, improve the patient's sense of security and well-being, as a minimum objective before a decision is made to extract teeth that are comfortable and healthy. Certainly teeth should not be removed solely because a younger member of the family seeks to bring about an improvement in the older person's appearance.

When age is factored into the decision-making process it is important to bear in mind the fact that individuals of the same age frequently differ over a wide gradient, both physiologically and in mental outlook. This may be explained by recognizing three "ages of man," i.e. chronological, physiological, and psychological. An individual who has lived 60 years might by 50 years of age physiologically and psychologically, and, unfortunately, the converse is true.

General Health. Except in unusual circumstances the patient who is in poor health should be spared the trauma of long, arduous dental operations. This may contraindicate extensive rehabilitation procedures which, under different circumstances, might be the ideal treatment. Radical disruption of the oral status quo should be avoided until the health of such a patient can be returned to a level that is, for him at least, optimal. The interim partial denture is sometimes the prosthesis of choice in preference to the complete denture, the temporary partial denture instead of the fixed partial denture. The rebase or reline, as well as the use of tissue treatment materials, may be a better approach than prescribing the con-

struction of a prosthesis requiring an extended series of lengthy appointments.

Sex. In general, the female tends to have a higher vanity index, i.e. to place a greater value on the esthetic excellence of the prosthesis, than does the male.

Generally it can be said that the female is more apt to equate loss of teeth with the process of aging or the state of old age. Accordingly, she may insist on retaining natural teeth of dubious value long after her male counterpart has accepted and grown accustomed to his complete dentures. Similarly, some compromise with mechanical excellence is sometimes warranted in order to effect an improved esthetic result. For example, a removable partial denture with precision attachments in lieu of clasps might be prescribed for the purpose of achieving an optimally pleasing appearance for a female patient even though this might mean some sacrifice in retention and stability.

It might be well to point out in this connection that when assessing the vanity index it is a mistake to give credence to the patient who professes little or no interest in the appearance of his prosthesis. This could well be the individual who, following insertion of his prosthesis, hurries to the privacy of his home for a critical inspection of his newly acquired "look," and who is inordinately disappointed if his appearance does not measure up to his self-image, or perhaps even worse, is not approved by his peers.

Economic Considerations. It may be posited on altruistic grounds that the "right" treatment, in a given instance, should always be the "ideal" treatment. From a practical standpoint, however, it must be conceded that the patient's ability to pay a reasonable fee for the service can hardly be ignored.

The complete denture is the least costly prosthesis to construct as well as to maintain. For this reason it must sometimes be prescribed in circumstances under which another type of prosthesis or combination of prostheses would be more nearly ideal were it not for economics. Partial denture service will inevitably require a higher fee initially than complete dentures, as well as higher follow-up maintenance. When removable partial denture service is prescribed, one or more restorations are usually needed, root canal therapy as well as crowns and inlays may be indicated, and periodontal therapy is a likely prerequisite, all of which add to the expense. Not to be overlooked is the possibility of abutment failure, an occurrence which would entail the additional expense of adding a segment to the prosthesis or perhaps of remaking it entirely. If the cost of the removable partial denture and its corollary treatment is beyond the patient's means, the complete denture might have to be substituted, even though the removable prosthesis might be more ideal. Certainly there can be little question but that an individual is better off with complete dentures, with which he can masticate comfortably, than with an inadequate number of unhealthy natural teeth with which he cannot properly supply his body with needed nutrients.

Socioeconomic Background. Closely related to the foregoing is the socioeconomic background of the patient. A familiar figure is the stenographer who takes meticulous care of her dentition and who seeks the finest dental care available irrespective of cost. Equally familiar is the affluent executive who is too preoccupied with business affairs to give more than cursory attention to his dental needs, who insists that any treatment which he receives be the most expedient available, and that it require only a bare minimum of time. The point thus illustrated is that the treatment recommended should not be based on a preconceived notion of the patient's presumed financial status.

The Desires and Attitude of the Patient. In prescribing the dental prosthesis, the patient's attitude toward his remaining natural teeth should not be overlooked since, in some circumstances, it may play a pivotal role in the decision-making process. This draws attention to the fact that the attitude of the public towards the retention or loss of natural teeth and the wearing of an oral prosthesis

covers a strikingly wide range of opinion. As an example, one patient may insist on the extraction of sound teeth despite recommendations to the contrary. Another may insist on retaining teeth whose potential as partial denture abutments is marginal at best, because he equates the loss of teeth with old age and even with a loss of virility. In between these two extremes is the patient who has no strong feelings one way or the other regarding his remaining teeth, and whose attitude toward his dental health can best be described as apathetic.

The weight assigned this factor must be tempered with clinical wisdom. Certainly the examiner should never permit it to dissuade him from recommending the service that is in the patient's best interests. However, borderline decisions must frequently be made in which the desires of the patient can be decisive. The patient who has only six maxillary anterior teeth remaining, when conditions are such that either a partial denture or a complete denture might be equally feasible, is a classic example. The patient who has no particular desire to retain the few remaining natural teeth will probably demonstrate little zeal in discharging his responsibility for home care and for this reason the complete denture would be a better choice than a partial denture. On the other hand, if the patient evinces a strong desire to retain his natural teeth under these circumstances, his wish should normally be granted by prescribing the removable partial denture.

Occupational Factors. The patient's vocation can be a pivotal factor in prescribing the prosthetic service. Individuals who hold public office, construction workers, farmers, and professional people, typically assign vastly diverse values to the various facets of prosthodontic service. For example, the professional person may require an immediate denture service while the construction worker might have a strong preference for having the denture made by conventional methods. A closely related aspect is the fact that the patient's dentition may play a critical role in his pursuit of a livelihood, the musician being a classic example. The musician who plays a wind instrument will probably be incapacitated by loss of anterior teeth which are essential to his embouchure. Heroic measures that would not be justifiable under different circumstances would thus be warranted in salvaging anterior teeth for such an individual.

Similarly, individuals who engage regularly in contact sports should be given special consideration when prescribing a prosthesis, since swallowing or aspirating a prosthesis, as a result of sudden impact, has been known to occur and is fraught with serious implications. The removable prosthesis has the advantage of being readily removed from the mouth while the person is engaged in the sport, while the fixed type of prosthesis has merit in the fact that under normal circumstances it cannot be dislodged and swallowed or aspirated. Generally the prosthesis that can be removed while the person participates in his sport is best for the anterior part of the mouth while the posterior teeth may best be replaced with the fixed type of prosthesis. The professional athlete may best be served with a removable prosthesis, while at the same time fitting him with a protective mouth guard to be inserted while he is an active participant.

The Time Factor. Under some circumstances the prosthesis that would be ideal is not feasible because sufficient time cannot be made available to accomplish all of the necessary treatment. An example is the school teacher who needs a complete maxillary denture, but who must postpone extractions until a time of the year when school is not in session. An interim removable partial denture might be the most suitable prosthesis in such an instance.

Conditions Which Militate for the Fixed Partial Denture

The fixed partial denture is probably the nearest to an ideal prosthesis to be found in the prosthodontic arsenal. It is small in bulk, hence seldom distracting or annoying to the wearer. When the full-coverage retainer is used, it affords a high degree of caries protection, esthetics are usually good, and breakage is not often a problem. And perhaps most important, because of its architecture masticatory stresses are directed principally along the long axis of the abutment teeth. From a biomechanical standpoint this is ideal.

Extensive cutting procedures, multiple visits, long appointments, and increased expense are the principal disadvantages which may be cited for the fixed means of replacement. Moreover, the fixed prosthesis must be rated somewhat less hygienic than a removable partial which can be removed from the mouth for more thorough cleaning. The following paragraphs call attention to situations in which the fixed partial denture is indicated.

Short Spans. The fixed partial denture is usually indicated for the one- or two-tooth unilateral space when the length of the span is not excessive. In determining the length of a span which should be restored with a fixed partial denture, Ante's rule may be applied. This rule states that there should be an amount of periodontal ligament surrounding the abutment teeth equal to or greater than the amount which surrounds the teeth that are to be replaced (Fig. 2.2). When the requirements of Ante's rule can be satisfied, the fixed partial denture will be adequately supported, assuming a healthy periodontal apparatus.

Replacing Anterior Teeth. Generally, anterior teeth are best replaced by fixed means. This is true, even when posterior teeth are programmed for replacement with a removable partial denture, for the following reasons. (1) If the removable partial denture is lost or becomes broken, the patient will not be incapacitated from a cosmetic standpoint during the time another prosthesis is being made or a broken one is being repaired. (2) The patient who wears a removable partial denture should leave it out of the mouth at night while sleeping. If the prosthesis includes anterior tooth replacements, it may be more difficult to overcome the patient's reluctance to being without cosmetic teeth during this eight-hour period. (3) Finally, it may eliminate an unfavor-

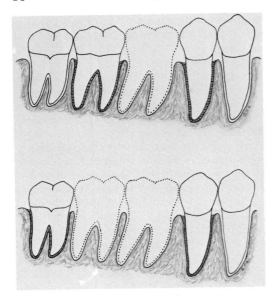

FIG. 2.2. Ante's rule states that for a fixed partial denture to be properly supported there should be an amount of periodontal ligament surrounding the abutment teeth equal to or greater than the amount that surrounds the teeth to be replaced. In the *top sketch*, the periodontal ligament which surrounds the second bicuspid and the second molar is greater than that which surrounds the first molar that is to be replaced, and support for a fixed partial denture will be more than adequate. In the *bottom sketch* the ratio is not as favorable and the use of double abutments should be given consideration.

able leverage factor which can be difficult to control when a segment must be attached to the partial denture anterior to the fulcrum line. However, the clinical wisdom of cutting unblemished anterior teeth for the sole purpose of replacing missing teeth by the fixed method certainly may be debated when the replacement teeth could be attached rather simply to a removable prosthesis.

As A Splint. A fixed prosthesis can sometimes be used to restore a small edentulous space, while at the same time improving the prognosis for the removable partial denture by increasing the strength and stability of one of the abutments. For example, the loss of a first bicuspid may result in the presence of an isolated second bicuspid which, because of an unfavorable crown/root ratio, will be a less than reliable abutment for a removable

partial denture. Such a tooth can be converted into a more adequate abutment by uniting it with the cuspid by means of a pontic (a fixed partial denture). The tooth becomes, in effect, a multirooted abutment (Fig. 2.3) with a vastly improved prognosis.

For the Handicapped Patient. All things being equal, the patient with a major handicap, such as the loss of an arm for example, may be better served with a fixed prosthesis which would not require manipulation into and out of the mouth.

Nervous Disorders. A nervous disorder such as epilepsy may predispose a patient to uncontrolled muscle spasms. Other factors being equal, he should be fitted with a fixed prosthesis in preference to a removable partial denture because of the danger of swallowing or aspirating the removable prosthesis during a convulsive seizure.

Conditions Which Militate for the Removable Partial Denture

In general, the removable partial denture is prescribed when the fixed type of prosthesis cannot be employed or when the attributes of the removable partial are considered advantageous in a particular set of circumstances. Advantages of the removable partial denture over the fixed partial denture are: (1) the fewer number of appointments needed, (2) the lessened

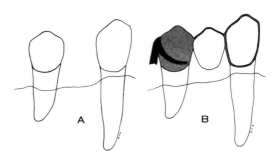

FIG. 2.3. When the first bicuspid has been lost and the second bicuspid has an unfavorable crown/root ratio or a short conical root (A) the second bicuspid can be converted into a more reliable abutment by splinting it to the cuspid with a fixed partial denture (B).

amount of intraoral instrumentation required, (3) the lower cost, and (4) the fact that it is possible for the patient to maintain a very high order of oral hygiene. More specific indications for use of the removable type of prosthesis are discussed in the following paragraphs.

The Distal Extension Base. Although a small pontic is sometimes cantilevered distally from the crown of a terminal abutment tooth, most edentulous spaces not bounded at both ends by teeth suitable as fixed partial denture abutments are best restored by a removable prosthesis.

Long Spans or Less Than Ideal Abutments. When the edentulous span is so long that Ante's rule cannot be satisfied, the removable partial denture should be prescribed. For example, a span from third molar to cuspid is too long for a fixed prosthesis because it places too much buccolingual stress on the abutment teeth. Generally, when the edentulous space "turns the corner of the arch" (e.g., bicuspid to incisor), the removable partial denture is the prosthesis of choice.

For Children and Adolescents. The removable partial denture is often the prosthesis of choice for the youthful patient whose pulp chambers are typically large, hence unusually vulnerable to injury from instrumentation.

For Cross Arch Bracing. When the two sides of a removable partial prosthesis are connected across the midline with a rigid connector all of the teeth involved receive support (in a buccolingual direction) from the prosthesis as well as from each other (Fig. 2.4). The result is a mutual sharing of stress, which is beneficial to all of the structures that play a role in supporting, stabilizing, or retaining the prosthesis. Hence the removable partial denture may offer advantages over the fixed type of prosthesis when periodontally weakened teeth must be stabilized by splinting. Splinting by fixed methods stabilizes the teeth well in a mesiodistal direction, but is not nearly as effective in stabilizing them buccolingually.

To Obturate a Palatal Cleft. When an opening in the palate communicates with

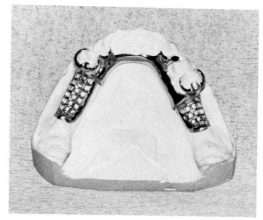

Fig. 2.4. When the two sides of a removable partial denture are connected across the midline by a rigid connector, all of the teeth involved will receive support from the prosthesis as well as from each other.

the nasal cavity (Fig. 2.5), it can best be closed by either the denture base or the major connector of a removable partial denture (Fig. 2.6). This draws attention to the fact that when there are natural teeth remaining in the mouth with a palatal cleft they should be salvaged if at all possible, because they can make an invaluable contribution to the support, stability, and retention of a prosthesis. The prosthesis that is retained by clasps is far superior to the complete denture because of the difficulty in obtaining adequate retention and stability with the latter. By any reckoning natural teeth are the finest retentive aids that a cleft palate patient can possess, and they should be retained for as long as it is possible to do so.

To Restore Facial Contour. A removable prosthesis can be used to provide a bulk of acrylic resin, in order to compensate for bone loss which has occurred as a result of an accident, or from excessive resorption. Such a requirement is encountered most frequently in the anterior part of the mouth where a bulk of acrylic resin is needed so that the anterior prosthetic teeth can be brought out labially to align them better with the remaining natural teeth. In addition, the flange provides needed support for the lip so that it can drape naturally over the replacement

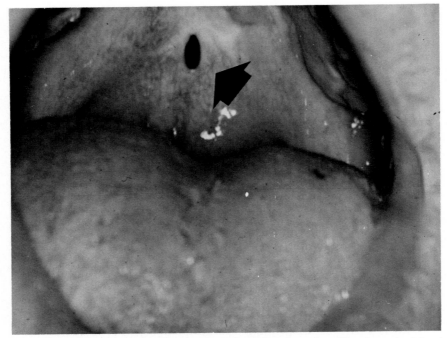

FIG. 2.5. When an opening in the palate connects the oral and nasal cavities, it can best be closed by either the denture base or by the major connector of a removable partial denture.

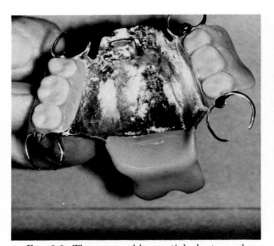

FIG. 2.6. The removable partial denture shown above closes the opening into the nasal cavity, while at the same time supplying a fixed type of obturator.

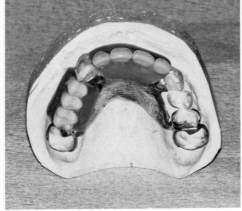

FIG. 2.7. When the labial bone has been lost through resorption or as a result of accident, the anterior replacement teeth can be brought into better labial alignment by means of an acrylic resin flange.

teeth (Fig. 2.7) thus restoring a pleasingly natural appearance.

As a Transitional Prosthesis. A removable partial denture may be best for the patient who, because of age or systemic illness, does not possess the physical stamina to undergo the operative trauma required for fixed replacements or the oral surgery needed for complete dentures. Similarly, the removable partial denture may provide a solution for the individual who, for psychological reasons, cannot face with equanimity the loss of the rest of his natural teeth even though it might be the treatment of choice from a clinical standpoint. A partial denture may enable such an individual to make the transition to complete edentulousness with a minimum of psychic trauma.

Shortened Life Expectancy. The removable partial denture may be the most suitable prosthetic service for the patient whose normal life expectancy has been drastically curtailed because of a systemic illness, such as leukemia, for example. The overriding objective in such an instance is to provide the patient with a prosthesis with which he can eat and function comfortably in the present and the immediate future.

Alteration of the Vertical Dimension. When an increase in the vertical dimension of occlusion is contemplated as a part of the overall treatment, the removable partial denture may play an important role in determining the exact amount of vertical opening that the patient requires. It is usually advisable to accomplish an alteration in the vertical dimension in not less than two steps. A temporary removable prosthesis is first made in which the vertical dimension is increased a tentative amount, and then the patient is closely observed for signs or symptoms of either over- or underclosure. If the increased opening proves to be a satisfactory amount, a more permanent type of prosthesis, fixed or removable, may be constructed at a later date.

Unblemished Abutments. The patient with a caries-free mouth may strenuously object to the mutilation of unblemished teeth for the sole purpose of serving as abutments for a fixed prosthesis. The removable partial denture may be the preferred treatment under the circumstances.

The Diabetic Patient. The diabetic patient, even though controlled by diet and drugs, may experience an immoderate amount of difficulty in wearing any oral prosthesis with comfort. This is due in large measure to the increased susceptibility of the mucosa to traumatic injury, and its propensity for delayed healing. Such a patient will probably fare better with a prosthesis that is at least partially stabilized and supported by natural teeth, than with a complete denture. This is par-ticularly apt to be true of the mandibular arch. Other things being equal, the partial denture will inflict less trauma on the mucosa, so that abrasions are fewer and less severe than with a complete denture.

The Extreme Atrophic Residual Ridge. The patient with an extremely atrophic residual mandibular ridge may fare better with as few as two natural teeth to stabilize, retain, and help support a removable partial denture, than he would with a complete denture. If the teeth are healthy and reasonably stable their use as abutments should be considered, even on a pro tem basis, in preference to extraction, because a complete denture will in all probability be more difficult for the patient to wear comfortably.

The Patient with a Previous Unsatisfactory Prosthetic Experience. The patient who has had an unsuccessful experience with a removable partial denture may have acquired a strong aversion to this type of prosthesis, and may insist that the remaining natural teeth be extracted and a complete denture inserted. If this course of action is clearly not in his best interests, an effort should be made to ascertain the reason for the dissatisfaction with the rejected prosthesis. Adroit questioning may disclose to an astute clinician that there are in truth two reasons: one volunteered by the patient and the second an underlying one of which he may be only dimly conscious. When the patient's reason for not wearing a prosthesis appears to be vague, or is obviously illogical, one may suspect that it is rooted in some cosmetic shortcoming. If the objectionable feature can be identified, and there is a reasonable hope of eliminating it by means of a design modification or an esthetic improvement, then construction of another removable partial denture may be warranted. Certainly this would be preferable to rendering the patient edentulous when it is not in his best interests to do so.

Conditions Which Militate for the Complete Denture

Sometimes the extraction of periodontally involved teeth is recommended under the mistaken notion that this will conserve bone, thus providing a better foundation or a complete denture. This is fallacious reasoning because the intrabony stimulation of natural teeth in function is far more beneficial to the alveolar bone than is the extrabony stimulation of the denture base. In fact, purely from a standpoint of bone preservation every healthy tooth should be retained and every unhealthy tooth treated, although obviously this is not a practical goal. Still, natural teeth should be retained whenever it is feasible to do so, because in general, the greater the number of healthy natural teeth and the fewer the artificial teeth which the patient has, the more efficient will be his masticatory apparatus. However, there are many circumstances under which it is best to remove the remaining teeth and construct complete dentures, this fact notwithstanding.

Inherently Poor Abutments. A complete denture may be the prosthesis of choice when the few remaining noninfected teeth that are salvable are poorly qualified as partial denture abutments, because of excessive bone loss, mobility, or perhaps inherently poor morphology (the lower incisors, for example).

Chronically Poor Oral Hygiene and Rampant Decay. When the patient has rampant decay, and demonstrates poor oral hygiene habits coupled with an unwillingness to renounce lifelong habits of oral indolence, complete dentures may be the most feasible prosthetic service to be recommended.

Cosmetically Unacceptable Anterior Teeth. When the few teeth which remain are confined to the anterior part of the mouth, and due to decay or malalignment are so poor esthetically that restoration by conventional means is not practical, the complete denture should be prescribed. This presumes, of course, that a better esthetic result is a reasonable expectation with the complete denture (Fig. 2.8).

Rejection of Professional advice. When a borderline decision must be made as to whether to extract or retain the remaining teeth, and the patient expresses a preference for extractions despite counsel to the contrary, the complete denture may

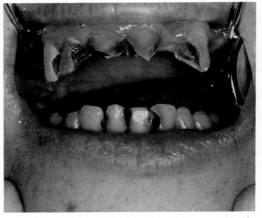

FIG. 2.8. When the few teeth which remain in the maxilla are in the anterior part of the mouth and are hopeless from an esthetic standpoint, the complete denture usually is the prosthesis of choice.

be the most prudent solution from all standpoints. The advantages of a prosthesis that is stabilized by natural teeth, over a complete denture, should be pointed out to such a patient. However, in the last analysis he retains the prerogative of exercising his own judgment.

Refusal of Mouth Preparation. A patient, for reasons of his own, may summarily refuse to have performed needed tooth alteration procedures which have been deemed essential to the success of a partial denture. Under these circumstances it may at times be best for all concerned, to construct a complete denture rather than to attempt construction of a partial denture without proper preparation. Every reasonable effort should be made to educate such an individual by pointing out the advantages of the recommended treatment and the reasons that the mouth preparation is essential to its success. However, the patient must make the final decision.

Poor Alignment. When the few remaining teeth are so extremely malaligned and so poorly distributed in the dental arch that a removable partial denture will create uncontrollable leverages, the prognosis for a clasp-retained prosthesis may be so poor as to make the complete denture a better choice (Fig. 2.9).

Radiation Therapy. When it is neces-

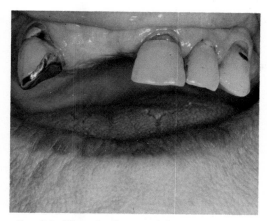

FIG. 2.9. When the few remaining teeth are badly aligned as well as poorly distributed in the arch, the prognosis for a removable partial denture is not favorable, and the complete denture is usually a better choice.

sary to apply radiation therapy in the treatment of a malignancy, and natural teeth are in the path of the therapeutic rays, a profoundly important decision must be made. If the teeth are allowed to remain and must subsequently be extracted, the probability of osteomyelitis is prohibitively high. For this reason most authorities recommend the removal of all the remaining teeth prior to the administration of radiation therapy. When these circumstances are encountered, the patient's physician, the oral surgeon, and the prosthodontist should reach a consensus before a final decision is made.

General Considerations in Selecting the Prosthesis

Certain types and combinations of oral prostheses have proven themselves clinically to be superior to others, because of such diverse factors as the type of occlusion, the effect of gravity, and the anatomical differences between the maxilla and the mandible. These factors, as well as the influence which they exert on the selection of a prosthesis, are discussed in the following paragraphs.

The Type of Occlusion as a Factor in Selection of the Prosthesis

The size and contour of the maxilla, as well as its relationship to the mandible, can be significant factors in selecting the most suitable type of prosthesis. In a mouth with a prognathic relationship, for example, the mandibular teeth tend to stabilize the maxillary occlusion, whereas the opposite is true with the Class II occlusion. Fortunately, the Class III relationship tends to be the rule more often than not, because of the normal pattern of bone resorption which is typical of the maxilla and mandible (Fig. 2.10). Following the removal of teeth, the bone of the maxilla resorbs superiorly and medially (upwards and inwards), while the bone of the mandible resorbs inferiorly and laterally (downward and outward). Thus, the resorptive process tends to create a Class III occlusion, which is favorable from a standpoint of mechanics for the stability of a prosthesis in either arch. However, it should be noted that the maxilla in the typical prognathic occlusion tends to be small, which must be counted an unfavorable factor from a standpoint of retention.

The mandibular teeth exert an upward, forward thrust on the maxilla in the mouth with a retrognathic occlusion (Class II), which has a tendency to dislodge a maxillary prosthesis. Hence, retention of maxillary teeth and construction of a partial denture might be preferable in a mouth with an extreme Class II

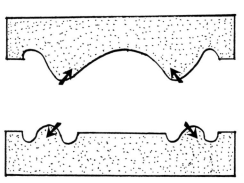

FIG. 2.10. This sketch depicts the typical pattern of resorption of the bone of the maxilla and the mandible that tends to produce a Class III relationship. The bone of the maxilla resorbs medially and superiorly, while that of the mandible resorbs laterally and inferiorly.

occlusion rather than to expose a complete denture to the disbalancing stresses generated by the mandibular teeth.

The Occlusal Plane as a Factor

In assessing the relative merits of the maxillary removable partial denture as opposed to the complete denture for the patient whose remaining maxillary teeth are tipped, rotated, and extruded a profoundly important consideration is the character and orientation of the occlusal plane. If it is markedly disarranged and irregular due to the migration and extrusion of the remaining teeth, it may be virtually impossible to restore a harmonious occlusion with a partial denture (Fig. 2.11). This means that the prognosis will be poor, not only for the maxillary teeth, but for the opposing mandibular teeth as well, because of the torsional stresses to which they will be subjected.

The Kennedy Class I Maxillary Denture. If the maxillary posterior teeth are extracted leaving only six maxillary anterior teeth, in the hope of realigning the

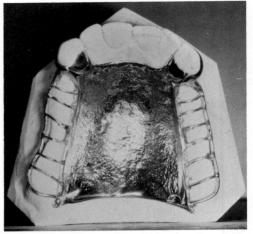

FIG. 2.12. The problem of restoring the maxillary arch with only six remaining anterior teeth is complicated by the fact that gravity becomes a potential dislodging force. Unless movement of the base is controlled, torsional stress will be transmitted to the abutment teeth.

hopelessly disoriented occlusal plane, the problem of both gravity and leverage must be contended with. The threat posed by gravity to the retention of a maxillary prosthesis that is retained only by anterior teeth is a serious one. If the denture is permitted to tilt downward posteriorly it will exert torsional stress on the abutment teeth, a stress which will be magnified by a leverage factor introduced by the distal extension base (Fig. 2.12). Unfortunately, the control of this leverage, unlike that in the mandibular partial denture, is difficult to achieve, and the problem does not end with the mechanical difficulties, formidable as they are. The crowns of anterior teeth seldom present good contours for clasping, nor do they, as a rule, lend themselves well to the preparation of proper lingual or incisal recesses for the clasp rests. If the tooth is covered with a crown for the purpose of improving the contour for clasping, the problem of displaying gold in the anterior part of the mouth must be met. If esthetically pleasing restorations are placed on the anterior teeth, the problem of displaying a labial clasp arm remains. Usually a clasp arm in the anterior part of the mouth is difficult to conceal and unsightly when displayed. If a precision rest is employed as a means to eliminate the display of a

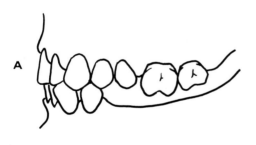

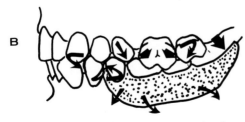

FIG. 2.11. The occlusal stresses transmitted to the abutment teeth and the residual ridge by an opposing occlusion in which the teeth are tipped, extruded, and rotated (A) will be largely horizontal and torsional as depicted by the *arrows* in B. The abutment teeth as well as the supporting tissues will not long withstand such a traumatic onslaught.

labial clasp arm, the stress transmitted to the abutment through the key/keyway device will be materially greater than the stress which would be exerted by a conventional clasp, unless a stressbreaking device is employed. Stressbreakers, of course, introduce problems of their own (see stressbreaker discussion, Chapter 18).

Advantages of the Complete Denture

The incisal guidance in the mouth with a deteriorated occusal plane has, almost invariably, evolved into a deep vertical overlap of the anterior teeth, and centric occlusion and centric relation rarely coincide. In addition, the vertical dimension of occlusion has typically been reduced. An important advantage of the complete denture is the fact that centric relation and centric occlusion can be made to coincide at the proper vertical dimension. The amount of both horizontal and vertical overlap can be reduced substantially with the result that the patient's appearance is enhanced, while at the same time the occlusion is improved. The occlusion can be developed so that the stresses are directed along the long axis of the mandibular teeth, which is in itself a major step towards increasing the longevity of natural teeth and preserving the supporting bone. Certainly the stresses generated by a complete denture with a harmonious occlusion will be less traumatic to the mandibular teeth than will extruded, tipped, and rotated natural teeth. As a consequence, retention of the remaining mandibular teeth, in a state of health over a longer period of time, would seem to be a reasonable expectation. Not to be overlooked is the fact that the amount of stress which the patient is able to apply to the dental structures is markedly reduced because of the limitations in biting force imposed by the artificial denture.

Finally, but not least, the need for a display of clasps on anterior teeth is eliminated thus improving immeasurably the esthetic opportunity. Clearly the maxillary complete denture has much to recommend it over the large maxillary partal denture, when the occusal plane is in an advanced stage of deterioration.

The occlusion should be so developed that there is no contact between the mandibular anterior natural teeth and the maxillary denture in centric position. The reason for this is that the structure of the maxilla is such that it cannot withstand the trauma of repeated impact from the natural mandibular teeth. The result of failure to observe this precaution will be hyperplasia of the mucosa, accompanied by rapid bone resorption of the anterior portion of the maxilla.

The Maxillary Complete Denture Opposed by the Mandibular Partial Denture

Generally it can be said that the average patient will experience more difficulty becoming accustomed to the mandibular complete denture than to the maxillary. Hence the conventional clinical wisdom is to go to greater lengths to retain mandibular teeth which can contribute to the retention and stability of the prosthesis, in preference to constructing a complete denture. Even when such teeth are lost after a relatively short period of service as abutments, the patient will have acquired a degree of neuromuscular skill in managing the prosthesis that will stand him in good stead as he takes on the more difficult challenge of controlling a complete denture. Fortunately the complete maxillary denture, as opposed to the mandibular removable partial denture, has proven itself in countless numbers of clinical cases to be a successful prosthodontic combination.

The Mandibular Complete Denture Opposed to Natural Teeth

There is a wide divergence of opinion concerning the wisdom of constructing a complete denture to oppose natural maxillary teeth. Because of the difficult mechanical problems which are posed, some highly regarded authorities consider such a procedure impractical. While it is true that the natural teeth have the potential of inflicting irreparable damage on the mandibular ridge, some cogent arguments can be mustered for giving the plan consideration.

For one thing it must be conceded that the procedure can succeed under the right combination of circumstances. Furthermore, there is an understandable reluctance to order the extraction of a complete, or nearly complete, arch of sound healthy natural teeth. Not unexpectedly, the patient may vehemently oppose such an approach to his problem of semiedentulousness.

The key to the problem is the occlusal plane of the maxillary teeth and the patient's health, or more precisely, his bone factor. If the occlusal plane has not deteriorated beyond reclamation and the patient is in good health, the complete mandibular denture is a feasible approach to this type of edentulousness. However, it is difficult to overestimate the importance of these two factors when making this decision. If the occlusal plane is markedly disarranged and cannot be restored to a near normal configuration by a combination of equilibration and restorative procedures, the prognosis must be considered very poor for the complete denture, and even less favorable for preservation of the mandibular residual ridge.

When a decision has been made to construct a complete denture to oppose natural maxillary teeth, the patient should be apprised of the problems inherent in the undertaking, so that he can assume a share of the liability. It is important, too, that such a patient be maintained in a state of optimal health and be nurtured with a balanced diet, that the fit of the mandibular denture be maintained, and that it be removed from the mouth for at least 8 of the 24 hours.

The patient for whom this service is rendered should be followed closely for signs of bone resorption, as evidenced by a too rapid loosening of the denture. If it is determined that resorption is occurring at a faster than normal rate, the maxillary teeth should be removed forthwith, in the patient's best interests.

Recommending No Prosthodontic Treatment

Occasionally, a patient seeks treatment whose loss of function is so minor as to cast doubt on the advisability of prescribing any prosthesis at all. The patient with a second and third molar missing in one quadrant of either the maxilla or mandible is a typical example. In order to restore such a unilateral space a prosthesis would have to be made up of a lingual (or palatal) bar and two or three clasps, in addition to the denture base and the replacement tooth. It is open to question whether the improvement in function, comfort, and oral health provided by such a prosthesis would justify, in the patient's mind, the inconvenience and annoyance of adapting to such a relatively large bulk of foreign material.

The Importance of Good Clinical Judgment

The wrong choice in prescribing the type of prosthetic service, besides demonstrating faulty clinical judgment, may be a gross disservice to the patient who must depend on the clinical wisdom of the dental profession for the preservation of his oral health. No matter how skillfully the wrong treatment is carried out, it is still the wrong treatment. It is critically important, therefore, that time be taken to gather all relevant data, and to bring to bear one's best clinical judgment in prescribing the prosthetic service that will best serve the patient over the longest period of time.

Bibliography

Applegate, O. C.: Conditions which may influence the choice of partial or complete denture service. J. Prosth. Dent. 7: 182–196, 1957.

Kennedy, E.: Partial Denture Construction, Ed. 2. Dental Items of Interest Publishing Co., Inc., New York, 1951.

Oesterling, B. O.: Complete dentures opposite partial dentures: Diagnostic factors. J. Amer. Dent. Ass. 63: 611–617, 1961.

Schuyler, C. H.: Elements of diagnosis leading to full or partial dentures. J. Amer. Dent. Ass. 41: 302–305, 1950.

Storer, R.: The effect of climacteric and aging on prosthetic diagnosis and treatment. Brit. Dent. J. 119: 349–354, 1965.

Tylman, S. D.: Theory and Practice of Crown and Bridge Prosthodontics, Ed. 5. The C. V. Mosby Company, St. Louis, 1965.

Wilson, J. H.: The general principles of diagnosis and prognosis of partial dentures. Dent. J. Aust. 11: 69–77, 1939.

Young, A. C.: Indications and the diagnosis for fixed partial denture prosthesis. J. Amer. Dent. Ass. 41: 289–295, 1950.

Chapter 3

TREATMENT PLANNING

This chapter focuses attention on the various clinical procedures which may be employed to upgrade the mouth to a status of optimum health while, at the same time, improving the design as well as the prognosis of the prosthesis. Each type of treatment is discussed as it relates specifically to removable partial denture design and construction. The material is organized according to the following format:

Introduction

When a firm decision has been made as to the type and design of the prosthesis that is to be prescribed, based on a careful assessment of all the accumulated data, the definitive treatment plan can be formulated. This will consist of enumerating in simple, concise terms each of the various clinical steps that need to be accomplished, in the sequence that they are to be performed, for the purpose of preparing the mouth to receive the prosthesis.

The Written Treatment Plan

It is not essential to the success of the treatment that the plan be recorded on paper provided the dentist who devises the plan personally accomplishes all of the prescribed treatment. A written plan is essential, however, if the patient is to be referred to another section of a large clinic, or to another dental office for a part of the treatment, or if two or more dentists are to assume, conjointly, the responsibility for the various phases of therapy (Fig. 3.1). There are definite advantages to be gained by establishing a written record, irrespective of how or by whom the treatment is to be accomplished. For example, a written record can be used as a check list to ensure that no phase of the therapy is overlooked or, what is much more apt to occur, be performed out of sequence. It is a convenience in explaining to the patient the clinical procedures that are to be accomplished so that appointments of the appropriate length can be scheduled at suitably spaced intervals, and in allowing sufficient time for healing, laboratory preparation, and similar unavoidable delays in the therapeutic continuum. Then too, a written treatment plan may be helpful to auxiliary personnel who must plan the chair and laboratory support that will be required as the treatment progresses. It can be kept on file if, for some unforeseen reason, the course of treatment must be temporarily postponed until a future date. In such a circumstance, when the patient subsequently returns for treatment, it represents an invaluable record of the recommendations made at the original visit. Parenthetically, it will be reassuring to the patient to receive precisely the same recommendations regarding his treatment, after an interval of several months, that he had previously been given, always provided, of course, that there has been no significant change in his oral condition

UNIVERSITY OF ALABAMA
SCHOOL OF DENTISTRY

DIAGNOSIS AND TREATMENT PLAN

Diagnosis

DEPARTMENT	TREATMENT PLAN	ESTIMATE
O.S.	1. EXT. #1 – #3	
PERIO	2. GTMY. #17	
OPER.	3. INLAY M.O. #14 AMAL. O. #15	
C & B	4. FX. BDG. #2 – #5 FULL CWN. #21 – #28	
	5. PRLX.	
PROS.	6. MAND. R.P.D.	

NAME SMITH, JOHN L.   REG. NO. 12961   TOTAL

STUDENT JONES, BEN   DATE   INSTR. DR. BROWN

FIG. 3.1. The use of a written treatment plan has much to recommend it. It should enumerate, in concise terms, each of the different clinical procedures that is to be accomplished, in the sequence that it is to be performed.

during the interval. When the plan is committed to paper the treatment procedures should be listed in simple, concise terms.

The Partial or Interim Plan

It may be necessary, at times, to prepare only a partial or interim treatment plan when the outcome of a key phase of the treatment is in doubt, and other required treatment, or perhaps even the type of prosthesis to be prescribed, may be contingent on the outcome of this particular therapy. For example, an extensively broken down molar may be an eminently desirable abutment and pivotal to the design of the prosthesis, provided it can be returned to a state of health and the contour of its crown satisfactorily restored. In this instance, the first step in the treatment plan would be to perform the needed therapy on this particular tooth, with completion of the overall plan held in abeyance until its state of health has been definitely established. When the status of this "key" tooth has been determined, the remainder of the treatment plan can be completed.

The Alternate Plan

It is usually a good policy to devise an alternate treatment plan when more than one therapeutic approach is feasible so that, should the patient feel compelled to reject one plan, because of financial considerations for example, another less expensive course of treatment can be recommended. However, it bears emphasis that a patient's financial status should never be permitted to interfere with his being advised of the ideal treatment and the reason it is recommended over any other.

Formulating the Plan

One method of managing the formulation and presentation of the treatment plan, that has much to recommend it, is to set aside an interval of time between appointments during which the planning casts, radiographs, and records can be leisurely reviewed and analyzed. In all but the most complex cases a tentative treatment plan can be prepared from the clinical data thus far accumulated. When the patient presents for the next appointment only a few confirmatory checks within the mouth will be all that is required, following which the treatment plan can be finalized and presented. The treatment plan need not be considered sacrosanct, obviously. Unforeseen exigencies may dictate some variation in clinical approach as the treatment progresses, or in some rather infrequent circumstances a change in the prosthesis may be prescribed. However, these cases are the exception rather than the rule. Generally, the clinical steps will be performed in the sequence prescribed by the treatment plan.

Sequence of Treatment

There are many clinical procedures that can be carried out to improve the prognosis for the removable partial denture. The treatment plan is, in effect, a blueprint which outlines the clinical steps that are to be accomplished in order to exploit the factors which favor the most ideal design, while eliminating, or at least minimizing, the effects of unfavorable factors. The very essence of good treatment planning is to devise a sequential arrangement of clinical procedures by means of which the overall treatment is accomplished in the most efficient and expeditious manner. Each step should logically follow the preceding one. Although the exact order of procedures will vary according to the patient's individual needs, certain imperatives should be recognized. Certainly, the chief complaint should be attended to with a minimum of delay, especially if it has been provoked by pain or discomfort. This may require the removal of gross decay, and placement of temporary fillings in one or several teeth, early in the treatment sequence, or an offending tooth may have to be extracted to allay pain. On the other hand, extractions of anterior teeth may have to be postponed for cosmetic reasons, and some palliative treatment instituted as a stop-gap measure to keep them comfortable. Occlusal adjustment must be accomplished early in the course of treatment because the occlusion is a keystone for all of the other treatment. The restoration of a tooth with a crown, for example, should be accomplished so that it is in harmony with the planned occlusal scheme as well as with the path of insertion of the prosthesis. Ideally, the occlusion will be one in which centric occlusion and centric relation coincide, although this cannot be achieved in every instance.

Surgical Procedures

The performance of various oral surgical procedures for one purpose or another will be required for many removable partial denture patients. The extraction of painful, infected teeth is, perhaps, the most common one, and should be one of the first operations to be accomplished. A number of other surgical procedures may be indicated which are capable of markedly improving the prognosis of the prosthesis, such as the smoothing of sharp bone, the ablation of bony overgrowths and undercuts, and the elimination of redundant hyperplastic tissue, to name a few. An awareness of the numerous oral surgical techniques which may be performed, coupled with an understanding of the circumstances under which they can most advantageously be employed, is an indispensable part of the prosthodontist's planning arsenal.

Surgery should be planned, whenever possible, so that all procedures needed in a quadrant of the mouth are accomplished at the same time, in order to eliminate unnecessary injections and to hold to a minimum the number of times that the patient is rendered incapable of performing normal masticatory functions comfortably. It is demoralizing to a patient to be required to submit to a second surgical procedure that had been overlooked in the same area of the mouth, because a thorough treatment plan was not devised beforehand.

A Philosophy of Bone Preservation

The patient and the prosthodontist share a mutual interest in having as substantial a bony foundation as possible for as long a period of time as it can be maintained. Indeed, the preservation of the remaining oral structures is a cardinal objective of partial denture prosthodontics. With an ever increasing life expectancy, the typical partial denture candidate can, on a statistical basis, be expected to wear a prosthesis during a time span of a quarter of a century and even more. Accordingly, the best surgical techniques are those which conserve a maximum amount of bone, thus providing the best residual ridges for support of the denture, for the longest possible duration. Clinical experience bears out the fact that the techniques which best conserve bone are oftentimes not the ones that ensure the most rapid healing and, in some instances, not the best denture foundation. Examples abound of severe undercuts which have been left undisturbed in an attempt to conserve bone, with the result that the patient cannot insert and remove the prosthesis and, in fact, may not be able to wear it without discomfort or pain. If the alveolar bone is carefully smoothed with files and rongeurs following extractions, healing will proceed at a maximum rate, and the prosthesis can be constructed and inserted in comparatively short order.

Extractions

Teeth which are hopelessly diseased or so badly destroyed as to be unsalvable should be removed and, as a general policy, this should be done early in the treatment sequence so as to allow ample time for healing. Extremely unesthetic teeth which cannot be restored to a state of cosmetic acceptability by restoration may also have to be extracted (Fig. 3.2). Anterior teeth may require removal when they are so badly aligned that they are a detriment to the patient's appearance as well as to the most ideal design of the prosthesis (Fig. 3.3).

Prosthetic Expediency. A tooth may have to be removed because its position in the arch is such that it interferes with insertion and removal of the prosthesis or with a desired design. Extreme lingual tipping of the mandibular bicuspids is a common example. In some instances a bicuspid may lean so far lingually as to make it impossible to position a lingual

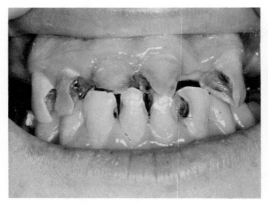

FIG. 3.2. Anterior teeth that are completely hopeless from an esthetic standpoint, as well as being poorly aligned in the dental arch, are candidates for extraction.

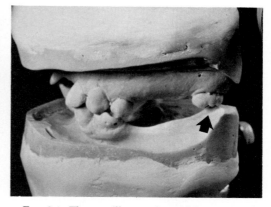

FIG. 3.4. The maxillary molar which contacts the mandibular ridge when the patient closes in centric position will interfere with the proper design of a mandibular prosthesis and must often be extracted.

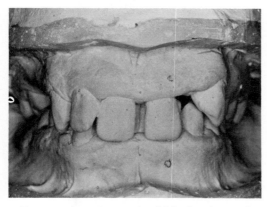

FIG. 3.3. Anterior teeth which deeply overlap their antagonists complicate the design of a prosthesis, and oftentimes must be extracted.

bar properly. The extruded molar that contacts the opposing ridge when the jaws are occluded is another example (Fig. 3.4), and buccal tipping of the maxillary bicuspids is still another, although less common, example.

Retained Roots and Tooth Remnants. The question of whether or not to remove embedded root tips or remnants (Fig. 3.5) prior to construction of a prosthesis may be a difficult one to answer, particularly if the patient is elderly or systemically below par and not expected to respond well to the surgery. Certainly there is no immutable rule stating that all embedded

bodies must be removed before a prosthesis is fitted. The age of the patient is clinically significant. The younger patient can be expected to heal more quickly, because normally the bone will not be as hard and his recupreative powers will be greater. Then too, there is more possibility of surgical complications when the bone is sclerosed around the embedded body, which is common in older individuals. Removing a root remnant from sclerotic bone may pose a very difficult surgical problem in the mandible, particularly when the mandible is atrophic.

Assuming the remnant to be asymptomatic, a key question is whether or not there is evidence of infection. If there is a reasonable doubt as to the presence of pathosis, the decision must be to remove it, unless there are valid reasons for not doing so. In the case of a retained root tip it must be conceded that it was once exposed to the oral fluids and that theoretically at least the root canal may still contain some pulpal tissue. This raises the possibility that it could be a source of infection.

In weighing the pros and cons of removing a root tip or tooth remnant it is profoundly important that its exact location be determined. A root tip that appears to be deeply embedded in the bone in a periapical radiograph, for example, may in fact, be located rather superficially

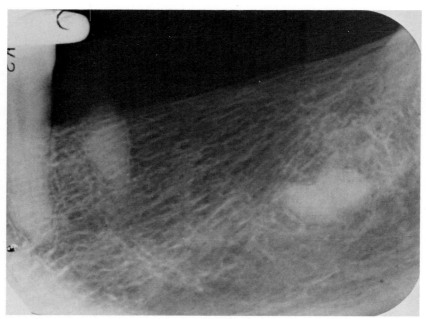

Fig. 3.5. The question of whether or not to remove deeply embedded root tips, or unerupted teeth, prior to the construction of a prosthesis is not always a simple one to answer, particularly if the patient is elderly or below par systemically. Each such instance must be decided on its own merits, following a careful evaluation of all relevant factors.

to the buccal or lingual plate of bone so that it would be pointless to agonize over a decision. The use of an occlusal radiograph to supplement the periapical radiograph should be routine in instances of this type.

Advising the Patient. When a decision has been made to leave an embedded root or remnant undisturbed this information should be conveyed to the patient with professional finesse so as not to evoke needless anxiety. The patient's record should be annotated to reflect that an embedded body is present, that a decision was made not to remove it, and that the pertinent facts have been explained to the patient.

Impacted and Unerupted Teeth. Impacted and unerupted teeth should, as a rule, be removed prior to construction of the prosthesis for three principal reasons: (1) if not removed the tooth may erupt beneath the denture, (2) the tooth may harbor pathosis, and (3) it might develop symptoms following a period of wear of the prosthesis. However, exceptions to the rule are sometimes made. Unerupted

maxillary third molars are usually not extracted for adolescents because to do so is to remove a major stimulus to bone formation in the tuberosity region. Since this particular area of the mouth is destined to play a key role in the support of a prosthesis of one type or another, over the many years of a normal life expectancy, the decision to remove or extract these molars may have far reaching implications and the evidence should be weighed very carefully. When a second molar is present along with an impacted third molar, the decision may be complicated by the fact that the impacted tooth can affect bone formation distal to the second molar and, in addition, may induce pocket formation between the two teeth. Thus, there is the threat of caries activity as a result of the communication with the oral cavity.

When evaluating the impacted or unerupted tooth from a standpoint of potential pathology, the possibility of dentigerous cyst formation from the follicular sac, which surrounds all developing teeth, should not be overlooked. Cyst formation is more often encountered around the third molar than any other tooth, and it is more common in the mandible than in the maxilla. When a decision is made to leave an embedded tooth undisturbed, the site should be examined radiographically at regular intervals. This inspection may conveniently be programmed to be accomplished at the same appointment that periodic maintenance is performed on the prosthesis.

Alveoloplasty

Ideally, the alveolar ridge will be prepared for load-bearing at the time the teeth are extracted. However, when a residual ridge is encountered that is rough and spinous, a decision must sometimes be made whether to wait for nature to smooth off the irregularities or to intervene surgically and smooth the bone with instruments. In making such a judgment, the length of time that the teeth have been missing is a key consideration. In some instances, additional healing time may be all that is required to bring about

a smooth, well contoured ridge. Under other circumstances, healing may be so slow, and accompanied by such discomfort, that it makes surgical intervention the only acceptable modality. Sometimes, smoothing the irregular atrophic ridge will reduce vestibular depth to a point where adequate support for the prosthesis is imperiled, in which case, a vestibular extension may be considered.

Teeth which have stood singly or in small groups, as a result of the extraction of adjacent teeth, are sometimes surrounded by a high island of bone which slopes steeply to join the adjacent resorbed residual ridge. When such teeth are extracted, the surrounding bone should be recontoured so as to blend as smoothly as possible with the adjoining residual ridge.

Palatal and Mandibular Tori

It may sometimes be necessary to remove the palatal torus (Fig. 3.6), but generally the maxillary prosthesis can be de-

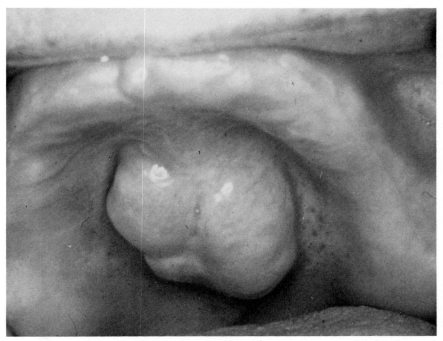

FIG. 3.6. The palatal torus seldom needs to be ablated unless it is massive, lobulated, or undercut, and the partial denture cannot be designed to circumvent it. If it is not too large in size and is not undercut, the maxillary connector, in most instances, can be designed to cover it. The reason that the palatal torus will tolerate contact with the prosthesis is that the mucosal covering is usually somewhat thicker and more resilient than is the case with a mandibular torus, and in addition there is usually much less movement of the maxillary denture than is true in the mandibular.

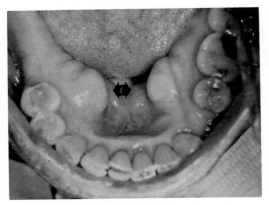

FIG. 3.7. The lingual torus is almost always an obstacle to successful wear of a mandibular prosthesis.

signed to avoid this bony overgrowth, if it is thought best not to cover it with the major connector or the denture base. Lingual tori (Fig. 3.7), on the other hand, are often formidable obstacles to comfortable wear of the denture, and should be ablated unless there is an overriding contraindication. When the torus, either maxillary or mandibular, must be removed, it should be remembered that healing will be more rapid and more comfortable and that there will be less chance of complications, if the wound site can be covered with a supporting stent. The healing time required for an operated torus is approximately 2 weeks when a supporting stent is used, and 3 to 4 weeks without one. The torectomy should be scheduled, whenever possible, so as to be carried out along with other surgical procedures that have been programmed for that area of the mouth.

Bony overgrowths may appear almost anywhere in the maxilla or the mandible (Figs. 3.8 and 3.9). Usually they are bulbous in form, and the overlying mucosa is typically quite thin. The area is thus a potential source of irritation and soreness if it is contacted by any part of the denture. In determining the wisdom of intervening surgically, each such area must be evaluated on its individual merits. Key considerations are whether or not the prosthesis will be in contact with the mucosa and, if so, whether or not it will be permitted, because of its design, to

move in function. If the answers to both of these questions are affirmative, the probabilities are that the mucosa covering the protuberance will be chafed, and become a source of discomfort and annoyance to the patient.

The Maxillary Tuberosity

The tuberosity may interfere with prosthesis construction by creating an undercut, by being overly bulbous, or by being so large (Fig. 3.10), that the prosthesis cannot be accommodated in the denture space. A tuberosity so formed is a stumbling block to proper partial denture design and should be surgically recontoured provided there are no contraindications to the needed surgery. One contraindication is the maxillary antrum which is in close proximity to the tuberosity, having accompanied the teeth and the bone as they descended into the space created by the missing mandibular teeth. Under such circumstances it may be unsafe to remove any maxillary bone at all, for fear of exposing the sinus, and an alternative solution must be sought.

Healing time for the surgically corrected tuberosity is approximately 10 days to 2 weeks for a fibrous excision, and 2 to 3 weeks for surgery which involves recontouring of the bone.

The Mylohyoid Ridge, the Lingual Shelf

Undercuts produced by ledges of bone often interfere with comfortable seating and removal of the denture and are always a potential source of soreness. An example of this is commonly encountered in the area of the mylohyoid ridge (Fig. 3.11), where an overly prominent ridge of bone may interfere with the ideal lingual extension of the denture base into its proper position in the alveolingual sulcus. If the ridge is sharp, and the undercut which it creates is extreme, it should be trimmed surgically. Failure to accomplish this surgery will mean that the denture flange may have to be designed short of its customary length in this region, a solution that the patient may find disconcerting if the truncated border attracts the attention of a curious tongue. On the

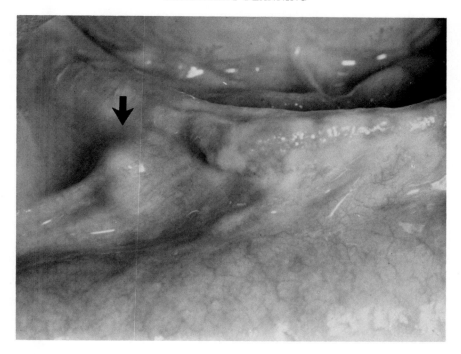

FIG. 3.8. Bony overgrowths (exostoses) may occur anywhere in either jaw. Usually they are bulbous in form and the overlying mucosa, particularly in the mandible, is typically thin and susceptible to trauma. When a prosthesis is fitted over such an area, the mucosa may be rubbed between the bone and the prosthesis, and abrasion and inflammation quickly ensue.

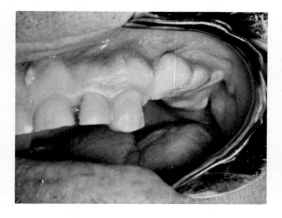

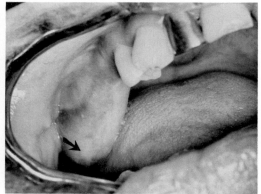

FIG. 3.9. The bony overgrowth shown here is on the buccal surface of the maxilla. In this location it is an obstacle to comfortable wear of a prosthesis and should be removed by surgery.

FIG. 3.10. An overly large tuberosity may create a lack of sufficient interridge space and usually requires surgical reduction. The location of the maxillary sinus must always be ascertained before surgery is performed in this area.

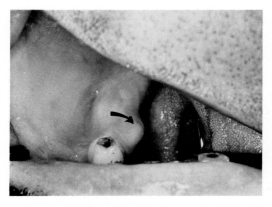

FIG. 3.11. The mylohyoid ridge region is a frequent site of bony outcroppings which interfere with ideal extension of the partial denture base. When the bony prominence is sharp and the undercut is extreme, alveoloplasty may upgrade the prognosis for the prosthesis substantially.

other hand, if the flange is extended into the alveolingual sulcus, it will be necessary to force it over the undercut each time the denture is inserted or removed from the mouth. In the latter instance, the thin mucosal covering over the crest of the undercut will be pinched between the bone and the denture, and soreness will quickly ensue. If the tissue surface of the denture is subsequently relieved in order to eliminate the contact between denture and mucosa, the void thus created may annoy the patient, is quite apt to be unhygienic, and is certain to affect the fit adversely. Conservative reduction of this lingual shelf of bone, before the prosthesis is constructed, is the only assurance that it will not create a problem. Although surgery of the mylohyoid ridge carries the risk of sublingual hemorrhage and swelling, which may cause delay, healing should be complete in approximately 3 weeks if it is uneventful.

The Genial Tubercle

Resorption of the mandibular ridge is sometimes so extensive that the genial tubercle becomes prominently located lingually to the residual ridge at the midline. Thus exposed it may be vulnerable to trauma from a prosthesis. Although this is rarely a problem in partial denture con-

struction, this bony structure can be ablated if comfortable wear of the prosthesis is prevented by its presence. Notwithstanding the fact that bleeding is a frequent complication of this operation, healing time may be as short as 3 weeks if it is uneventful.

Removal of Hyperplastic Tissue

The removal of hyperplastic tissue (Fig. 3.12) may improve immeasurably the foundation for the denture. While redundant tissue may appear in any area of the mouth, it is most commonly encountered on the residual ridges and in the palate. When a diagnosis of papillary hyperplasia of the palate (papillomatosis) has been established in a wearer of a prosthesis, it is usually best to remove the redundant tissue surgically. Although the acute inflammation may subside as a result of leaving the prosthesis out of the mouth, or of wearing a tissue-treatment material inside the prosthesis, the punctate tissue tends to remain. Largely for this reason, the area will be highly susceptible to a return of the inflammation, and generally, the favored treatment is to remove the hyperplastic tissue surgically.

Relief of Muscle Attachments

Muscle attachments, which attach near the crest of the residual ridge, may interfere with proper extension of the denture flange (Fig. 3.13) into the vestibule. Such an attachment may be surgically repositioned, a recommended procedure being to fabricate the framework prior to the surgery. An acrylic resin stent is then attached to the framework, which will serve to hold the vestibular tissue in its newly extended position while healing takes place (Fig. 3.14).

Frenoplasty

An overly large frenum, or one that attaches close to the crest of the ridge, always poses a potential threat to the snug fit of a prosthesis. This is particularly true of the maxillary labial frenum and the partial denture with a labial flange. The labial frenula (Fig. 3.15), either maxillary or mandibular, may be partially resected

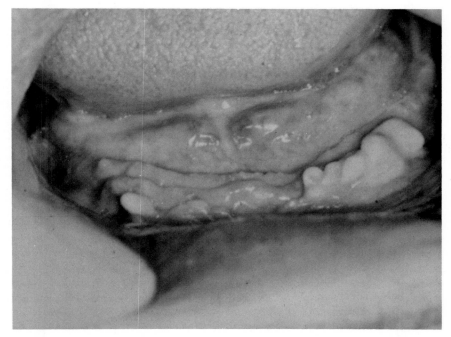

FIG. 3.12. Hyperplastic, redundant soft tissue provides an extremely poor foundation for the denture base and should be removed prior to denture construction, in the patient's best interests.

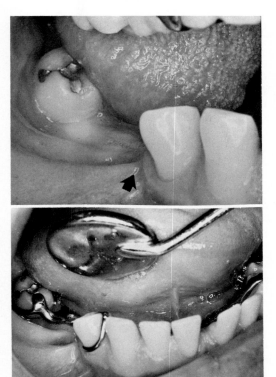

to provide additional room for the denture flange, if it interferes with ideal flange extension or with esthetics. This is a relatively minor procedure which may improve the wearability of the prosthesis out of all proportion to its simplicity. Deep resection or total frenectomy is never necessary, and indeed not even desirable. The objective is merely to raise the level of the frenulum attachment enough so that the vestibule will accommodate a normal extension of the denture border without the necessity of creating a deep, V-shaped slot in the flange, which may be uncomfortable, is usually unsightly, and always inter-

FIG. 3.13 (upper). The labial and buccal vestibules in edentulous areas should be deep enough to accommodate a reasonable extension of the denture flange. When muscle attachments or scar bands interfere, as shown in the photograph, they should be altered surgically.

FIG. 3.14 (lower). A framework was constructed and a temporary base of acrylic resin was attached to it, to hold the soft tissue in place after it was resected. When healing was complete, a new denture base was substituted for the original temporary one.

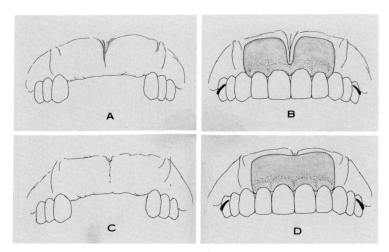

Fig. 3.15. When the labial frenum interferes with a properly extended labial flange, a frenotomy should be considered. *A*, a frenum which attaches near the crest of the residual ridge. *B*, the unsightly appearance of the flange which has been contoured to accommodate the frenum. *C*, a frenotomy has been performed raising the attachment of the frenum superiorly. *D*, a properly extended labial flange is stronger, contributes to the retention of the denture, and may be more hygienic, as well as consmetically superior.

feres with an optimum seal of the denture border in this area. As is true of many surgical procedures, healing will be more rapid, and there will be less likelihood of complications, if the wound site can be supported by a denture to act as a stent during the healing period.

The lingual frenum which attaches close to the crest of the mandibular ridge, or that is excessively large and fan-shaped, may interfere with proper positioning of the lingual bar and, in some instances, may impede speech. The condition can be corrected rather simply by a person trained in oral surgical techniques, and it may well spell the difference between success and failure in some circumstances. In common with all surgical procedures, the frenoplasty should be planned at the beginning of treatment so that it can be performed at the most propitious time in the treatment sequence, for example, during extraction of anterior teeth.

The Immediate Partial Denture

It may be desirable, under some circumstances, to construct a partial denture which replaces one or several anterior teeth as an immediate insertion. When this procedure is being followed, the teeth

to be replaced by the immediate technique should be restricted to the anterior part of the mouth. Immediate replacement of posterior teeth is seldom feasible. The technique of constructing an immediate partial denture is essentially the same as that for the immediate complete denture, with a few minor exceptions. Impressions are obtained in the usual manner. If there are large cavities in the teeth that are to be replaced, it is usually expedient to fill them with a sedative cement prior to introducing the impression material so as to avoid undue tearing of the material when the impression is withdrawn. The teeth to be extracted are cut from the stone cast and simulated sockets are prepared in the stone. When the framework has been fabricated, the replacement teeth are fitted into the residual ridge of the cast and attached to the retention latticework with wax. If a labial flange is to be used, of course, the teeth are set in the wax which will form the denture flange.

Usually denture teeth, either porcelain or acrylic resin, are used as replacements for the natural teeth, since they can be readily replaced and new teeth fitted, when the alveolar ridge resorbs and cre-

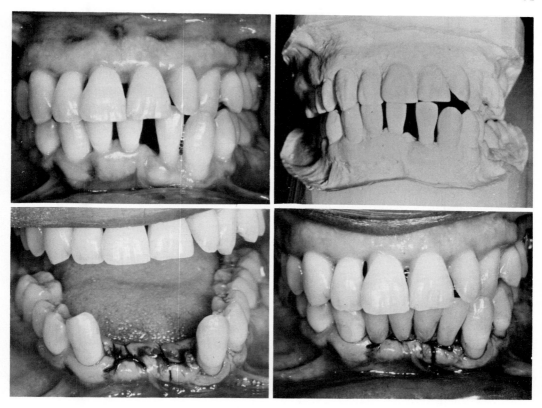

Fig. 3.16 (*upper left*). It is sometimes desirable to insert the prosthesis at the same appointment at which anterior teeth are removed. The three remaining mandibular incisors are to be removed and prosthetic teeth, attached to a removable partial denture, are to be substituted.

Fig. 3.17 (*upper right*). Shown here are the articulated casts of the mouth. The teeth to be extracted will be removed from the cast and a metal framework fabricated. The replacement teeth will be attached to the framework with acrylic resin.

Fig. 3.18 (*lower left*). The three remaining incisors have been removed and several loose sutures placed.

Fig. 3.19 (*lower right*). The prosthesis has been inserted.

ates a space between the tooth and the mucosa. When the teeth have been properly arranged, articulated with their antagonists, and attached to the framework with wax, the denture is processed in the usual manner. At the next appointment, the natural teeth are extracted and the denture is inserted (Figs. 3.16–3.19).

The advantages of the immediate technique are quite obvious for the patient who must appear before the public in pursuit of his livelihood. The disadvantages are that the resorption of the alveolar bone, which follows in the wake of extraction, must be compensated for by subsequent refitting operations. This entails additional expense as well as inconvenience for the patient. A second disadvantage of the immediate method is the fact that the replacement teeth cannot be tried in the mouth. Consequently, the first opportunity that the patient has to see the substitute teeth in place is after his natural teeth have been extracted and the denture inserted.

It is important to inform the immediate denture patient of the fact that refitting of the prosthesis will inevitably be needed from time to time as resorption occurs, and that when the refitting procedure is done it may be necessary to leave the prosthesis at the office during the time that the laboratory work is being accomplished. This is an opportune time to discuss with the patient the advantages of having more than one prosthesis. Certainly, a duplicate prosthesis should be given consideration by any patient who cannot carry on his routine affairs without the anterior substitute teeth which his denture provides.

Biopsy

Any suspicious lesion, for which a precise diagnosis cannot be made, should either be biopsied or referred to a tumor clinic for evaluation. The purpose of the biopsy is to establish an accurate diagnosis so that the appropriate therapy can be instituted with a minimum of delay when it is indicated. Although the performance of a biopsy is ordinarily not a difficult procedure, it should be performed only by an experienced professional, preferably one who practices one of the surgical specialties. A thoughtful analysis of the statistics on the incidence of oral malignancies makes it apparent that every practicing dentist (with the possible exception of those limiting their practices to orthodontics or pedodontics) will be given opportunities to detect cases of cancer. The dentist is professionally, as well as morally, obligated not to temporize with an oral lesion which he is unable to identify positively, in the hope that, given time, it may heal spontaneously.

Occlusal Adjustment

One of the early decisions to be made, in planning the construction of the removable partial denture, is whether to accept the occlusion as it is presented at the time of the examination or to modify it. Although often not feasible, the ideal occlusion is one in which centric relation and centric occlusion coincide. In instances where attainment of this goal is a reasonable expectation by means of equilibration procedures, this important phase of treatment should be given priority second only to making the patient comfortable and free from pain. It should follow very closely upon palliation of the chief complaint and accomplishment of the re-

quired surgical procedures. Whether or not centric occlusion and centric relation are made to coincide, equilibration should consist, at a minimum, of correcting interceptive contacts so that the patient has a comfortable, smoothly functioning articulation within his functional range. The objective in equilibration procedures is to create cuspal harmony, and not to develop the type of balancing contacts that are the goal strived for in complete denture construction. The emphasis should be on the elimination of traumatogenic interferences, i.e., interceptive and deflective contacts between opposing teeth when the mandible moves through the chewing cycle and terminates in centric occlusion.

The occlusal plane is crucial to the achievement of a harmonious occlusion, and the status of this plane should be given very early consideration, both in selecting the type of prosthodontic service to be prescribed and in formulating the plan of treatment. Many partial dentures do not achieve the degree of excellence which might otherwise be attained, because an attempt is made to develop the occlusion in the prosthesis to intercuspate with extruded, rotated, or malaligned teeth in the opposing arch (Fig. 3.20). A harmonious occlusion under such a handicap is a virtual impossibility. A para-

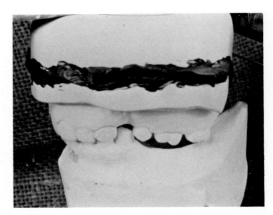

Fig. 3.20. The lost occlusal plane is a very common finding in the mouths of partial denture candidates. Attempting to develop a harmonious occlusion, by articulating the teeth of a prosthesis with misaligned, extruded teeth such as the ones shown in the photograph, is a virtual impossibility.

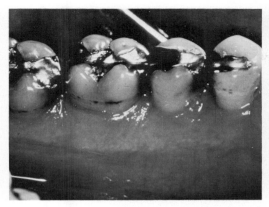

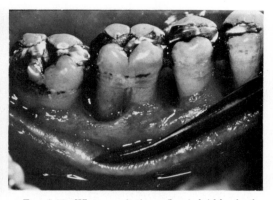

FIG. 3.21. The paramount objective of periodontal therapy is to eliminate, or at least to gain
control of, the factors which predisposed the patient
to the disease. The teeth and mucosa appear, from a
cursory inspection, to be in a state of health. However, Figure 3.22 depicts the cratering of the bone
which had taken place beneath the mucosa.

FIG. 3.22. When a soft tissue flap is laid back, the
bone cratering is apparent. Periodontal therapy is an
integral part of the overall treatment of many partial
denture patients.

mount objective in partial denture planning should be to coordinate restoration of
the occlusal plane, equilibration of the
existing occlusion, and articulation of the
prosthetic teeth to achieve a harmonious
relationship among all of the occluding
elements.

Periodontal Therapy

The objective of periodontal therapy is
the elimination, or at least the control, of
the factors which predisposed the patient
to the disease. This will consist, for the
most part, in elimination of the infection
and eradication of the periodontal
pockets. In addition to deep scaling and
root planing, treatment may consist of
gingivoplasty, gingivectomy, or osseous
surgery (Figs. 3.21 and 3.22). Since a high
percentage of patients with periodontal
disease are bruxists, this possibility
should not be overlooked. If there is evidence of bruxism, the fabrication of a
night guard should be considered to protect the remaining natural teeth during
sleep while the partial denture is not
being worn.

Periodontal procedures should precede
restorative work generally, because the
margins of inlay and crown preparations
can be better visualized and more accu-

rately established on teeth with a healthy
periodontium. Many times, periodontal
procedures can be combined with surgical
procedures so that all surgery required in
a quadrant of the mouth can be accomplished at the same sitting.

Salvaging the "Buried Crown"

The superior biomechanical excellence
of the all-tooth-supported removable partial denture, as opposed to the distal extension base type of denture, has been
well established. For this reason it is
usually in the patient's best interests to
press into service a distal abutment when
one is available. A rather common complication, however, is for the crown of a
second molar, or more commonly a third
molar, to be partly covered with an operculum of mucosa which substantially diminishes the tooth's claspability. Its potential as an abutment tooth can often be
spectacularly improved by means of a
gingivectomy which exposes more of the
clinical crown (Figs. 3.23–3.30).

Endodontic Procedures

A tooth with pulpal involvement or root
end pathology (Fig. 3.31) may be considered a candidate for endodontic therapy
when it is of pivotal importance to the

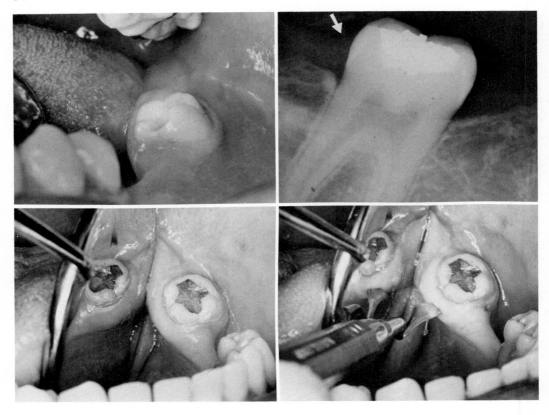

FIG. 3.23 (*upper left*). The claspability of the molar shown above is extremely poor because of the large cuff of mucosa which envelopes the anatomical crown.

FIG. 3.24 (*upper right*). A radiograph of a molar discloses the depth of the operculum (*arrow*) and the fact that the crown/tooth ratio is favorable. The tooth is potentially an excellent abutment, except for the fact that so little of the anatomical crown is available for clasping. A gingivectomy will improve the potential of the tooth immeasurably as a partial denture abutment.

FIG. 3.25 (*lower left*). The mucosa is anesthetized preparatory to the periodontal surgery.

FIG. 3.26 (*lower right*). An incision is made at approximately the depth of the mucosal cuff.

best design of the removable partial denture. Provided there is no contraindication and the tooth has an otherwise favorable prognosis, the pulpless tooth, properly treated, is perfectly reliable as a durable abutment for the partial denture. Although the tooth without a pulp may be slightly more brittle than the tooth which houses a vital pulp, all available evidence supports the view that the degree of brittleness is not clinically significant. Countless pulpless teeth have performed yeoman service as partial denture abutments over many years of service.

Employment of the pulpless tooth as an abutment for the removable partial denture may be considered under the following three sets of circumstances.

1. The pulpless tooth which has been treated endodontically is presented as a potential abutment in the mouth of a patient for whom a removable prosthesis is to be made.

2. A potential abutment with an infected pulp is present in the mouth of a partial denture candidate.

3. A tooth which has been serving as an abutment for a prosthesis has developed a pulpitis, and must be either treated endodontially or extracted.

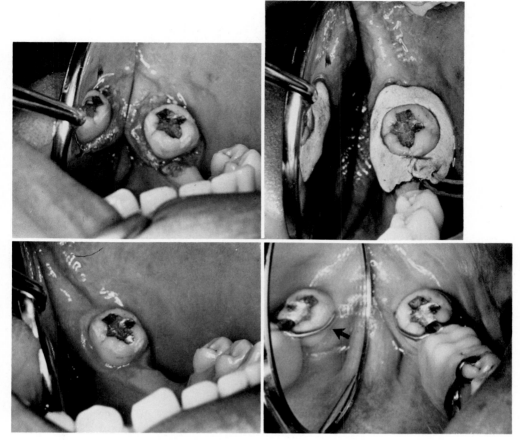

FIG. 3.27 (*upper left*). The mucosal cuff has been removed.

FIG. 3.28 (*upper right*). A periodontal pack is placed to protect the wound during healing.

FIG. 3.29 (*lower left*). The newly exposed crown, after healing has taken place, will make an excellent abutment for a prosthesis.

FIG. 3.30 (*lower right*). The photograph shows a clasp in place on the tooth (shown in FIGS. 3.23–3.29). Note the increased clinical crown, particularly the lingual surface shown in the mirror (*arrow*).

The Treated Pulpless Tooth. The objective in the case of the previously treated tooth is to determine the current health status of the tooth. If it passes this test satisfactorily, it can be evaluated for use as an abutment by the same criteria used for a tooth with a normal, healthy pulp. A status of health may be inferred if (a) the canals have been filled to the apex with what appears radiographically to be well condensed filling material, (b) there is no radiolucency at the apex, and (c) the tooth has been asymptomatic clinically since the therapy was accomplished. If there appears to be some radiolucency at the apex, the length of time that has elapsed since the therapy was performed must be considered, since a sufficient time may not have transpired for complete healing. If, on the other hand, the previously administered endodontic therapy does not meet acceptable standards, or the tooth has not been entirely asymptomatic, it should be viewed with considerable skepticism. Certainly it should not be placed into service as an abutment tooth until it meets, unequivocally, the requirements for a partial denture abutment tooth.

The Infected Tooth. A prime consider-

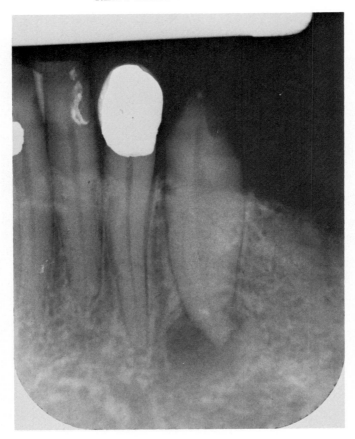

FIG. 3.31. A tooth that is strategically important to the design of a removable partial denture as an abutment, which has pulpal involvement or root end pathology, may be considered for endodontic therapy.

ation in the case of the infected tooth is its strategic importance to the design of the partial denture. If the loss of this tooth would materially downgrade the prognosis for the prosthesis, the feasibility of endodontic therapy should be considered. The criteria for feasibility follow.

1. Is there access to the canals?
2. If apicoectomy is needed, can it be performed without undue difficulty? If the apex is in the maxillary sinus, for example, the tooth would have to be ruled out as a candidate for endodontic therapy.
3. If an apicoectomy is performed, will it create an unfavorable crown/root ratio?

Abutment Tooth with Pulpitis. If a tooth develops a pulpitis while serving

actively as an abutment for a prosthesis, several factors must be considered in regard to treatment. Is the tooth healthy from a periodontal standpoint? Is the crown/root ratio favorable? Was it performing satisfactorily prior to the present episode? Is the prosthesis itself otherwise satisfactory? Is the mouth, as a whole, in a state of good health and repair? If the answers to these questions are affirmative, it may be assumed that the former state of comfort and function can be reestablished following endodontic therapy. If, on the contrary, the prosthesis has obviously outlived its usefulness, or the health of one or more of the other teeth is in doubt, a reappraisal of the entire oral mechanism may be in order. Under these latter circumstances, the tooth in question should be opened and treated palliatively until a treatment plan can be developed and definitive treatment instituted. If a decision is made to treat the tooth by endodontic therapy, then access into the pulp chamber, through the gold, acrylic, or natural tooth structure, as the case may be, will be needed. Before selecting the site for the opening, the position of the clasp on the tooth should be carefully noted so that appropriate care can be exercised to preserve the existing crown contour. The area under the occlusal rest should not be violated if it can be avoided, for obvious reasons, unless a decision has been made to place a restoration (crown) under the clasp following the endodontic therapy.

The Endodontic Implant

A root resection may create a tooth whose crown/root ratio does not meet acceptable standards for a partial denture abutment. When such a tooth is considered pivotal to the most ideal design of the prosthesis, an endodontic implant may be considered. The implant technique consists of placing a metal pin in the root canal, and extending it through the apex into the periapical bone. Obviously, this cannot be done on a tooth whose apex is close to the maxillary sinus or the mandibular canal. The pin increases the stability of the tooth and, in effect, improves the crown/root ratio dramatically. Such a procedure has the capability of transforming the prognosis for a tooth as a potential abutment from poor to excellent. However, it must be conceded that the technique is not time-proven, and its efficacy has not yet been corroborated by large numbers of clinical successes.

Orthodontic Treatment

Minor Tooth Movement

Anomalies in tooth position, which interfere with the ideal design of a prosthesis, are frequently encountered in the mouths of candidates for a removable partial denture. Although bodily tooth movement should not be attempted by one not trained in this branch of dentistry, very worthwhile results can be achieved in repositioning extruded, tipped, and rotated teeth by means of minor tooth movement techniques which do not require the expenditure of prohibitive amounts of time. When more complex orthodontic therapy is indicated, consultation with an orthodontist should be sought.

The Mesially Inclined Molar. The mandibular molar that has tipped mesially can be returned to a more nearly upright position, so that functional stresses will be transmitted to the periodontal apparatus in a direction more in line with the long axis. An additional benefit is that clasping will be facilitated as a result of the partial elimination of the overly severe undercut, which the tipped crown invariably creates. A simple, removable acrylic resin appliance can be employed with spring arms to effect this movement. The tooth cannot be moved, of course, if it is prevented from doing so by the opposing occlusion.

Teeth in Lingual or Buccal Version. Bicuspids (Fig. 3.32) which have moved out of alignment with the neighboring teeth may be difficult either to clasp or to splint. An acrylic resin stent with a small spring arm can be used to move such teeth into a more normal position in the arch.

Migrated Anterior Teeth. Anterior teeth which adjoin edentulous spaces frequently migrate into the space, often creating unsightly diastemas and making the arrangement of the replacement teeth into a pleasing alignment more difficult. Several techniques may be used to close up small anterior spaces or to realign a tipped anterior tooth. Perhaps the most common method is the use of the rubber dam elastic (Fig. 3.33). Movement is effected by enclosing the tooth to be moved inside the rubber elastic, with an adjacent tooth which has a larger, stronger root. Sometimes, two teeth may be pressed into service as anchor teeth. The tension created by the elastic is sufficient to bring about the desired closing-up movement. The band loses its tension at approximately 24-hour intervals, and must be

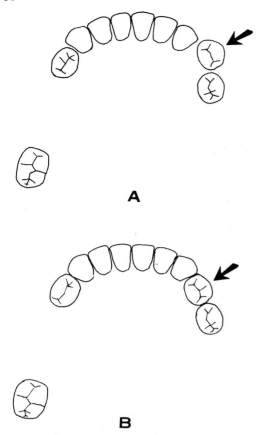

A

B

FIG. 3.32. Bicuspids which have migrated out of alignment with adjoining teeth sometimes create difficult clasping problems (*A*). A treatment prosthesis with a small spring arm can be used to return such a migrant tooth into a more normal position (*B*).

changed for a fresh one. This chore may be delegated to the patient, but the procedure must be supervised at frequent intervals by the dentist. Rubber ligatures have been known to slip down into the gingival crevice and wreak havoc on the periodontium when not supervised by a trained person. A Japanese hemp fiber known as "grassline ligature" may be employed for the same purpose (Fig. 3.34). A characteristic of this material is that it shrinks approximately 10% of its length in 24 hours (Fig. 3.35) when it is saturated with oral fluids. This property can be exploited to bring about a desired tooth movement (Fig. 3.36). The ligature should be changed every 24 to 48 hours until the desired amount of movement has been accomplished. When the teeth have been aligned, they can be held in position with wire ligatures until the prosthesis is inserted, so as to retain them in the newly created relationship. Although the action of grassline is gentle and well within physiologic tolerances, it should not go unnoticed that ligatures of any kind create conditions that make good oral hygiene difficult to maintain. It is important that the patient be forewarned of the need for increased vigilance.

Restorative Dentistry

Needed restorative work is, as a rule, best programmed to be accomplished following surgery and periodontal treatment.

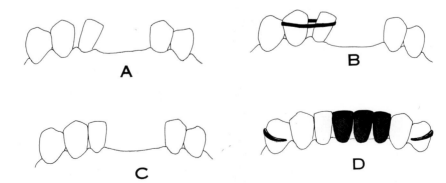

A

B

C

D

FIG. 3.33. Anterior teeth which adjoin an edentulous space frequently migrate into the space, thus making difficult an esthetic arrangement of replacement teeth. Rubber dam elastics may be employed to create a more favorable alignment. *A* shows the mandibular right lateral incisor migrated into the edentulous space. *B* shows the elastic in place between the lateral and the much stronger cuspid. In *C* the lateral has been returned to a more normal position. *D* depicts the replacement teeth fitted into the edentulous space.

When possible, it should be integrated with endodontic treatment when this type of therapy is a part of the treatment plan. It bears repetition that no permanent type of restoration should be placed until the design of the partial denture has been decided and the treatment plan formulated. All restorative work including crowns, inlays, and onlays should be programmed so as to contribute to the restoration of the best possible occlusal plane (Fig. 3.37). This is a profoundly important consideration.

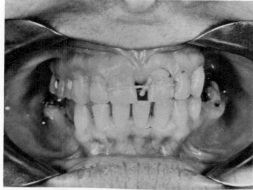

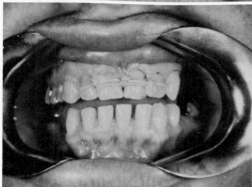

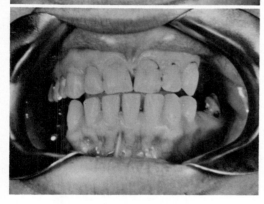

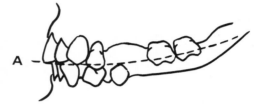

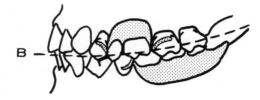

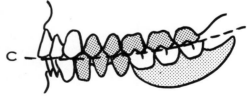

Fig. 3.34 (*top*). The grassline ligature can be used to effect a better alignment of anterior teeth that have migrated out of their customary positions. In this photograph the ligature has been secured around the two central incisors.

Fig. 3.35 (*middle*). The grassline ligature shrinks approximately 10% of its length every 24 hours when moistened by the oral fluids. Here, the lateral incisors have been included as anchor teeth to retain the central incisors in their new positions.

Fig. 3.36 (*bottom*). The ligature has been removed, showing the teeth in an improved alignment.

Fig. 3.37. All restorative work, including crowns, inlays, onlays, and fixed partial dentures, should be planned and constructed in a manner that contributes to restoration of the best possible occlusal plane. Restoring the occlusion shown at *A*, with the prostheses shown at *B*, would be foredoomed to failure. The proper approach is to coordinate all of the restorations with the prostheses in such a way that the occlusal plane is restored to as near normality as possible, as depicted at *C*.

Carious Lesions and Defective Restorations

Carious lesions should be treated with suitable restorations. Any existing fillings with ragged margins, broken contacts, leaks, overhanging margins, or other defects, should be repaired or replaced. As a general rule, teeth that are to support clasps should be restored with gold, although exceptions are sometimes made to this rule in the case of one-surface fillings. Each restoration should be planned so as to be consistent in contour with the path of insertion of the prosthesis. To illustrate, it is an exercise in futility to expend valuable time and effort restoring a classically ideal contour to the proximal surface of an inlay, if the same surface must subsequently be disked away to create a guiding plane for a removable partial denture. A frequently encountered defect, that may be corrected by means of a simple restoration or restorations, is the area of fibrous food impaction caused primarily by adjoining marginal ridges that are of unequal height, or that are poorly aligned because of rotation of one or both teeth. The placing of properly contoured restorations under such circumstances may avert subsequent breakdown of the periodontal apparatus.

The Retentive Restoration

When no usable undercut exists on a tooth, the conventional solution is to cover the tooth witn a crown into which an infrabulge is incorporated. However, there are circumstances when it is not feasible to construct a crown, and placement of a retentive restoration of either gold or amalgam may be a practical alternative (Fig. 3.38). The planning casts should be analyzed on the surveyor to locate the precise site on the crown of the tooth that is to be designated for the retentive clasp tip, so that the cavity can be prepared in the natural tooth to encompass the area. The gold or amalgam is then overcontoured to create an infrabulge of the desired depth. An undercut of approximately 0.020 inch should be created in the restoration, which is normally reduced to approximately 0.010 or 0.015 inch by pol-

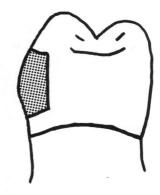

Fig. 3.38. When no natural undercut exists on the surface of a tooth, and it is not feasible to place a crown for one reason or another, a retentive restoration can be placed to create an infrabulge. The study casts should be analyzed on the surveyor to locate the site that is to be designated for the retentive terminal so that the cavity can be prepared to encompass this precise area.

ishing. It is important that the polishing not be overzealously done, so as not to reduce the undercut beyond the amount needed for retention. Gold is a more durable material than amalgam for this purpose, and is the material of choice. However, amalgam will serve the purpose satisfactorily when gold cannot be used for one reason or another.

Amalgam Splints

The amalgam restoration can be used to splint two teeth together to create what is, in effect, a multirooted abutment (Figs. 3.39 and 3.40). Although the use of the amalgam splint is limited to the bicuspids and molars, and the margins of this material are more friable than cast gold, the advantages of the amalgam splinting technique should not be overlooked. It can be used on teeth that are not in good alignment more readily than can the gold restoration, and it is less time-consuming to construct, and less costly to the patient. Splinting with gold requires that the cusps be covered with the gold to preclude loosening of the castings under the stresses of mastication. This sometimes creates a cosmetic problem that may be avoided by the use of the amalgam splint.

The amalgam splint is made by pre-

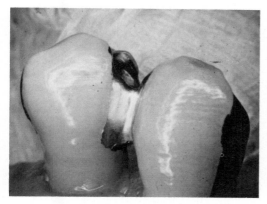

FIG. 3.39. When splinting of two or more teeth is desirable and gold crowns cannot be employed, an amalgam splint may be used.

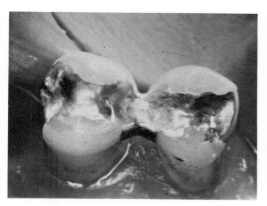

FIG. 3.40. Amalgam splints can be used on teeth that are not in good alignment, and the technique has the advantage of being less time consuming than splinting with gold. Another advantage over gold is that the amalgam splint may create less of a cosmetic problem, since the gold restoration normally covers more of the tooth surface than is necessary with amalgam.

paring contiguous cavities in the teeth that are to be united. If two bicuspids are to be splinted, it would typically be accomplished with a mesio-occlusal-distal cavity preparation in each tooth. A matrix of either compound or acrylic resin may be used to pack the amalgam. If compound is employed, it should be softened, placed in position, and chilled. If a resin matrix is used, an impression must be made of the quadrant of the arch which contains the teeth to be splinted, and a cast must be

poured in stone. The cavities of the stone teeth should be filled with wax and the wax built out to the contour desired in the fillings. A tinfoil substitute should be applied to the cast, and acrylic resin dough molded around and against the teeth to form the matrix. When the acrylic resin has polymerized, it can be divided into a buccal and a lingual segment. Small depressions may be placed in the matrix so that it can be held together in the mouth with a matrix retainer. With the matrix in place, the amalgam reinforcing wire (Markley Wire-Star Dental Mfg. Co., Philadelphia, Pa.) is laid across the cavities and the amalgam is packed.

The Inlay, the Onlay

The inlay or the onlay may be a more esthetic restoration, in some circumstances, than is either the full cast crown or the three-quarter crown. However, the margins are usually more vulnerable to recurrent decay and, for this reason, both the inlay and the onlay should be used sparingly in the caries-susceptible group of patients when the restoration is to be partially covered with a clasp. When the requirement is primarily for a durable tooth filling that will withstand the pressures of the denture and the frictional wear of the clasp, the gold inlay or onlay may serve the purpose surpassingly well. It is important that all margins of the restoration be carried out to self-cleansing areas of the tooth, and that the patient be encouraged to practice assiduous home care. A prosthesis with clasps which cover an inlayed abutment should, under no circumstances, be worn during sleep.

The Cast Crown

The gold crown comes very near to being the ideal covering for the abutment tooth for the removable partial denture. The only disadvantage of the gold crown, aside from its color, is the possible interference with the health of the gingival mucosa as a result of over- or underextension of the crown margins, or of faulty contouring of the crown surfaces. The crown can be veneered with a tooth-colored material (acrylic resin or porcelain) when there is an objection to the display of gold.

Crowning Anterior Teeth

Unesthetic or badly broken down anterior teeth, as well as teeth which are morphologically atypical (the peg lateral, for example), may be covered with crowns of gold, porcelain, acrylic resin, or a combination of these materials, to eliminate the cosmetic defect. The crown may also be used to realign a tooth that has migrated out of position in the arch. The design of a partial denture oftentimes is such that it requires a lingual or incisal rest on an anterior tooth, and when this is the case, the recess for the rest can be incorporated into the wax pattern of the restoration. A rest recess thus prepared in metal is far superior to one fashioned in the enamel surface of the tooth. If a precision type rest is to be employed, a gold crown is needed to house the female part of the key/keyway device.

Crowning Posterior Teeth

Crowns can be used to advantage in restoring and recontouring the posterior teeth, to improve both the design and function of the removable partial denture and, in the case of the bicuspids, the patient's appearance as well. Full-coverage metal crowns are indicated for use on the abutment tooth (1) when the patient's caries index is high, (2) when it is necessary to create an ideal retentive undercut on the precise area of the tooth where it is needed, (3) when tipped, rotated, and extruded teeth must be realigned, (4) when an ideal rest recess and guiding plane surface for the clasp must be provided, (5) the height of the tooth which is in slight infraocclusion must be increased, (6) when the embrasure clasp is to be employed (crowns on the two abutment teeth are an excellent solution to the problem of interocclusal space which so often attends the use of this particular clasp), and finally, (7) when the gold crown may be the restoration of choice for the abutment tooth which has been filled with multiple small amalgams or restored with one huge multisurface amalgam.

The Surveyed Crown

The full gold crown is the restoration par excellence for the abutment tooth which, for any one of a number of reasons, does not fully qualify as a partial denture abutment. In restoring the tooth with a surveyed crown the designer has virtually total control over the contour. He can create retentive undercuts and guiding plane surfaces in the wax pattern precisely where they will be most advantageous to the overall design. The surface of the tooth that is to support the reciprocal arm of the clasp can likewise be ideally contoured. In addition, the crown can oftentimes be made to intercuspate with its opponents more efficiently than was the case with the natural tooth.

The crown pattern should be fashioned on a full arch cast of the mouth, so that the cast can be oriented on the surveyor in the horizontal plane that was selected during the design and treatment-planning stage of construction. The crown may then be contoured with frequent reference to the surveyor spindle, to ensure that retentive and reciprocal areas, and the guide plane, are located precisely where they are needed. The occlusal anatomy should be developed so that the crown intercuspates properly with the teeth of the opposing arch. This, of course, requires an accurate counter cast. The recess for the occlusal rest needs to be prepared in the wax pattern in such a way as to ensure that the rest is of adequate thickness while, at the same time, not interfering with the opposing occlusion (Figs. 3.41–3.49).

The Veneered Crown

An oft-recurring problem for the prosthodontist is the patient who objects to a display of gold on the surface of an anterior tooth but who needs a full crown to create an infrabulge for the retentive clasp terminal. The conventional solution is to place an acrylic resin window in the labial or buccal surface of the crown, or to veneer the restoration with procelain. The physical properties of porcelain are such that it will stand up very well under the abrading action of a partial denture clasp, whereas acrylic resin has a very limited resistance to such wear and will suffer deterioration if the clasp is permitted to rub against it. If acrylic resin must be employed despite its low resistance to abrasion, it may be best to design the retentive arm of the clasp on the lingual surface of the tooth. The window can then be formed on the buccal surface of the crown in such a way that the buccal (reciprocal) arm rests only against metal (Figs. 3.50 and 3.51). Ideally, contact between clasp and acrylic resin should be nil. If contact between the clasp arm and the resin is unavoidable, the use of the combination clasp should be considered. Since the wrought-wire clasp arm of the combination clasp makes minimal (line) contact with the surface of the abutment, abrasion may reasonably be expected to be less than would be the case with a cast clasp. Moreover, the smooth, polished surface of the wrought wire is inherently less abrasive than is the surface of the gold casting.

The Lingual Ledge

The practice of creating a ledge in the lingual surface of the full cast crown (or of the three-quarter crown) to accommodate the lingual (reciprocal) clasp arm has merit under some circumstances. Perhaps the greatest advantage is the fact that the ledge provides a splendid guiding plane. Properly formed, it enables the reciprocal arm of the clasp to make and maintain contact with the tooth surface well before the retentive arm has had an opportunity to exert its whiplash effect as it flexes over the height of contour. Another advantage is the fact that, if the ledging operation is carefully planned and carried out, the lingual clasp arm can be inlaid into the lingual surface of the abutment, where it will be much less prominent than a conventional arm and so, presumably, less objectionable to the tongue (Fig. 3.52). It should be emphasized that the ledge must be planned in detail at the time the treatment plan is formulated, since the preparation of the abutment tooth for the crown must be made deep enough on the lingual surface to accommodate the width

of the ledge. The ledge should be positioned at approximately the junction of occlusive and middle thirds. The ledge width should decrease gradually as the area to be occupied by the clasp terminal is reached. Use of the wax carver of the surveyor, to form the axial surfaces of the wax pattern, will make simpler the task of creating the axial wall of the ledge so that it is parallel to the path of insertion. The ledging technique has special merit in the extremely close type of occlusion when, as a result of abrasion, it is difficult to provide for a sufficient thickness of gold in the crown to accommodate an occlusal rest of adequate depth. The lingual ledge, under these circumstances, can play a dual role as both rest recess and ledge for the reciprocal arm, thus making unnecessary a conventional occlusal rest in the customary site (the mesial or distal fossa) of the tooth.

Splinting with Crowns

Teeth may have a less-than-ideal prognosis as abutments for the partial denture when there is slight mobility or an unfavorable crown/root ratio, perhaps coupled with a conical root. Such a tooth may be transformed into a more durable abutment by uniting it with an adjacent stronger tooth, or teeth, by means of crowns which have been joined together (Figs. 3.53–3.55). The benefits of joining two or more teeth are that stresses are thus divided among two or more supporting units, rather than being concentrated on one tooth. Although splinting is a time-honored method of improving the status of the weak abutment, there are certain precautions that should not be overlooked. Certainly, it is not a method of salvaging a tooth with an otherwise hopeless prognosis, and indeed, the splinting technique should not even be considered for teeth that are not periodontially healthy. Its prime application is for the healthy tooth which does not fully qualify as an ideal abutment because of an unfavorable crown/root ratio, a short tapered root, or a slight degree of mobility. Rather than depending on two weak teeth splinted together, a third tooth should be added whenever possible. For example, a cuspid and a bicuspid might be splinted together, and the two attached to a lateral incisor. Full crowns should be employed for splinting rather than three-quarter crowns or inlays, since clinical evidence indicates that the stresses of mouth service frequently loosen the latter. The axial walls of crown preparations should be made as nearly parallel as pos-sible so as to exploit all possible retention and resistance form. Too great a degree of taper in an occlusal direction is apt to re-sult in loosening of the restorations and failure of the splint. It is important that interproximal embrasures be made cleans-able, and that the patient be taught the proper way to maintain the embrasure in a hygienic state. Accordingly, if the crowns are joined by the solder, the solder joint should be made small so as to encourage physiologic stimulation of the interproxi-mal mucosa. If they are cast together, the attachment between them should be made near the contact point, so that the natural configuration of the interproximal em-brasure is preserved. Because of the criti-cal importance of periodontal health, and the fact that a healthy interproximal em-brasure is an integral part of a healthy periodontium, the splinting technique should not be employed for crowns that are too short to be soldered without im-pingement on the interproximal papilla, or that will create a food trap.

Due to root morphology, the mandib-ular premolars are prime candidates for the splinting technique, with the maxil-lary premolars next in order. Mandibular incisors that must be pressed into service as abutments should, almost without ex-ception, be splinted together.

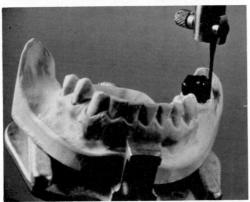

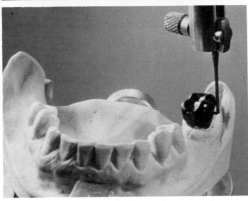

Fig. 3.41 (top). The tooth shown is needed as an abutment, but is unsuitable because it has no usable retentive undercut and is severely tipped mesiolin-gually. A surveyed crown can be made to transform the tooth into a near ideal abutment. When the crown must occlude with teeth in the opposing jaw, casts of both arches should be used and the occlusal surface fashioned to intercuspate with its antagonist. The crown shown will articulate with a complete denture. A guiding plane should be incorporated into the mesial surface of the wax pattern with the help of the surveyor.

Fig. 3.42 (middle). The wax pattern has restored the tooth to a more normal alignment, but there is still no retentive undercut on the distobuccal surface where it is desired that a retentive clasp arm be placed.

Fig. 3.43 (bottom). A retentive undercut has been incorporated into the wax pattern on the distobuccal surface.

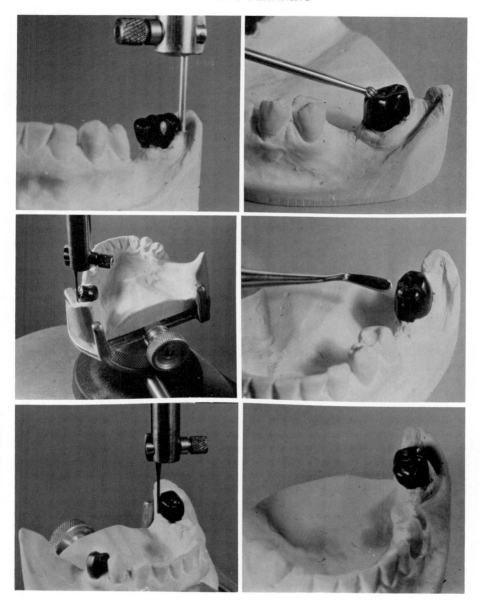

FIG. 3.44 (*top left*). The undercut is measured with the undercut gauge on the surveyor. As much as a 0.020 inch undercut may be incorporated into the wax to allow a slight surplus for finishing and polishing. An undercut of 0.010 or 0.015 inch will be employed in the final crown for retention.

FIG. 3.45 (*middle left*). The undercut on the distobuccal surface is shown from a distal view.

FIG. 3.46 (*bottom left*). The lingual surface is contoured to accommodate best the lingual or reciprocal clasp arm. No undercut is incorporated in this surface, so that the reciprocal arm can be placed at the same vertical height on the tooth as the retentive arm. It will thus be operant as a counterpoise for the retentive arm at the exact instant that it is needed.

FIG. 3.47 (*top right*). The recess for the occlusal rest can be outlined in the wax with a large round bur rotated between the thumb and forefinger.

FIG. 3.48 (*middle right*). The recess can be refined to the desired configuration with a rounded wax carver.

FIG. 3.49 (*bottom right*). The finished wax pattern ready for spruing and investing is shown in the photograph.

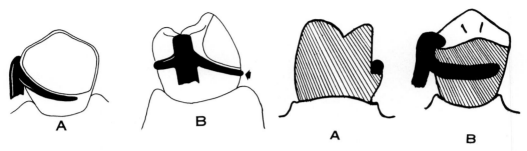

FIG. 3.50. If an acrylic resin window is employed rather than porcelain, it may be best to design the retentive arm of the clasp on the lingual surface of the tooth, and to place the reciprocal arm low enough on the buccal surface to be cosmetically acceptable. All of its contact should be with metal. *A* shows a buccal view of the tooth and the reciprocal arm. *B* is a proximal view showing the clasp arm (*arrow*) completely out of contact with the acrylic resin.

FIG. 3.52. The technique of ledging the lingual surface of a gold crown to accommodate the reciprocal arm of the clasp has certain advantages. It provides an excellent guiding plane (the axial surface) while at the same time positioning the clasp arm in the lingual surface in such a way that it is much less in evidence to the explorations of a curious tongue. *A* shows a proximal view of the ledge and *B* shows a lingual view.

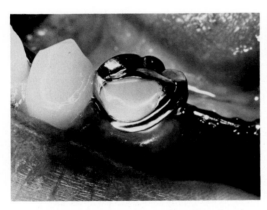

FIG. 3.51. If the retentive arm must be placed on the buccal surface, the wax pattern should be contoured to incorporate the retentive undercut while still keeping the retentive arm completely on the metal and out of contact with the acrylic resin.

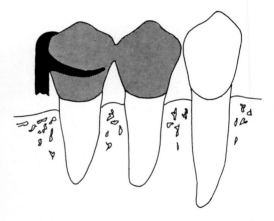

FIG. 3.53. Splinting is an excellent technique for converting a less than ideal abutment into a more nearly ideal one. Its prime application is for the tooth that is only marginally qualified as an abutment because of an unfavorable crown/root ratio, a short conical shaped root, or a slight degree of mobility.

The Three-Quarter Crown

The three-quarter crown may be ideal for use on an anterior tooth when a favorable retentive undercut already exists on the labial surface. Obviously, the three-quarter crown is of no avail on a tooth when a retentive undercut must be cre-

ated for a labial clasp arm. An ideal cingulum rest can be prepared in the wax pattern of the three-quarter crown, and this type of restoration is usually more acceptable cosmetically than is the full crown, owing to the fact that it can be fashioned in such a way as to display a bare minimum of gold.

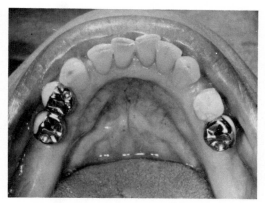

Fig. 3.54. The left mandibular bicuspids shown here have been united with gold crowns which have esthetic windows. They represent, in effect, a multi-rooted abutment for the removable partial prosthesis.

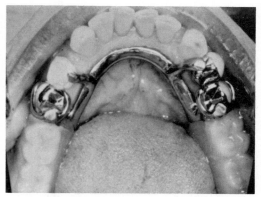

Fig. 3.55. The right mandibular bicuspids shown here have been united with gold crowns and the partial denture is in place.

The Fixed Partial Denture

When an edentulous space which is programmed to be restored with a fixed partial denture (a fixed bridge) opposes an edentulous space that is to be restored with a removable partial denture, the fixed prosthesis should, as a rule, be completed before fabrication of the removable partial denture is begun. The reason for this is that a better occlusion is usually possible if the occlusal plane is restored with the abutment restorations and pontics of the fixed prosthesis, and the teeth of the removable partial denture are then

arranged to articulate with them. More latitude is possible in positioning the teeth for the partial denture than is true with the fixed prosthesis. The important point is to study the existing occlusion of the planning casts, so that the restorations of both arches can be planned and coordinated to restore the best possible occlusal plane, and to create the most efficient, harmonious occlusion.

The Splint Bridge

The single bicuspid which stands alone with an edentulous space on either side of it is seldom an ideal abutment for a removable partial denture. The root is often conical in shape, especially in the case of the mandibular bicuspid, and typically, some bone loss has occurred, with the result that the crown/root ratio is marginal. In addition, the absence of tooth support from adjoining teeth tends to compound the problem. On the other hand, the alternatives to the employment of such a tooth as an abutment may be even less attractive. One solution to this apparent dilemma is to splint the bicuspid to the cuspid by means of a pontic which bridges the edentulous space (Fig. 3.56). This creates a more stalwart abutment, which is much better able to withstand the rigors of mouth service than could the isolated bicuspid alone. The crown of the bicuspid is usually well contoured for clasping so that, with the additional root supplied by the splint bridge, it becomes an eminently suitable abutment.

Cross Arch Stabilization

The Gingival Bar

When isolated teeth on either side of the arch are separated by an anterior edentulous space they can be united by a cross arch splinting technique, while at the same time being clasped in the conventional manner by a removable partial denture. This technique is used most commonly for two mandibular cuspids (Fig. 3.57) when labial alveolar bone loss contraindicates the use of a fixed prosthesis, and the additional stability and strength of splinting is needed by the cus-

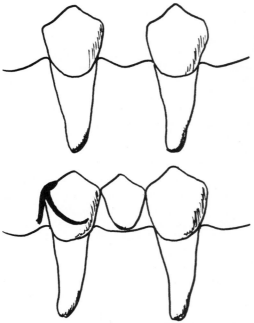

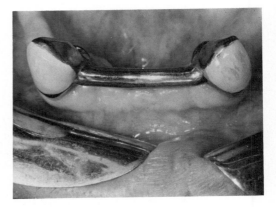

FIG. 3.57. When teeth on either side of the arch are separated by a large anterior edentulous space, they can be united with a gingival bar. The technique lends itself especially well for use with two mandibular cuspids. Crowns are made for each tooth and a 10 gauge gold bar is waxed, cast, and soldered to each crown to unite the two teeth.

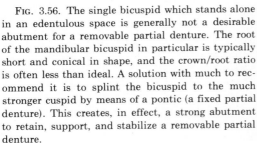

FIG. 3.56. The single bicuspid which stands alone in an edentulous space is generally not a desirable abutment for a removable partial denture. The root of the mandibular bicuspid in particular is typically short and conical in shape, and the crown/root ratio is often less than ideal. A solution with much to recommend it is to splint the bicuspid to the much stronger cuspid by means of a pontic (a fixed partial denture). This creates, in effect, a strong abutment to retain, support, and stabilize a removable partial denture.

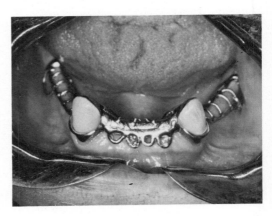

FIG. 3.58. The partial denture framework is made to fit over the gingival bar and to clasp the abutments. Teeth so splinted will have much greater stability than teeth which do not stabilize each other.

pids. Crowns are made for each abutment and a gold alloy bar of approximately 10 gauge is cast to fit between the two crowns along the crest of the residual ridge. The cast bar is soldered to the proximal surfaces of the crowns, and the partial denture framework is made to fit over the bar (Fig. 3.58). Teeth so splinted will have maximum stability since the bar is attached low on the tooth, close to its center of rotation.

This technique has much to recommend it since, in effect, it combines the esthetic advantages of the removable partial denture with the splinting effect of the fixed prosthesis.

Tooth Alteration Procedures (Odontoplasty)

Various alterations can be made to the

contours of the natural teeth, over and above the usual conventional restorative procedures, to eliminate interferences and troublesome undercuts, to make clasping more effective, and to make insertion and removal of the prosthesis easier for the patient. These alterations should be planned during the survey and analysis of the study cast, and should be programmed as an integral part of the treatment plan, to be accomplished at the most propitious juncture in the treatment sequence. Notations can be made on the study cast of tooth alterations that are to be carried out. A method with much to recommend it is to indicate the proposed tooth alteration with colored pencil on the planning cast, so that it can serve as a blueprint. The planning cast should then be available at the chair, for reference when the clinical procedures are being carried out. It bears emphasis that one of the purposes of a carefully formulated treatment plan is to ensure that all needed treatment is accomplished in the most efficient sequence, with a minimum amount of discomfort to the patient. Accordingly, all treatment of whatever type, that is programmed for a quadrant of the mouth, should ideally be accomplished at the same sitting, if at all feasible. As an example, recesses for occlusal rests and guiding planes should be prepared in a quadrant of the mouth at the same time that the area has been anesthetized for a cavity preparation. Tooth alteration procedures are considered in more detail in Chapter 6.

Treatment of Abused Oral Tissue

Patients who have worn a prosthesis for a considerable period of time may present for a new prosthesis with inflamed, hyperplastic tissue under the denture. This irritated tissue results from a combination of deteriorated fit and neglected oral hygiene. It would obviously not be good clinical procedure to perpetuate this condition by taking impressions and placing new or refitted dentures over such irritated, distorted tissue. The immediate objective should be to restore the oral mucosa to a state of health, after which the refitting or reconstruction of the prosthesis can be accomplished.

The Pros and Cons of Constructing Two Partial Dentures Simultaneously

When the patient requires both a maxillary and a mandibular removable partial denture, the question may be raised as to the advantages of completing one partial denture first, followed by the second, as opposed to making the two partial dentures concurrently. Each method has advantages, and cogent arguments can be marshalled to support either viewpoint. Perhaps the most important criteria to be considered are, the type and design of the prostheses, the time requirements, and the emotional make-up of the patient.

The Advantages of Making One Partial Denture at a Time

1. It is considerably less wearing on the patient's spirit to adapt to one prosthesis than to two.
2. Adjustments can be accomplished on the first prosthesis while the second one is being made.
3. An occasional patient will be found who is simply unable to make a satisfactory adjustment to an oral prosthesis. Treatment can be stopped or modified for such a patient, with an obvious saving of time, money and, in some circumstances, good will.
4. The generated path method of establishing the occlusion may be employed in instances where it would not otherwise be feasible.
5. It might be desirable to modify the design of the second partial denture because of some idiosyncrasy brought to light by wear of the first.
6. The results of the patient's efforts to establish good oral hygiene habits can be better assessed. The encouragement, advice, and moral support, provided by the dentist over the longer period of observation, might be more effective in keeping the patient on a good oral hygiene regimen.

The Advantages of Making the Two Dentures Together

1. Overall, there would be fewer clinical steps performed, hence less duplication of effort.
2. Two partial dentures can be completed in less time than would be required to make them separately.
3. When the patient has adapted to the two partials, he is completely adjusted and need not look forward to a repetition of the awkward break-in period.

Bibliography

Alloy, J., and Motohiko, K.: The amalgam splint. J. Amer. Dent. Ass. *65:* 381–384, 1962.

Gershater, M. M.: Orthodontic diagnosis for the general practitioner. J. Amer. Dent. Ass. *44:* 194 –203. 1952.

Goldman, H. M., and Burket, L. W.: *Treatment Planning in the Practice of Dentistry.* The C. V. Mosby Company, St. Louis, 1959.

Hirschfield, L.: *Minor Tooth Movement in General Practice.* The C. V. Mosby Company, St. Louis, 1960.

Kruger, G. O.: *Text of Oral Surgery*, Ed. 2. The C. V. Mosby Company, St. Louis, 1964.

Rudd, K. D., and Dunn, B. W.: Accurate removable partial dentures. J. Prosth. Dent. *18:* 559–570, 1967.

Somner, R. F., Ostrander, F. D., and Crowley, M. C.: *Clinical Endodontics*, Ed. 2. W. B. Saunders Company, Philadelphia, 1961.

Weinman, J. P., and Sicher, H.: *Bone and Bones*, Ed. 2. The C. V. Mosby Company, St. Louis, 1955.

Chapter 4

OBTAINING THE IMPRESSION
AND FORMING THE CAST

*This chapter deals with the principles involved
in impression making for the removable partial
denture. The materials and techniques for
obtaining the impression and forming the
master cast are described and discussed. The
chapter is organized in this fashion:*
Introduction
Techniques of Impression Making
Pressure and Non-Pressure Impression
   Techniques
Impression Materials
The Impression Procedure
Management of the Patient with a
   Hypersensitive Gag Reflex
Care of the Impression
Methods of Forming the Cast
Trimming and Caring for the Cast
Types of Partial Denture Casts

Introduction

The critical need for finely detailed and
meticulously accurate impressions in the
practice of partial denture prosthodontics
scarcely needs elaboration. Unless the cast
upon which the prosthesis is to be constructed is an exact replica of the mouth,
the prosthesis cannot be expected to fit
properly, and, of course, an accurate cast
can be obtained only from an accurate
impression. The impression for a removable partial denture differs from one for a
complete denture in two important respects. The complete denture impression
records soft tissue only. The partial denture impression must accurately register
the relatively soft, yielding tissue (the oral

mucosa) at the same time that it records a
hard unyielding substance (the remaining
teeth). The procedure is further complicated by the fact that the hard structures
are irregular in contour as well as varying
in their vertical postures relative to the
occlusal plane. Because of this bell-shaped
contour and variance of vertical alignment
of the teeth (Fig. 4.1), the impression
material must be capable of entering into
intimate contact with each crown surface
of each tooth, withstanding the momentary distortion which occurs as the impression is withdrawn, and then instantly
springing back to its original form without
rupture or distortion. This elastic rebound
of the impression material is an essential
physical property which ensures that the
teeth on the master cast are precisely accurate reproductions in every detail of
their counterparts in the mouth. A partial
denture made to fit such an exact replica
will also fit the mouth.

Techniques of Impression Making

Techniques of obtaining the impression
may be classified, according to the
method used to record the tissues, into (1)
the open mouth method, and (2) the
closed mouth method. The open mouth
technique consists in introducing the tray
containing the impression material into
the mouth and holding it in place until
the material has gelled or set. The closed
mouth method, on the other hand, entails
placing the impression tray in the mouth
and having the patient hold it in place by
occluding on it. Usually this technique is
employed with a denture that is to be re-

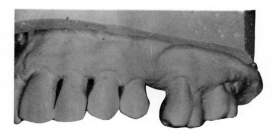

FIG. 4.1. In addition to registering the relatively soft oral mucosa, the impression for the removable partial denture must record structures which are bell shaped in contour (the teeth), and which are in varying vertical postures relative to the horizontal plane. The impression material must be capable of entering into intimate contact with each crown surface of each tooth, withstanding the momentary distortion which occurs as the impression is withdrawn, and then instantly springing back to its original form without rupture or distortion.

fitted (a reline), or by means of a customized impression tray. If a custom tray is employed, an occlusion rim of modeling composition is attached to the tray upon which the patient can comfortably close as the impression is being registered.

Types of Impression Trays

For the purpose of conveying the impression material into the mouth and over the teeth, and holding it in this position until it hardens, specially designed impression trays are customarily used. Impression trays can be classified broadly into stock trays and custom trays. Stock trays (Fig. 4.2) are made by the dental manufacturers, most commonly of metal, in a variety of sizes to fit large, medium, and small mouths. Stock trays may be dentulous for use with the dental arch which has some remaining natural teeth (Fig. 4.3), or edentulous for the mouth with no remaining teeth. Another category is the depressed anterior tray, designed especially to be used for the mouth which has only anterior teeth remaining. Stock trays for partial dentures may be perforated to retain the impression material in place better, or they may be constructed with a rim lock for this purpose. The rim lock retains the impression material in

position in the tray by means of an overlapping edge which wedges it in place. Another type of stock tray, designed for use with the reversible type of hydrocolloid, is the water cooled tray (Fig. 4.4). It contains tubes through which water can be circulated for the purpose of cooling the agar. Custom trays are sometimes needed for mouths that are abnormally large or small or of unusual configuration. Another indication for the custom tray is the case where all of the peripheral borders must be precisely delineated in the impression.

The Custom Impression Tray. The custom impression tray (Fig. 4.5) has certain advantages over the stock impression tray, and it may be desirable in some circumstances to take the extra steps, and expend the additional time, required for its fabrication. One major advantage of the custom tray is that the thickness of the impression material can be precisely controlled. This is an important consideration when using the rubber-base type materials which should not exceed a thickness of 2 to 4 mm., since sections thicker than this are more subject to distortion as the material polymerizes. Another advantage of the custom tray is the fact that a well fitted tray will better support the impression in the palate, thus avoiding the ever present danger of the material slumping in this vital area. The custom tray is sometimes heralded as being less of an ordeal than is the stock tray for the apprehensive patient, but this may be open to question in light of the fact that a prerequisite to use of a customized impression tray is an impression with a stock tray. Hence, the patient must be exposed to two impression procedures when the custom tray is employed.

The custom tray is especially recommended for the impression in which it is desirable to establish precise borders, as for example, in the case of the Kennedy Class I maxillary partial denture, when an accurate post dam is an important requirement. The peripheries including the post dam can be established with a high degree of accuracy with the customized tray.

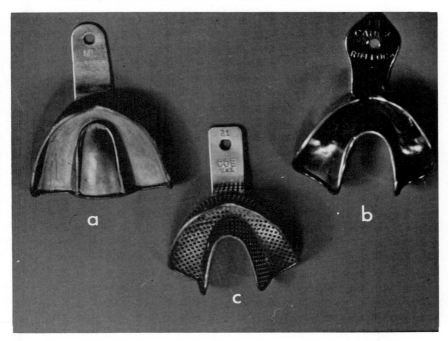

FIG. 4.2. The photo shows three types of stock impression trays. The tray shown at *a* is a rim lock tray for the maxillary arch. The one shown at *b* is a depressed anterior tray for the mandibular arch with only anterior teeth remaining. The tray at *c* is a mesh tray for the mandibular arch with some or all of the natural teeth remaining.

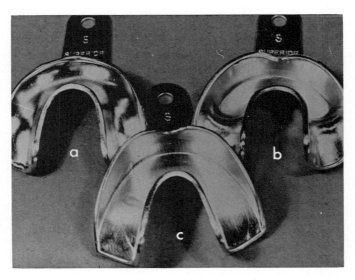

FIG. 4.3. The trays shown here are all of the rim lock type for the mandible. The one shown at *a* is for an edentulous arch (note the shallow flanges). A depressed anterior tray, *b*, is for an arch with only anterior teeth remaining. The tray shown at *c* is for an arch that is either fully or partially dentulous (note the deep flanges).

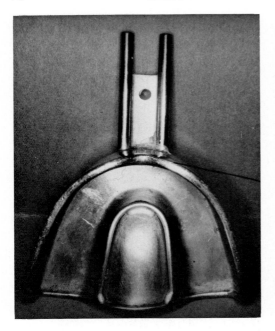

FIG. 4.4. Shown here is a water cooled tray for use with agar type hydrocolloid impression material. Rubber tubes are attached to the openings in the handle so that the water can enter one side and exit through the other, thus cooling the material and hastening the set.

The custom tray may be made of acrylic resin, or of either guttapercha or shellac baseplate material. When baseplate material is used for the tray, it is customary to employ two layers of the material to impart needed rigidity and strength. Nevertheless, a tray made of acrylic resin is generally more durable, as well as more stable, than one made of either of the baseplate materials.

The Modified Stock Tray (Individualized Tray). The stock tray can be modified with modeling composition or with wax to create a very accurately fitting tray which, for want of a better name and to distinguish it from the conventional custom tray, may be termed the "individualized tray." The technique has an important advantage over the use of a customized tray in that an alginate impression, in a stock tray, need not precede fabrication of the tray. The prime indication for the individualized tray is the mouth with edentulous spaces which are not tooth-bounded, the Kennedy Class I and II in particular.

Technique. Softened modeling composition is placed in the stock impression tray in such a way that it may capture the edentulous areas of the mouth and include one or two teeth adjacent to the space (Fig. 4.6). The tray is positioned in the

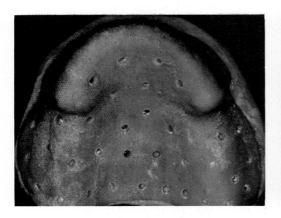

FIG. 4.5. This photograph shows a customized tray for a maxillary impression made of acrylic resin. Perforations have been made in the resin with a bur, to assist in retaining the impression material securely in the tray.

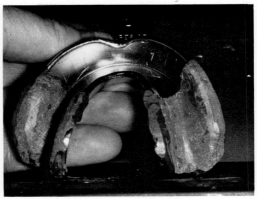

FIG. 4.6. An individualized tray can be made by modifying a stock tray with modeling composition. The modeling composition is scraped to a depth of 2 to 4 mm. to provide space for the elastic corrective material.

mouth and the compound is allowed to cool, but it is not permitted to harden completely, so that it is prevented from becoming locked around the adjacent teeth. When it has hardened sufficiently to maintain its contour, it is removed from the mouth and thoroughly chilled. The compound is trimmed so that it does not contact the adjacent teeth, and the surface of the compound in the edentulous areas is scraped to a depth of 2 to 4 mm., to provide space for a uniform layer of impression material. In the maxillary impression, the compound should cover the edentulous ridges and the palate, and should be accurately fitted to the post dam area. Before placing the corrective material into the tray, the compound must be made adhesive so that the elastic material will adhere to it. If the impression material to be used is either alginate or agar, this can be accomplished just prior to introducing the material into the tray, by heating the surface of the compound with a flame. An alternate method is to paint the surface of the compound with a solvent such as chloroform to make it "tacky," and then to embed cotton fibers in it. The impression material will become enmeshed in the cotton fibers, which will serve to retain it firmly against the surface of the compound. If rubber base material is to be employed, a rubber adhesive is painted on the compound for the same purpose.

Wax may be employed to create a customized tray, instead of modeling composition, if desired. When wax is used, it should contain perforations to help retain the elastic impression material, thus preventing its lifting or shifting (Fig. 4.7).

Advantages. The individualized tray technique is especially useful for the mouth that is either exceptionally large or small, or the one of anomalous contour which cannot be accurately fitted with a conventional stock tray. A decided advantage of the technique over the custom tray method is the fact that it can be accomplished in one appointment. Another advantage over the conventional impression procedure is that the posterior border (the post dam) can be established with precise

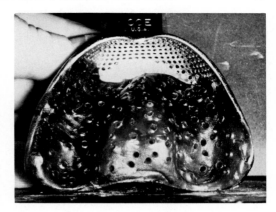

Fig. 4.7. An individualized tray can be made by adding wax to a stock tray, as shown here. Perforations are added to the wax to guard against movement of the impression material as the impression is removed from the mouth.

accuracy. A further advantage is the fact that the modeling composition can be molded into place in the stock tray in increments, by means of a series of add-on-and-try procedures. This has special merit for the patient with a tendency to gag, since it tends to repress his fear of a foreign body entering the throat.

Disadvantages. The disadvantages of the technique are the fact that the peripheral borders, with the exception of the post dam area, cannot be accurately established, and the fact that the tray is considerably more bulky than is a custom tray.

Pressure and Non-Pressure Impression Techniques

An impression technique may be described as being either pressure or non-pressure in type. The explanation for this is that both the maxilla and the mandible are covered with oral mucosa which is made up of epithelium and connective tissue of varying degrees of thickness. This soft tissue covering differs enormously in degree of displaceability from one area of the mouth to another. It is markedly displaceable in the region of the retromolar pads for example, yet is normally not displaceable to any discernible degree in the midline of the palate. As a consequence, impression techniques are

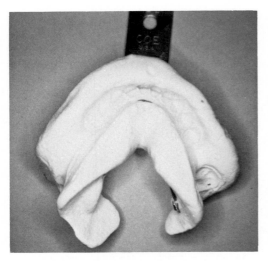

FIG. 4.8. The alginate hydrocolloid impression shown here is an example of a pressureless type of impression.

often referred to as being pressure or nonpressure in type, according to the amount that the mucosa is compressed or displaced under the pressure of the impression.

The Negative Pressure Impression. An impression that is registered with a very minimum of pressure is sometimes referred to as a mucostatic impression. An impression obtained with a hydrocolloid material is an example of this type of impression (Fig. 4.8).

The Controlled Pressure Type Impression. A controlled pressure technique is one in which the tissue is compressed or displaced to some degree. One obtained with zinc oxide-eugenol paste in an individualized modeling composition tray would be an example of this type of impression. A variation of the pressure technique is the functional impression, in which an effort is made to capture the tissue in its working, or functional, form. Low fusing wax, in an acrylic resin tray under normal bite pressure (closed mouth technique), would displace tissue in a manner similar to the way it is displaced in function, and is an example of a functional impression.

The Two-Piece Impression (Composite Impression)

It is sometimes desirable to exploit the advantages of more than one technique or material in an impression by using two different materials in two separate steps. This is referred to as a two-piece impression, and the technique can be employed to advantage in the maxillary arch which has only six anterior teeth remaining. A custom tray is fabricated of acrylic resin, to fit the edentulous portion of the mouth, this portion of the impression is border molded with modeling composition (Fig. 4.9), and an impression is registered with zinc oxide-eugenol paste or rubber base material (Fig. 4.10). A second impression of the teeth is taken with hydrocolloid (Fig. 4.11), and the composite impression is poured to form the master cast. Although this technique is employed most commonly for the maxillary immediate complete denture, it lends itself very well for use with the Kennedy Class I partial denture in the maxillary arch. The advantage over the conventional procedure is that the areas to be occupied by the denture borders, including the post dam, can be accurately delineated in the impression.

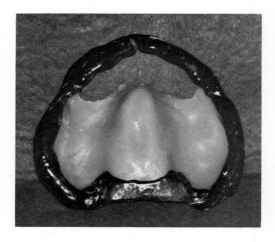

FIG. 4.9. An impression of a partially edentulous arch may, for greater accuracy, be taken in two separate steps. The custom-acrylic resin tray shown here has been border molded with modeling composition.

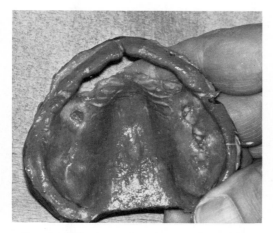

FIG. 4.10. The impression shown in Figure 4.9 has been used to register an impression of all of the mouth, except the teeth, with rubber base as a corrective material.

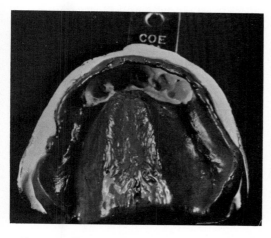

FIG. 4.11. The impression shown in Figure 4.10 is placed in the mouth and an impression of the teeth is taken with alginate type hydrocolloid. A cast is then poured into the composite impression.

Impression Materials

It is often said that there is no perfect dental material, and certainly, when applied to impression materials, few would take issue with this assertion. There are, however, several excellent materials available for registering the partial denture impression that will yield an eminently satisfactory result provided they are properly manipulated. The elastic group of impression materials is employed almost exclusively for this purpose although plaster of Paris and modeling composition were once widely used, the latter as a sectional impression. Materials classified in the elastic group are the hydrocolloids, both reversible (agar) and irreversible (alginate) types, and the rubbers, both mercaptan and silicone. Each of these materials possesses strengths as well as weaknesses; each offers advantages and also has limitations. Because of its unique combination of physical properties, the irreversible type of hydrocolloid—or alginate as it is more commonly referred to —is more extensively used in dentistry than any other material for the partial denture impression. However, other materials of the elastic group may be used for this purpose, and when properly handled will yield excellent results.

In the assessment of a dental material for a specific purpose, it is undeniably true that no material can be expected to yield an optimal result unless it is manipulated in precisely the manner that the manufacturer intended, and recommends, that it should be. Each of the elastic group of materials is compounded by the manufacturer with a unique combination of physical properties, which enables it to accomplish a specific clinical task or tasks with distinction, provided it is properly manipulated. Thus it follows that, in order to employ one of these impression materials to maximum advantage, one should be intimately familiar with the physical properties of the group to which it belongs, in addition to having a thorough understanding of the manufacturer's directions for handling the specific material being used. One must know the variables that can affect its behavior, and adhere religiously to a technique which ensures rigid control of each variable.

Each one of the elastic impression type materials has physical properties which make it especially suitable for accomplishing a specific clinical procedure. One who is familiar with the properties of each of the elastic materials can select, with discernment, the one best suited for a given task. The following discussion is not intended to give a full account, but only to give salient characteristics of each material as they pertain strictly to the partial denture impression. For a detailed comparison of the physical properties of the elastic materials, the reader is referred to one of the textbooks which deals exclusively with dental materials. (Impression materials of all types, together with the most common usage of each, are listed in Table 4.1.)

The Reversible Type of Hydrocolloid (Agar)

The agar type of hydrocolloid is classified as reversible, which means that it can be heated to become a viscous liquid and then cooled to form a rubber-like gel, and the process can be repeated again and again with the same material. It is an extremely accurate impression medium and its ability to reproduce surface detail is excellent. An agar type impression can be stored for periods of up to 1 hour without fear of dimensional change, provided it is maintained in an environment of 100% humidity. (Wrapping in a wet towel will provide this environment.) Although an agar impression can be obtained without the use of a water cooled tray, it is an inordinately cumbersome procedure to do so. Preparation of the material for use in the mouth requires a water bath, and manipulation of the agar in obtaining the impression demands, perhaps, more expertise than any of the other elastic materials. Moreover, the heat of the material may stimulate the flow of secretions from the palatal glands, which must be counted a disadvantage.

Although it must be conceded that the agar type of hydrocolloid does possess some advantages, it is questionable whether they are of sufficient weight to override the many advantages of the irreversible type of hydrocolloid. Certainly, when properly handled, the latter will consistently yield a dimensionally accurate master cast.

The Rubber Base Impression Materials

Two types of synthetic rubber impression materials, mercaptan and silicone, have gained rather wide acceptance in clinical dentistry in recent years. Both are used extensively in restorative dentistry for the fabrication of inlays, crowns, and bridges. One reason for their popularity in this phase of prosthodontics is the fact that they are the first elastic impression materials against which a metal die can be made, although there are other reasons to justify their widespread use as well.

The dimensional accuracy of both types of rubber is excellent, although in terms of yielding an accurate cast for the removable type of partial denture no clear superiority over either alginate or agar has ever been demonstrated. Nevertheless, the ability of the rubbers to reproduce surface detail is unsurpassed and, in fact, they are superior to alginate and at least the equal of agar in this respect.

Another advantage of the rubbers is the fact that a gypsum material poured against them will be smoother and have a denser surface than one poured against a hydrocolloid. Still another advantage of the mercaptan type of rubber is that pouring does not have to be done upon removal from the mouth with the same urgency that is a requirement when using the hydrocolloids. Indeed, the mercaptan impression may be stored for periods of up to 1 hour without fear of dimensional change. However, this is not true of the silicone impression which, like the hydrocolloids, should be poured as soon as possible.

Both rubber materials require that the bulk of material in the impression be rather closely controlled, so as not to exceed 2 to 4 mm in thickness in order to ensure dimensional accuracy. This makes it necessary to employ a custom tray, which requires an additional appointment, as well as two separate impression procedures, and raises the question: Does the advantage which accrues from the use of a rubber impression material for the removable partial denture justify the ad-

TABLE 4.1.
Impression Materials

Materials	Removable Partial Dentures	Complete Dentures	Crown and Bridge	Form Used	Example	Remarks
Modeling composition (compound)	1. To contour borders for the functional impression	1. For trays 2. Used to border mould the custom tray	1. Tube impression for crown or inlay	Cakes and sticks		Marketed as low, medium, and high fusing
Plaster of Paris	1. Check bites 2. Sectional impression (now passe)	1. Check bites 2. As corrective 3. As a rebase impression	1. Bridge impression	Powder mixed with water	Plastigum	Requires a separator prior to pouring cast
Metallic oxide paste	1. Check bites 2. As rebase impression material	1. Check bites 2. Corrective impression 3. Rebase impression	1. Bite registration	Base and hardener supplied in tubes	Coe-Trans; Opotow	No separator required
Impression wax	1. Functional impression 2. Rebase impression	1. Corrective impression 2. Rebase impression		Wafers (also in bulk)	Iowa University wax; Korecta	No separator required
Reversible hydrocolloid (agar)	1. Impressions	Rarely used	Full arch impressions	Tubes and in bulk	Surgident	Widely used for cast duplication in the laboratory
Irreversible hydrocolloid (alginate)	1. Widely used in a stock or custom tray for obtaining the impression	1. As a corrective impression 2. As an impression material for the immediate denture	Full arch impression (not widely used for this purpose)	Single units of powder or in large container of 24 units	Super Gel	Can be used for cast duplication in the laboratory
Mercaptan rubber base (polysulfide rubber)	1. Impressions in a custom tray	1. Corrective impressions	Full arch impressions (widely used)	Tubes (base and hardener)	Elasticon; Plastosil	Requires a tray adhesive. Should not exceed 2-4 mm. in thickness
Silicone	1. Impressions in a custom tray	1. Corrective impressions.	Full arch impression (not commonly used)	Tubes (base and hardener)	Elasticon; Plastosil	Requires a tray adhesive. Should not exceed 2-4 mm. in thickness.
Tissue treatment material	1. Tissue treatment 2. Rebase impression	1. Tissue treatment 2. Rebase impression		Powder and liquid	Soft-Tone; Hydrocast	Primarily a tissue conditioner for inflamed or hyperplastic mucosa

ditional time and inconvenience imposed by the double impression procedure?

Irreversible Hydrocolloid (Alginate)

Irreversible hydrocolloid, or alginate as it is more commonly referred to, is a salt of alginic acid in powder form. When it is mixed with water, a chemical reaction takes place, in which the material gels or congeals into a rubber-like solid. In technical terms the sol is transformed into a gel. This is not a reversible reaction, in contrast to the agar, and hence the term "irreversible." It is far and away the most commonly used material in dentistry for the removable partial denture impression, and its physical properties are such as to warrant fully its position of preeminence. Besides being reliably accurate, it is not objectionable to the patient, requires no special equipment or lengthy preparation (as does agar), and is less expensive than either mercaptan or silicone rubber. To all this can be added the fact that it may be conveniently stored in the dental operatory, so as to be instantly available when needed.

Types of Alginate Impression Material. Two different types of alginate are marketed by most manufacturers, the distinction between the two being the differing times required for the material to gel. The regular material sets in approximately 3 minutes and the quick-set material gels in approximately half this time, or 90 seconds. The regular material is recommended for routine use. The quicker setting material may have advantages for use with children, or for problem patients who require special management for one reason or another.

The Accuracy of Alginate. In judging an impression material, it is axiomatic that, irrespective of any other consideration, the ultimate criterion must be how accurately it can reproduce, in the cast, every detail of the dental arch. Many research studies have been carried out in an effort to assess the relative accuracy of the irreversible hydrocolloids, as compared to the other elastic materials, since the material was first introduced to dentistry

late in the decade of the 1930's. The results of this investigative effort have been so inconclusive that few categorical statements can be made, other than to say that no one material can demonstrate any clear-cut superiority over the others. The work of some investigators has shown the alginate type hydrocolloid to be superior in accuracy to the agar type material. Other workers have shown it to be equal in accuracy to agar, while still other research has indicated that the alginate material, while equal in dimensional accuracy to either the agar type materials or the polysulfide rubbers, is slightly inferior in reproducing surface detail. Certainly, the alginates have proven themselves thoroughly accurate for clinical use in literally millions of practical cases, and none of the other elastic materials offers any challenge to the alginate for ease of handling and convenient availability. While it may be argued that the superior ability of the rubbers to reproduce surface detail justifies the additional appointment and the extra effort of obtaining two impressions, a very persuasive case can be made for the use of alginate, all things considered.

Types of Inaccuracies and Distortions. Although there is no lack of evidence that a properly manipulated alginate impression will yield a cast upon which a partial denture casting, that will fit the mouth with precise accuracy, can be fabricated, it must be conceded that it is a tempermental material. It will perform commendably for the person who manipulates it with understanding and respect, but it can be treacherous and unreliable when handled carelessly. The following paragraphs discuss the characteristics, and point out the peculiarities, of alginate impression material in general, and offer suggestions for avoiding certain of the more commonly overlooked pitfalls.

Surface Inaccuracies. The material is subject to small ruptures and tears, particularly in areas where it has been removed from an excessively deep undercut. Then too, it may also show small voids and pits caused by air bubbles or droplets of saliva. A more serious defect occurs when a layer of thick mucinous saliva is allowed to interpose itself at the interface of the mucosa and the alginate. Proper mixing and timing of the impression procedure will ensure a tough, strong impression, which will eliminate all but clinically insignificant minor tears and ruptures of the material. The defects caused by the mucinous saliva can be controlled by mouth washes and proper impression technique.

Dimensional Distortion. Dimensional change can take place either while the impression is in the mouth or following its removal. If the discrepancy is gross, it may be readily detected by careful examination of the impression but, more often than not, it will be so subtle as to escape notice. The first inkling that distortion has occurred may be when the framework does not fit the mouth although it fits the master cast. Again, dimensional inaccuracies can be virtually eliminated by meticulous adherence to good impression technique, and careful handling of the impression after it is removed from the mouth.

Intraoral Distortion. Gelling of the material begins first in the alginate which is directly in contact with the oral mucosa, because the chemical reaction is accelerated by body heat. Hence, any movement of the tray while the gel reaction is taking place is very apt to result in distortion of the impression. To avoid this type of error, the tray should be held absolutely immobile, with light but firm pressure from the time it is seated in position until it is removed from the mouth.

Extraoral Distortion. It is possible for the impression to become distorted as a result of careless handling. For this reason it should be grasped only by the handle of the impression tray and when stored temporarily, it should be propped up on a cotton roll or suspended by the handle in such a way as to avoid contact of the impression with any hard object.

Shrinkage. So sensitive is alginate to its environment that it will begin to change form to a measurable degree within 12 minutes of the time it is removed from the mouth. Accordingly, any impression which is to be used for construction of a prosthesis should be poured within this time period. As a further precaution the impression should be wrapped in a moist towel or cloth as soon as it has been removed from the mouth and rinsed off. An alginate impression should never, at any time, be placed directly under an incandescent bulb, in direct sunlight, or close to any source of heat.

Variables that Affect Dimensional Accuracy. It is important to remember that the physical properties of all alginates are such that the material is extremely susceptible to variations in handling technique. Even a slight change in procedure from one mix to the next, such as water of a different temperature, or a different water/powder ratio, for example, can bring about erratic, ofttimes unpredictable, behavior.

Timing. The proportions of the various constituents contained in the different brands of alginate are balanced by each manufacturer to allow ample time for mixing of the powder and water, and spooning the mixed material into the impression tray, within a time frame in which gelation will begin to occur shortly after it has been positioned in the mouth. This necessarily precise timetable is highly desirable from a clinical standpoint, so as not to subject the patient to an unnecessarily prolonged period of tedium, as well as to reduce to a minimum the muscle fatigue which may result from an awkward holding position. Precise timing is obviously critical to success in manipulating such a sensitive material, hence it is customary for the manufacturer to list a setting time in the directions which he provides. Setting time extends from the time that the powder is introduced to the water in the mixing bowl, to the point at which gelation takes place in the mouth. The setting time specified is predicated on all variables being constant. The mixing time customarily recommended is in the range of 45 seconds to 1 minute. Given these basic guidelines, a technique may be worked out by the dentist and his assistant which is geared to their individual work tempos, and comfortably within the time frame allotted by the manufacturer. To illustrate, if 45 seconds is used to spatulate the material in the bowl, then approximately 45 seconds may be taken to place the material into the tray and onto the abutment teeth, and to insert the tray into the mouth, well before gelation begins. It should be obvious that all variables must be kept constant or the timing will not serve its intended purpose. A timing device such as a sandglass or an interval timer is a useful adjuvant to the armanentarium for the impression procedure.

The Water. The temperature of the water which is used to mix the material is critical, a temperature of 68–70° F usually being considered optimal. A temperature lower than this will slow the set (increase the setting time) while a higher temperature will have the opposite effect. A thermometer should be available so that this factor can be rigidly controlled. Ice cubes can be used to lower the temperature, while warm water will elevate a temperature which is too low.

Tap water varies greatly in mineral content in different geographic regions, and various kinds and quantities of minerals can affect the behavior of the alginate in an unpredictable manner. For this reason, distilled water should be used if available. It may be stored in a demijohn on a shelf in the laboratory, a modus operandi which at the same time makes available water of a reduced mineral content and a constant room temperature, generally in the neighborhood of 70° F.

Water/Powder Ratio. It is very important that the exact amount of water and powder recommended by the manufacturer be used. Research has shown that there will be less variation in physical properties if the powder is measured by weight (in grams) rather than by volume (in a measuring cup). If the material is purchased in individual units, the quantity is more apt to be a precisely accurate weight, since it is weighed by the manufacturer prior to packaging. If the larger

cans of alginate (containing material for approximately 24 maxillary impressions and up to twice that number of mandibular impressions) are used, however, the difference in the amount of powder which may be contained in each measuring cup can vary substantially, depending on how densely it is packed into the cup. If a volume measure is used, it should be routine practice to roll the large can of alginate back and forth on its side so as to "fluff" the powder before filling the measuring cup, and also to smooth off the powder with the spatula, the edge of which must be level with the top of the measuring cup (Fig. 4.12). Although this will not guarantee a precise quantity of powder by weight, it will go far towards ensuring a reasonably constant amount of powder for each succeeding mix. An insufficient amount of water will produce a grainy mix, which will not possess maximum strength and may result in a cast with a rough surface. Too great an amount of water will produce an overly thin mix, retard the setting time, and may weaken the material. A few drops more of water, over that recommended by the manufacturer, will not affect the strength of the material appreciably, but research has shown that more than a few drops in excess of that recommended will result in an impression of less than maximum toughness and strength.

Mixing Technique. In mixing alginate type hydrocolloid, the solid should always be carried to the liquid, i.e., the powder to the water. When the powder and water are mixed, a chemical reaction takes place in which the sol is converted into a gel. In order to develop the optimal properties of the material, every bit of the powder should react with all of the water, and the two should be mixed together for the exact period of time prescribed by the manufacturer. Alginate which has been thoroughly mixed will have a smooth, shiny appearance. An under-spatulated batch will be weak and vulnerable to tearing, while over-spatulation incurs the risk of breaking up some of the gel after the gelation has begun. This, too, may be respon-

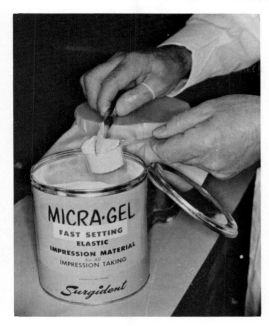

FIG. 4.12. When mixing alginate type hydrocolloid, it is important that the powder/water ratio recommended by the manufacturer be observed, because the behavior of the material is profoundly affected by the relative amounts of each that are used. A technique should be developed in which a uniform amount of each material is used for each impression.

sible for a weak material. If spatulation is continued after gelation has started, it may prolong the setting time. Although some authorities have advocated that the material be mixed only in a plastic bowl, clinical evidence indicates that the rubber mixing bowl is entirely satisfactory for this purpose. Research studies have demonstrated, however, that an alginate that has been mechanically mixed is stronger, more homogeneous, and less porous, than is hand-spatulated material. Hence, mechanical spatulation is preferred, if the means are available. If the material is stirred by hand, it should be mashed frequently against the side of the mixing bowl, to force bubbles of air out of the mix.

The Effect of Age. Alginate which has been stored for long periods of time is very apt to behave in an erratic manner, and for this reason only material of known vintage should be used. Overage material may set too rapidly, thereby upsetting the timetable of impression registration or, even more disconcerting, it may fail to harden altogether. For this reason it is unwise to keep large quantities on hand.

Contamination of the Alginate. The alginate material can be contaminated by moisture so that its physical properties are altered and its behavior affected. The individually wrapped units of alginate, in addition to ensuring a uniform quantity of material by weight, are protected from contamination by the foil in which they are contained, a fact which recommends them for use in the average dental office. If the larger sized units of alginate are used, care should be exercised to keep the lid tightly on the can at all times that the material is not actually being removed from it, so as to protect it from the moisture of the atmosphere as well as any other contamination. Perhaps the best modus operandi, when the alginate is being used in substantial quantity, is to purchase the larger units of material, and then weigh out individual units and store them in tightly stoppered bottles, instantly available for future use. This method should eliminate the variation in the amount of powder that may result when the powder is apportioned by means of a measuring scoop.

Variations in Alginates. Although the alginates of the different manufacturers are basically alike, they do vary somewhat in handling characteristics from one brand to another. One may be more viscous than another, or smoother, or more grainy, without affecting the accuracy or overall merit of each material in any way. Because of these slight differences, each nanufacturer may recommend slightly different manipulative procedures for the material which he markets. Therefore, when a switch is made from one brand of alginate to another, the directions which accompany the new material should be carefully noted and followed to the letter.

The Impression Procedure

Obtaining the impression for the removable partial denture can be a thoroughly unpleasant experience, from the patient's point of view, if it is not accomplished with skill and finesse. The dentist who prepares himself with an intimate knowledge of the impression material with which he is working, and who follows a technique which is consistent with its physical properties, can eliminate most of the unpleasant aspects for all but the most squeamish of patients. Moreover, he will be successful in obtaining accurate impressions with simple routine procedures in perhaps 98% of patients.

Patient Management

Many dental operations are totally new experiences to the patient, and the clinician should not lose sight of the fact that all human beings are subject, in some degree, to what the psychologists term "fear of the unknown." The impression procedure, besides engendering the trepidation of a new experience, may activate a subconscious fear of having the airway blocked. This can give rise to a feeling of mild panic in a patient who is already apprehensive. It is time well spent, therefore, to devote a few moments to explaining to the patient, for whom an impression is to be made, that it is basically a simple procedure, and to reassure him that there is no need to feel anxiety. Such psychological conditioning, accomplished with professional finesse, can transform an apprehensive, restless patient into a more relaxed, cooperative one.

It is quite common, too, for people to have preconceived notions concerning dental procedures, perhaps stemming from some dimly remembered experience of the past. Merely reassuring such an individual that there is nothing in the procedure to cause him more than mild discomfort will usually suffice to relax him and restore his confidence and sense of security. Permitting the patient to smell the impression material while it is being mixed has merit, the implication being that a material with such a pleasant odor and innocuous appearance (like cake frosting) could not be too disagreeable to have in the mouth, and then too, famil-

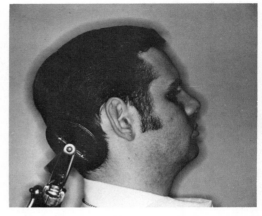

FIG. 4.13. Proper positioning of the patient is an important prerequisite of good impression procedure. He should be comfortably seated in the chair, with the head firmly supported by the head rest and the plane of occlusion approximately parallel to the floor.

iarity tends to dispell misgivings and uncertainties. The word "gag" should not be used in the presence of the patient. It has an unpleasant connotation to many people, and is better left unsaid in the prosthetic operatory. If the patient volunteers the information that he is a "gagger," he should be reassured that there will be no reason to be concerned about it, and the subject should not be pursued at the time. However, a mental note should be made of this fact, and the management of the patient may be modified slightly, as recommended in a later section of this chapter. Another term that is not recommended for use in conversing with the patient is "load." The dentist who instructs the assistant to load the impression tray may unwittingly unnerve the hypertensive patient who associates the word "load" with syringes, needles, and injections.

Positioning of the Patient

The patient should be seated comfortably upright, with the head firmly supported in the headrest (Fig. 4.13). The plane of occlusion should be approximately parallel to the floor. The head of the patient shown in Figure 4.14 is tilted too far back. He should be instructed to

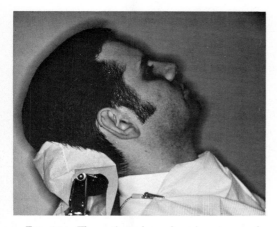

FIG. 4.14. The patient shown here is not properly positioned in the chair for an impression; his head is tilted too far back. Besides being uncomfortable, such a position may be disconcerting to some individuals who are apprehensive that some of the impression material will find its way into the throat.

sit quietly and to relax. The average patient who has no nasal obstruction may be instructed to breath through the nose while the impression tray is in place. It makes little difference, of course, whether he breathes through the nose or the mouth, but the slight distraction provided by his concentration on one or the other breathing method may be helpful in diverting his attention for the brief period that the impression is in his mouth. Certainly the patency of the airway will not be obstructed by the impression procedure. He should be instructed not to swallow while the impression is in place, because of the danger of causing a shift in the tray. He may be advised not to be concerned about the excess saliva that may accumulate in the floor of his mouth. This can be removed by the assistant with an aspirator, or a chin basin can be used if an aspirator is not at hand. If neither one is available, a towel held under the chin will suffice to maintain the patient in an acceptable state of comfort for the short period of time it is required. Not to be overlooked is the fact that the patient should be suitably draped to protect his clothing from accidental spillage of impression material or saliva.

Mouth Preparation and Prophylaxis

All mouth preparation should have been accomplished prior to impression taking, and the teeth should be clean. It is not recommended that a prophylaxis be accomplished immediately prior to obtaining the impression, however, as this will sometimes cause the alginate to stick to the teeth. The prophylaxis should ideally be accomplished 24 hours, or more, prior to the impression appointment.

Saliva Control

The saliva may at times become an obstacle to obtaining an accurate impression, if it is either excessive in amount or thick and ropy in character. The former type tends to produce pits and voids in the impression. The latter (mucinous) type may obscure tissue detail by filling in minute wrinkles, folds, and declivities, so that they are not accurately recorded in the impression medium.

Copius Saliva. The fact that the patient has an overabundance of saliva will be evident early in the therapeutic sequence. Typically, the floor of the mouth will fill with saliva during the visual-digital examination or as the radiographs are being taken. Excessive volume can usually be controlled by having the patient rinse with ice water just before the impression tray is inserted, in order to close the orifices of the salivary glands partially. Another approach is to place gauze packs or cotton rolls opposite Stensen's ducts, as well as in the floor of the mouth under the tongue, just prior to mixing the impression material. The packs should then be removed immediately prior to inserting the impression tray. In the rare case that cannot be controlled by either of these methods an antisialagogue such as Pamine (The Upjohn Company, Kalamazoo, Mich.) may be prescribed.

Thick, Mucinous Saliva. More than 350 palatine glands are located in the posterior third of the palate. In some mouths these glands secrete a profuse supply of a thick, mucinous type of saliva that can interfere with registration of an accurate impression (Fig. 4.15). The patient who

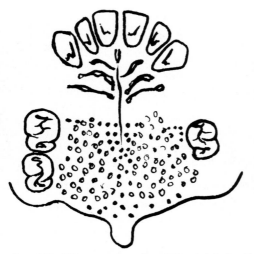

Fig. 4.15. There are more than 350 palatal glands located in the posterior part of the palate, beginning at the mesial area of the first molars. When these glands are active, they secrete a highly mucinous type of saliva that may interfere with registration of an accurate impression.

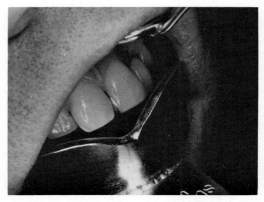

Fig. 4.16. The impression tray should be carefully fitted to the mouth. The flanges of the tray should clear the teeth by approximately ¼ inch, as shown in this photograph.

has this thick viscous type of saliva can usually be identified by rubbing the ball of the finger over the posterior third of the palate. A mucosa which feels exceptionally slippery indicates that it is coated with a layer of thick mucin. If the comparatively rough texture of the palatal mucosa can be felt with the finger tip, the viscosity of the saliva need not be an item of concern. The mucinous type of saliva can usually be controlled by means of a mouthwash consisting of ½ teaspoon of bicarbonate of soda in a half glass of water. This preimpression rinse has a thinning effect on the saliva, so that it is much less likely to obliterate tissue detail by intervening at the impression-tissue interface. If a mouthwash is not at hand, the problem may be overcome by employing the "tandem" impression technique, in which one impression is taken to "soak up" the bubbles and mucinous saliva, followed immediately by a second impression which will record the tissues in a relatively saliva-free state.

Tray Selection

Selection of a proper tray, and fitting it to the mouth, are the keystones of the impression procedure. The tray should be moistened with water prior to trying it in the mouth, so as to reduce to a minimum frictional contact with the lips and oral mucosa. The sides of a properly fitted tray should avoid direct contact with the buccal and labial surfaces of the teeth by approximately ¼ inch (Fig. 4.16). The tray shown in Figure 4.17 is too small, the one shown in Figure 4.18 is too large. The maxillary tray should extend posteriorly to include the hamular notches. The mandibular tray should be extended to include the retromolar pads. An important objective in impression making is to control, as nearly as possible, the thickness of the impression material so that there is a reasonably uniform thickness of material between the surface of the tray and the structure being registered. A relatively uniform thickness of material will tend to minimize differences in behavior between a thick section and an overly thin section, although it is obvious that the thickness will be somewhat greater in the palate than it will be over the biting surfaces of the teeth. When fitting the trays to the mouth, a comfortable holding position should be rehearsed so as to obviate the need for a shift in finger position during the time that the impression is being recorded.

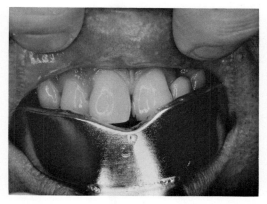

FIG. 4.17. The impression tray shown here is too small for this mouth.

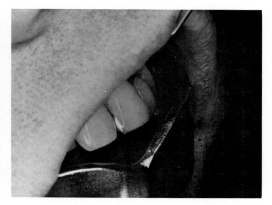

FIG. 4.18. The tray shown here is too large for this mouth.

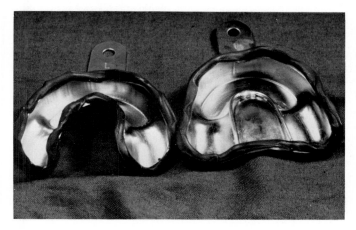

FIG. 4.19. The fit of the tray should be refined by rimming the peripheries with some readily moldable wax, such as utility wax. The wax will be more comfortable for the patient than the edge of the tray, will provide a stop for the impression in the vestibules, and will reduce the possibility of the tray border cutting through the soft alginate as it is seated over the teeth.

When fitting the mandibular tray, it is generally best not to give the patient any instructions concerning the position of the tongue. The reason for this is that if he is instructed to lift the tongue upon insertion of the tray when it is being fitted, he may reflexly raise it when the filled impression tray is being introduced into the mouth, and this is very apt to interfere with visibility as well as with proper placement of the tray.

Tray Preparation

The fit of the stock tray should be refined by rimming the peripheral borders with some readily moldable wax, such as utility wax (Fig. 4.19). This will, of course, include the post dam area of the maxillary tray, where the wax will serve to confine the material to the tray and impede its entry into the oropharynx. In addition to improving the fit of the tray and being more comfortable to the patient, the wax peripheries provide a stop in the vestibule for the impression. Another purpose of the wax is to reduce the possibility that the edge of the tray will penetrate the soft alginate as the impression is pressed into position over the teeth. The tray should be modified with wax in any area of the mouth that it does not encompass reasonably well. The labial vestibules (both mandibular and maxillary), for example, often will not be properly recorded unless the labial border of the tray is recontoured with wax so as to provide an accurate matrix to support the impression material in the area in question. If the vault area is unusually deep (high), the palatal region of the maxillary tray should be built up with utility wax (Fig. 4.20) or modeling composition, to prevent slumping of the impression material as it responds to gravitational pull. When wax is added to this area, holes should be punched in the wax at approximately ¼ inch intervals, to help in holding the impression material in place. Another reason for building up the palate of the tray when registering a high vault is that alginate shrinks towards the center of its greatest bulk as it gels. Thus, a large mass of impression material in the vault may slump, and the clinical result will be an inaccurate cast and a faulty fit of the partial denture.

Tray Release Compounds

Various compounds are marketed for the purpose of providing easy release of the material from the tray, following the pouring of the cast. These preparations are not recommended, because of the danger of premature release of the alginate material from the tray at some point in the procedure before the cast has been poured, which would introduce an inaccuracy that might go undetected until the try-in of the casting. The probable result of such a mishap would be that the framework would fit the cast but not the mouth.

Impression Sequence

Since the average patient accepts the registration of the mandibular impression with more equanimity than he does the maxillary, it is usually preferrable to obtain the mandibular impression first, all else being equal. On the other hand, when the prosthesis is to be made for the mandibular arch, it may be best to register the

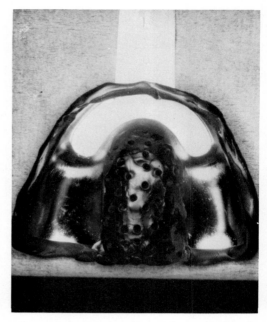

FIG. 4.20. If there are areas of the mouth that the stock impression tray does not encompass reasonably well, they should be modified with utility wax to effect a better fit. The labial vestibules of both arches often require some recontouring with wax, so that the tray will support the impression material and thus make possible a more accurate registration of the area. When the palatal vault is immoderately deep (high), the palatal region of the tray should be built up with wax to carry the impression material into place better, as well as to preclude slumping of the material because it is unsupported. Holes have been placed in the wax in this photograph to retain the impression material better.

impression for the opposing cast (the maxillary first, so that the mandibular cast can be poured immediately following removal of the impression from the mouth.

Filling the Tray

The tray should be dry when the impression material is placed in it. The alginate is best spooned into the tray with the spatula, using a spreading motion against the bottom and sides of the tray, in order to squeeze out air and force the material into the perforations or under the rim lock. Alginate possesses no adhesive properties whatever, and for this reason locking the material into the perforations or under the rim lock is necessary to ensure that it will not pull loose from the tray when the impression is forcibly disengaged from the teeth. Even a slight shift of the material, in relation to the tray, will result in an inaccurate cast. The material should be packed into the tray with a spreading motion which distributes it evenly throughout the tray and onto the borders. When a sufficient quantity has been spooned into the tray, a shallow gutter should be formed with a moist finger to correspond with the alveolar ridge. One of the hallmarks of inexperience in impression making is a tendency to overfill the tray. In all but unusual cases, a level, full tray is slightly more material than is needed. When there are prepared recesses in the teeth to be registered, care must be exercised to avoid the entrapment of tiny air bubbles in the rest seats. This is an ever-present problem for which there is no foolproof solution. One method that is generally successful is to dry the recess with a gentle blast of air, and then to apply a small amount of alginate to the recess with the finger (Fig. 4.21), just prior to inserting the filled tray (Fig. 4.22). Rest areas, whether in gold or

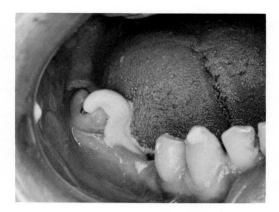

FIG. 4.22. In this photograph, the rest seat has been dried with air and a small amount of alginate has been daubed onto the rest just prior to introducing the tray.

enamel, should be smooth and highly polished, to counteract the affinity of saliva for a roughened surface.

Inserting the Tray

Immediately prior to inserting the tray, alginate should be applied to any area of the mouth where the fit of the impression tray is less than ideal, and there is reason to doubt that it will be properly registered in the impression. The labial vestibule frequently requires this treatment (Fig. 4.23). Alginate should be applied to the vault with the finger in any mouth that has a palate of more than average height, to minimize the possibility of trapping air which would, of course, result in a faulty impression. (Note: the following directions are for a right-handed individual.)

Mandibular Impression. Standing to the right and in front of the patient (Fig. 4.24), he is instructed to open wide, and the tray is inserted sideways into the mouth (Fig. 4.25). With a rotary motion it is lined up with the area to be registered, with the tray handle approximately parallel to the occlusal plane and in line with the midline. The patient is instructed to close slightly, so as to increase the space in the vestibules, and the tray is guided gently but firmly into place. When the

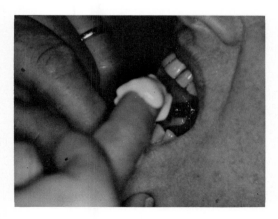

FIG. 4.21. A good method of avoiding the entrapment of air in the prepared rest seats of the abutment teeth is to dry off the recess with a gentle stream of air, and then to apply a small amount of impression material to the recess with the finger just prior to introducing the impression tray into the mouth.

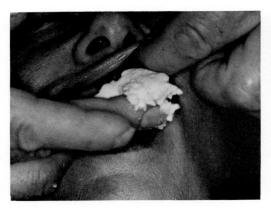

FIG. 4.23. Immediately prior to inserting the tray, some impression material should be applied to any area of the mouth where the fit of the tray is less than ideal. The labial vestibules of both arches frequently require this added material in order to be accurately registered in the impression. Alginate should be applied to the palate with the finger when the vault is of more than average height, unless the palatal area of the tray has been built up with wax or compound.

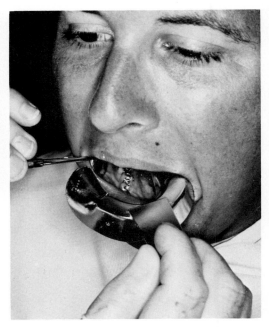

FIG. 4.25. The impression tray should be introduced into the mouth sideways and then rotated into position over the teeth. Maximum space will be made available for the tray if a mirror is used to retract the cheeks, rather than the finger.

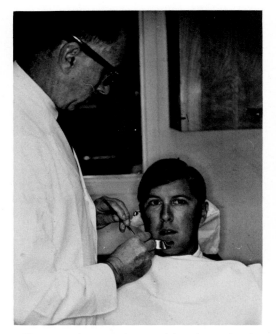

FIG. 4.24. A convenient position for registering the mandibular impression is to the right and in front of the patient. This affords maximum visibility and, in addition, makes possible a comfortable holding position.

tray is seated, the patient is instructed to lift the tongue and touch the roof of the mouth with it. The purpose of lifting the tongue is to elevate the floor of the mouth, thus bringing the mylohyoid musculature out from under the flange of the tray, so that the residual ridge in this area can be accurately recorded in the impression. This is an important step which should not be overlooked, since failure to accomplish it may result in an impression which includes the lateral surfaces of the tongue. It is worthy of note, too, that the impression should never be registered with the mouth stretched open, since the mandible is actually capable of flexing a slight amount in the wide open position.

Maxillary Impression. From a position to the right of, and slightly behind, the patient (Fig. 4.26), he should be instructed to open wide, and the tray is inserted sideways into the mouth (Fig. 4.27). The tray should then be rotated so that

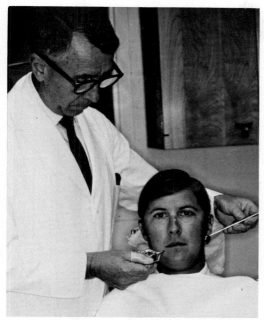

FIG. 4.26. In registering the maxillary impression, a convenient position is to the right and behind the patient.

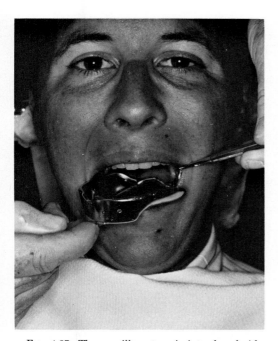

FIG. 4.27. The maxillary tray is introduced sideways and then rotated into its proper position over the structures to be registered, with the tray handle lined up with the midline.

the handle is approximately parallel to the midline. In registering the maxillary impression, it must be remembered that when the mandible is open wide, the coronoid process of the mandible is brought forward, and may enter the buccal space, thus interfering with proper positioning of the impression tray in some mouths (Fig. 4.28). Accordingly, the patient should be instructed to close slightly from the wide open position, so as to increase the space in the vestibules, as well as to withdraw the coronoid process from the buccal space. The posterior border of the tray should first be guided into place until the impression material begins to exit from the posterior border. At this juncture the upward pressure should be directed so as to guide the anterior part of the tray up into its seated position. When the tray has been seated, the upward pressure is released and the tray is held with firm, steady pressure until the material has gelled.

Holding the Impression

The impression should be held in place, without movement of any kind, until the material has completely set. The patient should never be permitted to hold the tray. Besides the likelihood of jeopardizing the accuracy of the impression by slight movement, there are legal implications in such a procedure as well. Moreover, it is very poor psychology to treat such an important step in such cavalier fashion. No attempt should be made to border mold the impression, since the overextended tray flanges make such a procedure of dubious value at best. A small sample of the alginate may be placed on the bracket table where the progress of gelation can be tested with the finger, although it will gel more rapidly within the mouth because it is accelerated by body heat. When the material is no longer sticky or tacky when touched with the finger, it may be considered gelled. Following initial gelation, the tray should be held an additional 2 or 3 minutes to allow the alginate to attain maximum strength. If a sandglass or an interval timer is placed on the bracket table, the

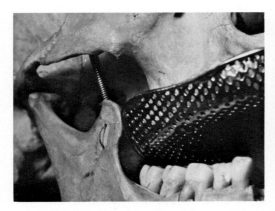

FIG. 4.28. When the mouth is opened wide, the coronoid process of the mandible travels forward and, in some mouths, it may so fill the buccal space that it interferes with proper placement of the tray in the tuberosity area. If interference is encountered in this area with the mouth open wide, the patient should be instructed to close slightly, which will retrude the coronoid process sufficiently so that the space will accommodate the tray.

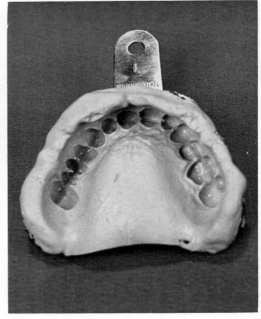

FIG. 4.29. The impression should be blown off with a gentle stream of air and inspected under a good light for imperfections.

patient can participate in the experience of "watching the time pass," a diversion which seems to make the waiting period a bit less tedious and may even encourage a mood of relaxation.

Removing the Impression from the Mouth

The internal structure of the alginate material is such that it will resist a sudden unidirectional force without distortion or fracture better than it will a twisting or rocking force applied gradually or intermittently. Rocking the tray applies stresses which alternately stretch and compress the material, and may very well lead to a dimensional inaccuracy. To remove the tray, a finger of the free hand should be wedged gently between the peripheral border of the impression and the adjacent tissues of the vestibule in the bicuspid-molar area, at the same instant that direct pressure is exerted downward and slightly forward (for the maxillary impression).

Properly applied, and coordinated with a downward thrust, the finger will allow air to enter between the mucosa and the impression, thus breaking the seal created by the interfacial tension between the

two, and making possible ready withdrawal. The direction of removal of the mandibular impression should be upward and in a slightly labial direction.

Inspecting the Impression

The impression should be blown off with a gentle stream of air and inspected under a good light (Figs. 4.29 and 4.30). If there are no obvious defects, such as voids or a section of material loosened from the tray, attention should be focused on the areas around the abutment teeth for tears in the material, and on the rest preparations for tiny bubbles. A bubble in this critical area (the rest recess) must disqualify the impression, because it is virtually impossible to remove the resulting bleb of stone from the master cast and have an occlusal rest that fits the tooth with accuracy. Minor imperfections, such as wax showing through the alginate in noncritical areas (i.e., those which will not be contacted by the prosthesis), do not warrant rejection of an otherwise acceptable impression. If the impression mate-

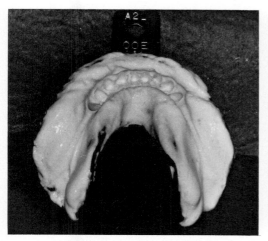

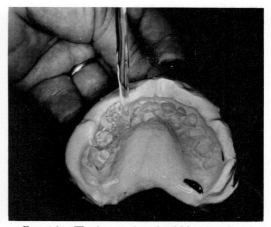

FIG. 4.30. The rest preparations, in particular, should be carefully scrutinized for bubbles, since a bubble in this critical area must disqualify the impression.

FIG. 4.31. The impression should be rinsed under a gentle stream of water to remove surface debris and saliva.

rial lifts away from the tray, however, an event that is prone to occur with the mandibular impression in a rim lock tray, no attempt should be made to reposition it. Repositioning a section of impression material that has broken loose from an impression tray is a risky undertaking, and the most prudent course is to obtain another impression. And similarly, alginate which extends unsupported beyond the confines of the impression tray, in addition to casting doubt on the accuracy of the impression, is evidence of a faulty fit of the tray, or of failure to center it properly over the teeth.

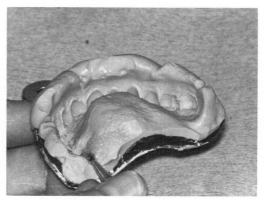

FIG. 4.32. If saliva tends to cling to the surface of the impression, it may be necessary to introduce some soapsuds to loosen it, followed by a rinse with water.

Washing the Impression

The impression should be rinsed under a gentle stream of tap water (Fig. 4.31) to cleanse it of saliva and mucous. If the saliva tends to cling to the material, it may be necessary to flow some soapsuds into the impression to loosen it (Fig. 4.32). In the case of extremely adhesive saliva, dry stone, or plaster, (Fig. 4.33), may be sprinkled into the impression, or introduced with a fine brush and then rinsed out with water. The latter method will loosen any saliva, however tenacious. When the impression has been rinsed, it should be wrapped in a wet towel preparatory to

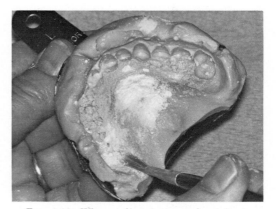

FIG. 4.33. When saliva is immoderately tenacious, some dry stone, introduced into the impression and then rinsed with water, will remove it.

pouring of the cast. It should not be laid down on a bench top without support, for fear of distorting it.

Management of the Patient with a Hypersensitive Gag Reflex

A patient with a hypersensitive gag reflex will occasionally be encountered in dental practice, and may require special management. As a rule, the person with a gagging tendency will in one way or another make the fact known early in the treatment continuum. He may describe a past experience in which he gagged and retched or, perhaps more commonly, it will be discovered during some phase of the examination or while some other procedure is being performed. The gag reflex is associated very closely with the vomit reflex, which is a protective mechanism devised by nature to prevent noxious substances from entering the intestinal tract or the airway. The nerve pathways which activate the reflex are located in the parasympathetic portion of the autonomic nervous system. The reflex is present at birth and is manifested differently in each individual, depending on a myriad of factors, principally psychological. It is most commonly triggered by tactile stimulation of the soft palate, the fauces, the posterior wall of the pharynx, or the posterior third of the dorsum of the tongue. In addition, to touch any one of the other four senses, taste, visual, olfactory or auditory, may provide the stimulus, and certainly not to be lost sight of, the psychological component is always a potent factor to be considered.

When complete dentures are to be made for such a patient, the problem resolves itself into phases: (1) the problems associated with obtaining the impressions and intraoral records, and (2) the problems which confront the patient in adjusting to wearing the prosthesis. The candidate for a partial denture, on the other hand, presents a far less formidable challenge. Once the impressions and intraoral records are obtained, the prosthesis can almost always be designed in such a way that the patient can adjust comfortably to it.

The patient should be seated as upright as the chair will permit (Fig. 4.34). If the gag reflex is unusually acute, the head should be pitched still farther forward and downward, so that the chin contacts the chest as soon as the impression tray is seated (Fig. 4.35), and held in this downward-forward position until the material has gelled. The maneuver should be explained to the patient, and it may be rehearsed beforehand, so that he will not be alarmed by the unorthodox head position. Except in extreme instances, this head-forward procedure will not be necessary when obtaining the mandibular impression.

The sight of the impression material being spatulated and loaded into the tray may add to the patient's apprehension, and for this reason all preparation of material should be carried out behind the chair insofar as it is possible to do so. A quick-set alginate material is recommended for the patient who demonstrates gagging tendencies.

If the first attempt at obtaining the impression is less than completely satisfactory in spite of the additional precautions, it might be well to consider the use of a customized tray constructed on a cast of the impression, if it is accurate enough for this purpose. A custom tray of acrylic resin is usually more acceptable to the hypersensitive patient than is the bulkier stock tray. On the other hand, if the first impression is not accurate enough for construction of a customized tray, an individualized tray may be employed in which the stock tray is modified with modeling composition or with wax.

Psychological Conditioning

The approach to the problem gagger should be sympathetic but positive and firm. An equivocal attitude by the dentist will only complicate the problem. The patient should be told that neither the tray nor the impression material will contact any part of the mouth which is not

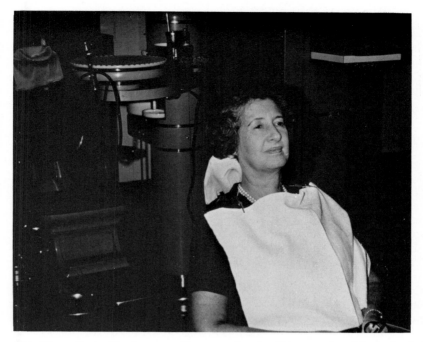

FIG. 4.34. The patient with a hypersensitive gag reflex should be seated upright in the chair.

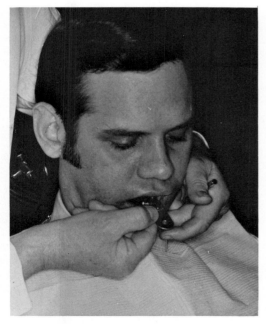

FIG. 4.35. As soon as the maxillary tray has been introduced, pitch the patient's head forward so that the chin touches the chest, and hold it firmly in this position until the impression has gelled.

contacted by food every time that he eats. He may be assured that he is no different from any other person, insofar as the anatomy of his mouth is concerned, and that upwards of 25 million of his fellow Americans have weathered the experience with no ill effects. Further, he may be told that the procedure is identical to the one employed by orthodontists for children of all ages, who rarely have any problem accommodating to the procedure. Children are, in fact, typically quite casual and unconcerned about the matter. This may arouse the patient's ire to some extent, which in turn is almost sure to increase the flow of adrenaline. This seems to enable some individuals to face up to the challenge and to endure the "ordeal" with an equanimity which may even astonish the patient himself.

Anesthetics

The soft palate may be anesthetized with a topical anesthetic to suppress the gag reflex. Cetacaine spray (Cetylite Industries, Long Island City, N.Y.) is a useful one since it can be applied without touching the trigger zones with an applicator. A few drops of local anesthetic may be injected into the posterior palatine foramen, if no suitable topical is on hand. This is unpleasant from the patient's point of view, however, and is rarely necessary.

Premedication

Various drugs may be helpful, such as sedatives (Nembutal, Abbott Laboratories, North Chicago, Ill.), antihistamines (Benadryl, hydrochloride, Parke, Davis & Company, Detroit, Mich.), antiemetics (Thorazine, Smith Kline & French Laboratories, Philadelphia, Pa.), and antinauseants (Tigan, Roche Laboratories, Nutley, N.J.).

The administration of drugs should be planned beforehand, never used on a spur of the moment basis. The use of some drugs, such as tranquilizers, should ideally begin several days prior to the appointment. Of course, the patient who is under the influence of sedatives or antihistamines should be accompanied to the office by a responsible adult.

Distraction

The gag reflex is so highly conditioned by psychological factors that anything which takes the patient's mind away from the area of the mouth and throat, and concentrates it on another object, will tend to diminish the tendency to gag or retch. An ingenious expedient, which is usually as effective as it is simple, is to instruct the patient to lift one foot off the foot rest and to keep it elevated from the time the impression tray is introduced until the material has set and the impression is removed. The concentration by the patient on another part of the body (and away from the mouth) which this stratagem requires, seems to sublimate the gag reflex, temporarily at least, so that the impression can be obtained without untoward incident.

Control of Tongue Position

There seems to be a close relationship, in some individuals, between an extended tongue position and a gagging tendency. The explanation postulated for this phenomenon is that when the tongue is thrust upward and forward, it causes a contraction of the palatoglossus muscle which, in turn, produces tension in the soft palate, and this is thought to trigger the reflex mechanism. To counter this tendency, the patient with a gagging problem should be trained to carry the tongue low and flat behind the lower anterior teeth, and to refrain from lifting and thrusting it forward. As might be expected, this has considerable psychological value as a distracter, whether or not it is anatomically and physiologically tenable.

Postdelivery Medication

The patient who is convinced in his own mind that he is going to have a problem with gagging and nausea as he becomes accustomed to the prosthesis, may be given an antinauseant drug to tide him over the difficult "break in period." Tigan, which is a specific antinauseant, is a very useful drug for this purpose. One 250 mg. capsule, three times daily, may be prescribed for a period of 4 or 5 days. The patient should not operate a motor vehicle during this period.

Care of the Impression

Protection Against Distortion

Following removal from the mouth, the impression must be carefully protected from any form of distortion. The two greatest hazards are from direct contact with a hard object, and shrinkage from dehydration. To avoid the first, the impression should be protected from contact with any object, with the exception of the materials used to rinse it out (see next paragraph) and the stone that will be introduced into it during pouring of the cast. To avoid the second, the impression should be poured within 12 minutes of the time it is removed from the mouth.

Hardening Solution. The impression may be stored for a few moments in a solution of 2% potassium sulfate prior to pouring the cast, to give it a harder, denser surface.

Drying. The impression should be dried out with air, but the surface of the material should not be desiccated. In short, it should retain a thin, surface film of moisture, but should contain no pooled droplets of liquid in the deeper crevices. A properly dried impression will not have a dull appearance but, on the contrary, will glisten.

Methods of Forming the Cast

The gypsum and water should be employed in the proportions recommended by the manufacturer for all cast pouring. Too thin a mix will produce a weak, fragile cast which is vulnerable to breakage in the laboratory. Too thick a mix can cause inaccuracy in the cast by distorting the alginate as the stone is introduced into the impression. Care should be exercised not to over-vibrate the material, as this, too, can cause distortion of the alginate. Any one of the following techniques described may be used to pour an accurate cast. However, the technique of filling the impression with stone and then immediately inverting it onto a mass of soft stone should never be employed, because to do so is to risk distortion from either of two causes: (1) if the stone is quite stiff, the pressure of forcing the impression down onto the patty may distort the alginate, or (2) if the stone is soft, it may slump away from the impression by force of gravity. This method is fraught with too much risk to be recommended for construction of a prosthesis that must fit the mouth with precision.

The Two-Step Inverted Method

The two-step inverted method is the recommended way to pour the cast into the alginate impression. The stone is vibrated into the impression (Fig. 4.36), and *allowed to reach its initial set with the impression face up*. A second mix of stone, approximately 4 x 4 inches square, and 1 inch thick, is made and placed on the bench top (Fig. 4.37). The impression, filled with the hardened stone, is inverted onto the soft stone (Fig. 4.38), and con-

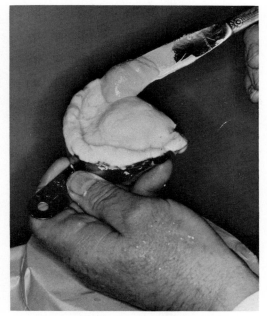

FIG. 4.36. The stone is vibrated into the impression. When the impression is filled, it is set aside, face up, until the stone has reached its initial set.

toured to the desired shape, and the edges of the two mixes of stone are bonded together with a wet plaster spatula. The tongue space of the lower impression should be contoured while the stone is soft. Excessive vibration should be avoided when pouring a cast in any hydrocolloid material, because of its flexibility which makes it susceptible to distortion.

The Boxed Method

It is difficult to box an alginate impression in the conventional manner, because the wax will not stick to the alginate. However, the alginate impression may be boxed with the help of complaster, which is a mixture of 2 parts plaster and 1 part coarse pumice.

The complaster is mixed, a mass approximately 4 x 4 x 1 inches is placed on a clean, smooth surface, and the impression is partly embedded, face up, in it (Fig. 4.39). While the complaster is still soft, it is formed into the shape of a cast and the tongue space is formed with a spatula.

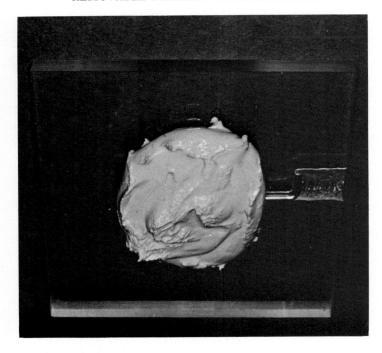

FIG. 4.37. A second mix of stone is made in the form of a patty 4 x 4 inches square and 1 inch thick, and placed on the bench top. The stone has been placed on a split remounting plate in this photograph.

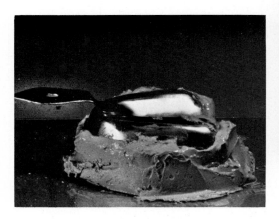

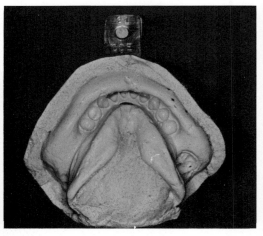

FIG. 4.38. The stone-filled impression is inverted onto the patty and contoured to the desired outline form with the spatula. A moistened spatula is used to bond the two mixes of stone together.

FIG. 4.39. When the impression is to be boxed prior to pouring the cast, it should be embedded, face up, in a mixture of 2 parts plaster and 1 part coarse pumice. While this "complaster" is still soft it is formed into the desired outline form of the cast. Note the treatment of the tongue space in the photograph.

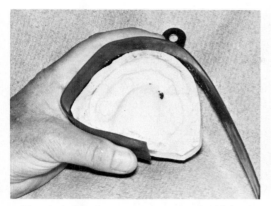

FIG. 4.40. The impression is wrapped with boxing wax, the wax is sealed to the complaster, and the complaster "land" and tongue space are painted with a separating medium.

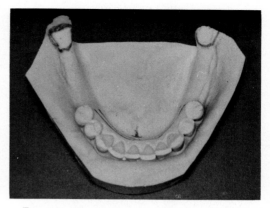

FIG. 4.41. The cast shown here has been over-trimmed on the model trimmer. The retromolar pads have been outlined in pencil to show that the pad on the left side of the cast (reader's right) has been partly trimmed away.

When the complaster has set, it is trimmed to suitable cast outline and wrapped in boxing wax (Fig. 4.40), which is sealed to the gypsum with hot wax. The complaster "land" is painted with a separator and the cast is poured. A split remounting plate may be positioned in the base of the cast, if desired.

The One-Step Upright Method

The upright method is a useful one, but it requires more than average skill to control the thickness of the base as well as the overall size, contour, and appearance of the cast. The cast material (stone or plaster) is carefully vibrated into the impression until it is filled. The impression is then laid on the bench top (face up), and more material is added until the base and art portions of the cast have been built up to the desired form.

The lower impression is prepared by filling the tongue space with either wax or a mixture of plaster and pumice. When the latter is used, a separator must be applied prior to pouring the cast. The mandibular cast is poured in the same way as was the maxillary.

Trimming and Caring for the Cast

Trimming the Cast

The clinical skill and meticulous atten-

tion to detail, which is required to register accurately all of the necessary mouth structures in the impression, can be completely nullified by careless trimming of the cast in the laboratory. The maxillary cast, in addition to representing an accurate replica of the remaining teeth and areas of edentulous ridge, should contain also a full peripheral roll opposite each edentulous area, and should include also both tuberosities as well as the hamular notches. Similarly, the mandibular cast, besides being an accurate replica of the teeth and areas of edentulous ridge, should contain the buccal shelf and, when the posterior teeth are missing, the retromolar pads. The mandibular cast should show, in addition to the buccal and labial peripheral roll, a lingual peripheral roll indicating the junction of the floor of the mouth and the lingual surface of the alveolar ridge. The area of the mylohyoid ridge should also be clearly delineated. The mandibular cast shown in Figure 4.41 has been overtrimmed on the cast trimmer and a part of the retromolar pad on the left side (reader's right) has been lost. The maxillary cast shown in Figure 4.42 has been overtrimmed in the hamular notch area and, in addition, the peripheral roll is not entirely present on the left side of the mouth (reader's right).

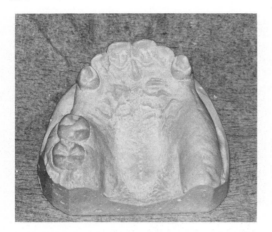

FIG. 4.42. The maxillary cast has been overtrimmed on the cast trimmer. The left (reader's right) hamular notch is completely missing.

Care of the Cast

When a dry cast is immersed in ordinary tap water, the surface of the stone will immediately begin to dissolve, because all gypsum materials are soluble in water. Although so slow as to be imperceptible, this dissolution is as insidious as it is inevitable. It can be demonstrated by immersing part of a cast in water overnight. The immersed part of the stone will show a "water line," indicating an erosion of the surface, the next morning. Running tap water is even more damaging than standing water. It will erode the cast at a rate of 0.1% loss of linear dimension for each 20 minutes of immersion. Therefore, when it is necessary to moisten the cast for any of the various laboratory proce-

TABLE 4.2.
Common Causes of Faulty Casts

Obvious Deficiencies	Possible Causes
Soft chalky surface	1. Impression not separated from cast soon enough 2. Water in deep parts of impression
Rough cast surface	1. Water in impression when casts was poured 2. Grainy mix of impression material
Voids	1. Insufficient vibration 2. Water in impression when cast was poured
Elongated teeth	1. Movement of the impression before gelation was complete
Broken teeth	1. Impression not separated from cast soon enough (within 45 min to 1 hr.) 2. Careless separation

Dimensional Inaccuracies (Cause not Apparent)	Possible Causes
Metal framework fits the master cast but not the mouth	1. Impression moved during gelation 2. Impression material loosened from tray 3. Shrinkage of impression material (not poured within 12 min.) 4. Expansion of impression material from inhibition. Note: Expansion of the material results in smaller teeth since it expands into the tooth space of the impression 5. Film of mucinous saliva or materia alba left on teeth 6. Impression stressed during removal by rocking or twisting 7. Impression distorted by contact with a hard object (sink, plaster bowl, lab bench) 8. Stone so thick that alginate was distorted as cast was formed 9. Impression inverted onto a mass of soft stone during pouring of the cast, causing soft stone to slump away from impression 10. Impression inverted onto a mass of stiff stone. Pressure distorts impression

dures which require it, it should be done with slurry water, which is a saturated solution of calcium sulfate. The stone or plaster will not dissolve in such a solution. Slurry water can be made in the laboratory by placing several discarded stone casts in ordinary tap water and allowing them to dissolve for approximately 48 hours, so as to create the saturated solution of calcium sulfate.

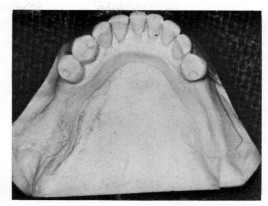

Fig. 4.45. The refractory or investment cast is the one on which the pattern for the framework is formed, and to which the metal is cast to produce the framework. It is made of a refractory material that is capable of withstanding the heat of the burnout oven. Note the relief which has been provided for the retention latticework and for the lingual bar.

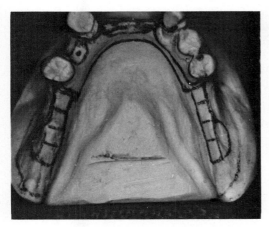

Fig. 4.43. The study or planning cast is used for three major purposes: (1) for cast analysis and treatment planning, (2) as a blueprint for the tooth alteration that has been listed on the treatment plan, and (3) as a supplement for the laboratory authorization to aid in clarifying instructions to the laboratory technician.

The Faulty Cast

Careless technique in either the impression making procedure or in forming the cast may result in a cast that is inferior for one reason or another. For convenience in discussion, the faulty cast may be classified into one of two categories: (1) the cast that has deficiencies that are readily apparent, and (2) the cast that appears to be accurate but obviously is not, as evidenced by the fact that the framework fits the cast but not the mouth. The more common causes for faulty casts are listed in Table 4.2.

Types of Partial Denture Casts

Five different types of casts are used for various purposes in the construction of a removable partial denture.

The Study Cast (Fig. 4.43). The study or planning cast has three major uses: (1) for cast analysis and treatment planning, (2) as a blueprint for tooth alterations, and (3) as a supplement to the prescription or laboratory work authorization form for directing the dental laboratory.

The Master Cast (Fig. 4.44). The master cast is made from an impression of the mouth when all mouth preparation

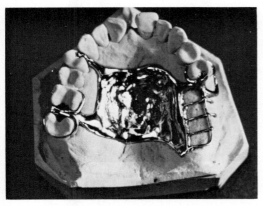

Fig. 4.44. The master cast is made from an impression of the mouth after all mouth preparation has been completed. It represents an accurate replica of the mouth for which the prosthesis is to be made.

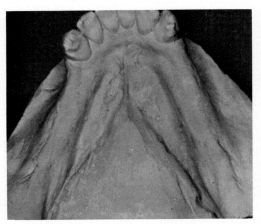

FIG. 4.46. The processing cast is made by duplicating the master cast after the saddle relief wax has been removed from it. The acrylic resin portion of the denture is customarily processed to the framework on this cast, so as to preserve the master cast.

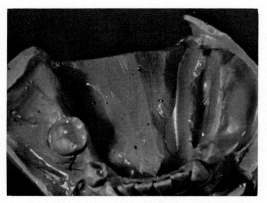

FIG. 4.47. The altered cast is made by attaching the functionally recorded distal extension base(s) to the master cast. In this photograph, the distal extension base area has been registered with fluid wax.

has been completed, and represents an accurate replica of the mouth for which the prosthesis is to be made. It is used to make the refractory cast, and the finished

prosthesis is customarily returned on it from the laboratory.

The Refractory Cast (Fig. 4.45). The refractory cast is made by duplicating the master cast, following the blockout and design procedure. It is made of a refractory gypsum material that is capable of withstanding the heat of the burnout oven, since this is the cast upon which the casting is made.

The Processing Cast (Fig. 4.46). The processing cast is made by duplicating the master cast after the saddle relief wax has been removed. The acrylic resin can be processed onto the framework on this cast if desired, so that the master cast can be preserved.

The Altered Master Cast (Fig. 4.47). The altered cast is made by substituting the distal extension base areas of the master cast, with base areas that have been captured by a functional impression.

Bibliography

Ayers, H. D., Jr., Phillips, R. W., Dell, A., and Henry, R. W.: Detail duplication test used to evaluate elastic impression materials. J. Prosth. Dent. *10:* 374–380, 1960.

Jordan, L. G.: Alginate impression materials. J. Amer. Dent. Ass. *32:* 985–986, 1945.

Phillips, R. W., and Price, R. R.: Some factors which influence the surface of stone dies poured in an alginate impression. J. Prosth. Dent. *5:* 72–79, 1955.

Shippee, R. W.: Accuracy of impressions made with elastic impression materials. J. Prosth. Dent. *10:* 381–386, 1960.

Skinner, E. W., and Carlisle, F. B.: The use of alginate impression materials in Sears hydrocolloid impression technique. J. Prosth. Dent. *6:* 405–411, 1956.

Skinner, E. W., and Hoblit, N. E.: A study of the accuracy of hydrocolloid impressions. J. Prosth. Dent. *6:* 80–86, 1956.

Skinner, E. W., and Pomes, E. C.: Alginate impression materials: technic for manipulation and criteria for selection. J. Amer. Dent. Ass. *35:* 245–256, 1947.

Chapter 5

THE CAST SURVEYOR—
THE SURVEYING PROCEDURE

This chapter deals with the important role that the dental cast surveyor and the surveying process play in the planning, design, and construction of the removable partial denture. Terms used in the surveying process are defined, and the two major steps in the surveying process are discussed: the preliminary analysis of the study cast and the definitive design of the prosthesis. The chapter is organized under these subject headings.

Introduction

An essential key to success in the practice of removable partial denture prosthodontics is thorough, knowledgeable planning of each structural detail of the prosthesis. The surveying procedure is an integral part of the planning process. A typical dental arch, for which a partial denture is to be planned, consists of asymmetrical, disparate clusters of teeth, separated by areas of edentulous, residual alveolar ridge of varied lengths, breadths,

and contours. The long axes of the standing teeth usually lack parallelism with each other, while the surfaces of the crowns of the teeth are irregularly convex in shape. The challenge which confronts the designer is to create a prosthesis that will go smoothly into place on the teeth and over the edentulous ridge, and that when in place, will resist dislodging forces that tend to unseat it. Since the problem involves both biological and engineering components, bioengineering principles may be applied to its solution. The cast surveyor is an instrument by means of which these principles may be applied.

The Development of the Cast Surveyor

Dr. A. J. Fortunati is generally given credit for being the first to employ a mechanical device for determining the relative parallelism of two or more tooth surfaces, having demonstrated the principle with a bridge parallelometer in 1918. The first commercial dental surveyor to be offered to the profession was designed 5 years later by engineers at the J. M. Ney Company of Bloomfield, Conn.

During the succeeding few decades, following the introduction of the Ney instrument, a number of different surveying instruments were marketed by various dental manufacturers. The number subsequently dwindled, however, to a point that there are, at the present time, less than half a dozen being manufactured in the United States. Although the surveyors offered by the various manufacturers differ to some extent in minor detail, all are structured on the same basic principle

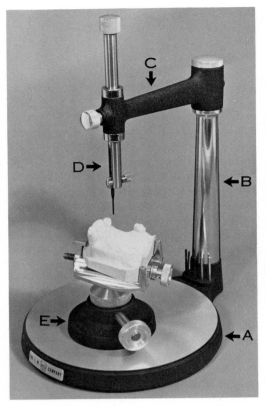

FIG. 5.1. The Ney surveyor shown here illustrates the essential elements of all dental cast surveyors. The working parts consist of a vertical column (*B*), mounted on a horizontal platform (*A*). From the vertical column extends a horizontal arm (*C*) and from this arm extends a tool holder (*D*). The cast holder (*E*) is simply a table and clamp mounted on a ball-and-socket. (Courtesy of The J. M. Ney Company, Bloomfield, Conn.)

of the parallelometer (Fig. 5.1). The essential components of each one consists of a platform which is parallel with the bench top, from which a vertical column extends perpendicularly. Extending at right angles from the vertical column is a horizontal extension, from which extends a movable, vertical part that is capable of a limited degree of movement in the vertical plane. The cast to be surveyed is held in a cast holder, which consists of a table equipped with a clamp that is mounted on a ball-and-socket joint. The ball-and-socket permits the cast to be oriented in various

horizontal planes, so that axial surfaces of the teeth, as well as other areas of the cast, can be analyzed in relation to the vertical plane (Fig. 5.2–5.4).

Although the surveyor was made available to the profession during the third decade of this century, many years passed before the practice of surveying the dental cast, as an integral part of the design procedure, became standard practice. During the era which preceded its routine use, the practice of dividing a supposedly finished partial denture into two or more parts, and then reassembling it with solder so that it would go into place on the teeth, was commonplace. For every partial that had to be cut into segments and reassembled, there were others that were, by one means or another, forced onto the teeth by a resourceful dentist and worn by a determined patient, until it finally had to be abandoned, either because of loosening

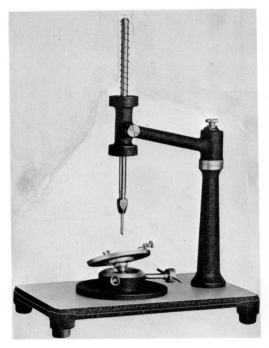

FIG. 5.2. The Jelenko surveyor is shown above. A feature of this instrument is the spring-mounted tool holder. (Courtesy of the J. F. Jelenko & Co., Inc., New Rochelle, N.Y.)

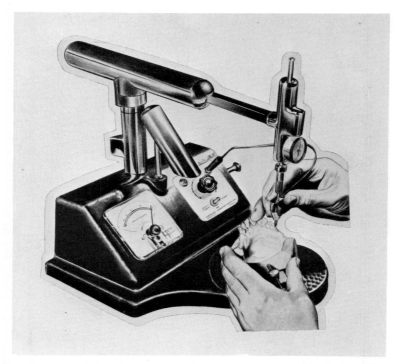

FIG. 5.3. Shown here is the Micro-Analyzer. This is a somewhat more sophisticated instrument than the previous ones, and is capable of measuring the amount of undercut electronically in millimeters. (Courtesy of the Howmet Corporation, Chicago, Ill.)

and premature loss of abutment teeth, or because frequent episodes of breakage ultimately rendered it irreparable. Undoubtedly there were still others which were never successfully worn because the patient simply refused to tolerate the excessive pressure and discomfort, with the consequence that the prosthesis was laid aside and forgotten. Many of these failures were due to the fact that, without the benefits of a surveying instrument, the design of each of the different structural units of the partial denture could not be accurately correlated with one another. The various segments were, in effect, designed and constructed as individual entities. When united as a single unit, the assemblage could not be seated in the mouth, because the individual units could not go into place along their separate pathways. The surveyor makes it possible to design a removable partial denture so that resilient and nonresilient sections go into place in the mouth as a single unit, free from interferences from either tooth or soft tissue convexities, and so that, when in place in the mouth, it resists dislodging forces that would tend to unseat it (Fig. 5.5).

The Objective in Surveying

The objective in the surveying procedure is to reveal to the designer those physical characteristics of the mouth which favor the design of a successful prosthesis, as well as those which will be deterrents to the most favorable result. Knowledgeable survey of the study cast will identify the structures that will need to be modified in order to make possible a design of the prosthesis that (1) can be easily inserted and removed by the patient, (2) will contribute optimally to ap-

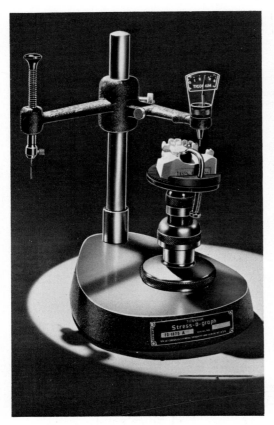

FIG. 5.4. The Stress-o-graph is pictured here. Note the two vertical tool holders. This is a more elaborate instrument than either the Ney or the Jelenko instruments. (Courtesy of the Ticonium Company, A Division of CMP Industries, Inc., Albany, N.Y.)

Design Responsibility

It is worthy of note that all of these factors are directly under the control of the dentist, and that generally he has one or more alternatives in coping with a given factor. The hallmark of the skilled designer is his ability to create a successful prosthesis, by prescribing the most effectual combination of clinical mouth preparation and structural detail of the prosthesis. A carefully planned removable partial denture should require of the labora-

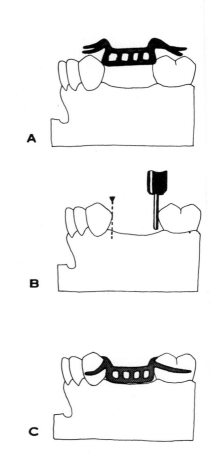

FIG. 5.5. In this illustration, the prosthesis at A cannot be seated because of interferences created by the convex surfaces of the teeth which adjoin the edentulous space. At B the axial surfaces of the teeth are analyzed by the surveyor. At C necessary alterations have been made on the teeth and the design of the prosthesis has been modified so that the prosthesis now goes smoothly into place without interference.

pearance, (3) will resist unseating forces to a reasonable degree, and (4) will create no undesirable food traps when in place in the mouth. The degree of success achieved will depend, in large measure, upon the designer's judicious management and correlation of four factors: (1) retentive undercuts, (2) interferences, (3) esthetic considerations, and (4) guiding plane surfaces. When these four factors have been assessed, the path of insertion can be decided and the design of the prosthesis established. This procedural sequence is depicted diagrammatically in the chart, Figure 5.6.

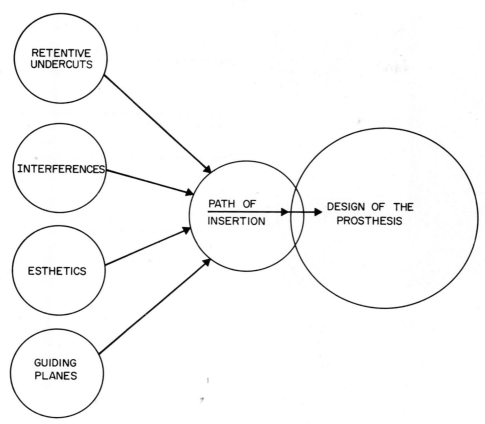

FIG. 5.6. The surveying procedure focuses attention on the four factors which are the keystones of partial denture design: retentive undercuts, interferences, esthetic problems and opportunities, and guiding plane surfaces. When these factors have been evaluated and correlated, a path of insertion can be selected and the design of the prosthesis can be devised.

tory technician only that he faithfully follow the directions given him by the dentist, and use only dental materials of the highest quality in his fabrication of the prosthesis.

The Two Stages of the Surveying Procedure

The surveying procedure takes place in two distinct stages. First, the preliminary analysis of the diagnostic cast, to determine the most advantageous path of insertion and to decide upon the various types of mouth preparation that will be required, and second, the definitive design in which the guidelines are drawn, undercuts are measured and marked, soft tissue undercuts are delineated, and the design of the framework is outlined on the planning cast.

The Preliminary Analysis

Evaluating the Claspability of Potential Abutments

The surveyor may be used to determine which of the remaining teeth are most suitable for clasping (Fig. 5.7), and to identify the precise area of each tooth that will provide the required amount of retentive undercut. Often no undercut can be found on a tooth that would otherwise be ideally located to act as an abutment. Solutions to this problem might be re-

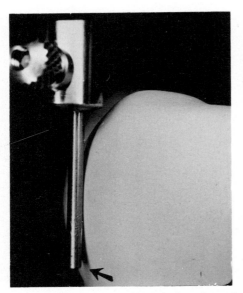

FIG. 5.7. The surveyor can be used to determine which of the remaining teeth are most suitable for clasping and which surfaces of the teeth that are selected, present the most ideal retentive undercuts. The analyzing rod shown here discloses a usable undercut on the buccal surface of a molar (*arrow*).

be dealt with by (1) elimination (extraction-ablation), (2) alteration (disking, surgery, restoration), (3) avoidance (modification of design), or (4) exploitation (using an undercut to help retain the prosthesis). For convenience of discussion, these areas of interference may be divided into soft tissue obstacles (the mucosa and bone), and hard tissue obstacles (the teeth).

Soft Tissue Obstacles. Soft tissue redundancies and bony exostoses, which have the potential of interfering with insertion and removal of the prosthesis, may occur randomly in either jaw. However, certain areas of the mouth are especially prone to present troublesome interferences. One of these is the area of the mylohyoid ridge (Fig. 5.8), which tends to become excessively angular and prominent following removal of mandibular molars, and which is subject to the atrophic change that typically follows in the wake of extractions. The tuberosity is another (Fig. 5.9). It may become excessively prominent, as a result of the buccal plate of bone being sprung laterally during extraction of the maxillary molars,

storing the tooth with a properly contoured gold crown, placing a retentive filling, or altering the tooth surface so as to create an undercut for the clasp tip (see The Retentive Restoration, Chapter 3, and Dimpling, Chapter 6). When the undercut area on the tooth has been selected, the surveyor can be employed to measure the exact amount of undercut to be engaged by the clasp tip. If the surveying procedure is accurately carried out, the partial denture will go into place with moderate pressure, and when in place will resist reasonable dislodging forces.

Identifying Interferences and Undesirable Undercuts

Certain areas of the mouth may present interferences to easy insertion and removal of the prosthesis. These can be identified and evaluated with the surveyor, so that solutions to the problems which they create can be integrated into the treatment plan during the planning stage. Once identified, an interference can

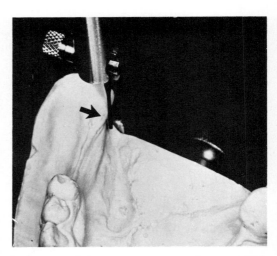

FIG. 5.8. Certain areas of the mouth are prone to harbor soft tissue undercuts, which are potential obstacles to smooth insertion and removal of the partial denture. The mylohyoid ridge area shown here is such an area. Focusing attention on these potential problem areas is an important objective in the surveying procedure.

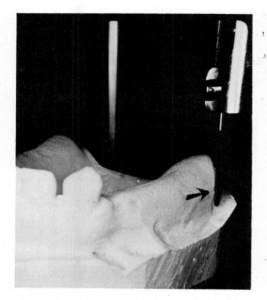

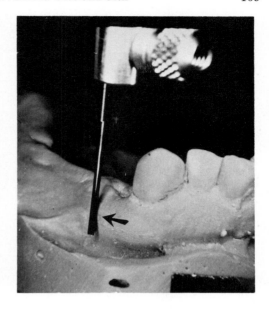

FIG. 5.9. Another area of the mouth which may present interference to unimpeded insertion and removal of a prosthesis is the tuberosity region. The tuberosity may be undercut so that the denture flange cannot be comfortably seated in the buccal vestibule along the chosen path of insertion.

FIG. 5.10. The mandible is typically thinner in the vestibule than it is at the crest of the ridge in the mandibular bicuspid area. This often creates a problem in fitting a denture flange so that it fits snugly but does not abrade the mucosa.

or it may be naturally bulbous. A third area often involved is the mental region of the mandible (Fig. 5.10). The typical mandible is not as wide in the bicuspid region as it is in the molar area, and it is usually thinner in the apical region than it is at the crest of the residual ridge. A problem may thus arise in attempting to fit the buccal flange of the denture, so that it will pass over the area of the greater width at the crest of the ridge and down into the area of lesser width in the vestibule (Fig. 5.11). Finally, the alveolar ridge with a severe labial undercut may present a problem when the denture must include a labial flange. The surveyor can be used to determine the best means of correlating the path of insertion of the prosthesis with the slope of the undercut.

Hard Tissue Obstacles. Migrated, tipped, and rotated teeth may be found anywhere, in either jaw, and may interfere with the most ideal design of the prosthesis. Examples are lingually inclined mandibular teeth (Fig. 5.12), which oft-times also tip mesially, as well as "splayed," maxillary molars and bicuspids which tip buccally (Fig. 5.13). In addition, there are areas on the surfaces of certain teeth which, either because of their natural contour or as a result of atypical alignment in the arch, present obstacles to ideal clasp design. A frequently encountered problem is the crown of a tooth which presents an abnormally high height of contour on one surface, thus requiring that the body and shoulders of the clasp be placed higher (occlusally) than is desirable from a standpoint of either esthetics or mechanics. Tooth surfaces which are common offenders in this regard are the distobuccal line angles of the maxillary bicuspids, the mesiobuccal line angles of the maxillary molars, mesiolingual line angles and, less commonly, the mesiobuccal line angles of the mandibular molars.

Esthetic Considerations

The configuration of anterior edentulous spaces can be studied, with the help of the

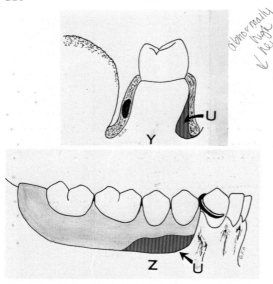

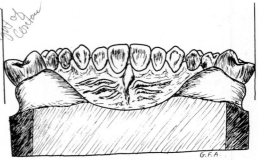

abnormally high ↓ region of contour

FIG. 5.13. "Splayed" maxillary teeth may present a difficult problem in partial denture design. The potential problem should be recognized during the surveying procedure, and steps for its correction incorporated into the treatment plan.

FIG. 5.11. A problem is often encountered in fitting a denture flange so that it will pass over an area of greater buccolingual width into an area of lesser width as it follows the path of insertion of the denture. In the illustration a cross section of the mandible, *Y*, is shown with an undercut, *Z*. In sketch *Z*, a buccal view shows schematically the relationship of the denture flange to the undercut, *U*. The surveyor enables the designer to identify such an undercut in the early planning stages, so that it is not discovered unexpectedly at the time of insertion of the prosthesis.

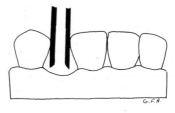

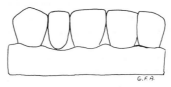

FIG. 5.14. The surveyor can be used to study the configuration of anterior edentulous spaces, in order to evaluate the cosmetic opportunity and/or problems that are posed.

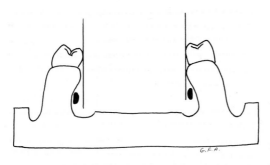

FIG. 5.12. When mandibular teeth have a pronounced lingual inclination, they may interfere with proper placement of a lingual bar. This fact will be divulged by knowledgeable analysis of the cast during the surveying procedure.

surveyor, to assess the cosmetic potential, i.e., the problems and the opportunities which the space presents. The axial walls of these spaces frequently lack parallelism because the teeth which adjoin the space are bell shaped (Fig. 5.14), and perhaps, in addition, are tipped or rotated. The surveyor is indispensable in determining the amount of recontouring that will be necessary to improve the alignment of these surfaces.

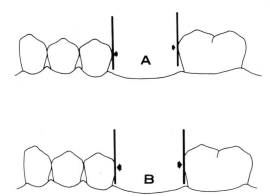

F<small>IG</small>. 5.15. The surveyor will delineate existing or potential guiding plane surfaces that will assist in providing unimpeded passage of the prosthesis along the chosen path of insertion.

Identifying Potential Guiding Plane Surfaces

Guiding planes are the axial surfaces of teeth which are contacted by the rigid elements of the prosthesis as it is seated and removed from the mouth. The surveyor can be used to locate existing or potential guiding plane surfaces so that they will assist (or can be altered to assist) in providing unimpeded passage of the appliance along the established path of insertion (Fig. 5.15).

The Path of Insertion

The path of insertion may be defined as "the direction in which the restoration is inserted upon, and removed from, the abutment teeth." The terms "path of insertion" and "tilt of the cast," although not synonymous, are nevertheless inseparably linked. The tilt of the cast refers to the position of the cast on the surveyor table relative to the horizontal plane, at the time that the prosthesis is designed. Thus it follows that the path of insertion of the prosthesis is always parallel to the surveyor spindle. Although it is customary to refer to "the" path of insertion as though it were always a single entity, the reality is that only under certain rather rigidly prescribed conditions is there a single path of insertion. With many designs of partial dentures there are two or

more paths. The dominant influencing factor, affecting the number of paths of insertion that a prosthesis has, is whether the edentulous space is tooth-bounded or a distal extension type. If the space is tooth-bounded, the prosthesis will typically have a single path of insertion. If a prosthesis has a tooth-bounded edentulous space on one side of the arch and a distal extension base on the contralateral side, the path of insertion will be governed by the tooth-bounded side because the major connector is rigid. The partial denture with two distal extension bases will have two and sometimes more paths of insertion—one perpendicular to the plane of occlusion, the other an arcuate path which it follows as the clasps rotate on the abutment teeth (Fig. 5.16). The partial denture with an anterior edentulous space usually has a single path of insertion, which is parallel to the guiding planes adjoining the anterior space.

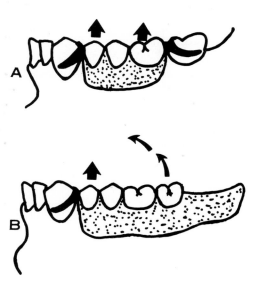

F<small>IG</small>. 5.16. The prosthesis may have a single path of insertion or it may have two and sometimes more. In *A* the edentulous space is tooth-bounded and the prosthesis has a single path of insertion as indicated by the arrows. In *B* the distal extension base partial denture may be inserted or removed along a path of insertion which is perpendicular to the plane of occlusion or by an entirely different, arcuate path which is indicated by the curved arrows.

The structural unit of the prosthesis which governs the direction of insertion and removal more than any other is the clasp, since it is generally the only segment of the prosthesis that contacts the guiding plane surfaces of the teeth unless anterior teeth are being replaced. The part of the clasp which exerts a dominant influence is the truss arm which fits snugly against the guiding plane surface. The influence which the truss arms exert is directly proportional to the amount of areal coverage of the guiding planes and to the amount of contact between tooth and clasp. The body and shoulders of the clasp exert some influence on the path of insertion, although it is limited because they are positioned above the guideline and usually lie on sloping tooth surfaces. The retentive clasp arm normally exerts only a minor influence because the terminal is flexible whereas the remainder of the clasp lies above the guideline. The reciprocal arm of the clasp can exert considerable influence, particularly on a cast crown that has been properly contoured.

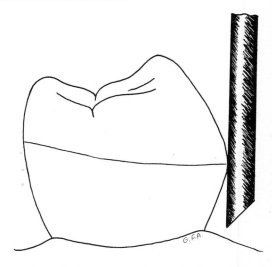

FIG. 5.17. The survey line is the line which is marked on the tooth with the surveyor to indicate its greatest circumference in that particular horizontal plane. It should always be marked on the tooth with the side of the marker as shown here, never with the point of the marker.

The Height of Contour, The Survey Line

The "height of contour" is the greatest circumference of a tooth in a given horizontal plane. The "survey line" is the line which is marked on the abutment tooth by the surveyor spindle, to indicate its greatest circumference in a given horizontal plane (Fig. 5.17). The survey line divides the crown of the tooth into two zones: an undercut area (everything below the line), and a non-undercut area (everything above the line). Sometimes the area above the line is known as the suprabulge area and the area below the line as infrabulge area. The terms "guideline" and "breadth of contour line" are synonyms for "survey line." *The significance of the survey line is that any rigid, nonflexible part of the prosthesis must be designed to lie above the survey line, and only flexible parts may be designed to go below it* (Fig. 5.18). The only part of a removable partial denture that is flexible is the terminal of the retentive clasp arm.

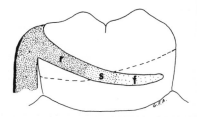

FIG. 5.18. The significance of the survey line to the designer is that all rigid parts of the prosthesis must be designed to lie above the line and only flexible parts (the retentive clasp tip) may lie below it. In the sketch, the portion of the clasp, *r*, is rigid, the portion *s*, has a limited flexibility, and the terminal, *f*, is flexible.

When marking the survey line, care must be taken not to mark the line with the end of the graphite rod, because such a line will be inaccurate. The contact should always be made between the side of the marker and the greatest convexity of the tooth as the survey line is marked on the crown.

The Retentive Undercut

The retentive undercut on an abutment tooth that is to be occupied by the retentive terminal of a clasp may be visualized as having three dimensions: (1) a mesiodistal dimension, (2) an occlusal-gingival dimension, and (3) a dimension that is essentially in a buccolingual plane. Of the three, the buccolingual dimension is by far the most significant because when the clasp terminal enters or leaves the infrabulge area of the tooth it must flex an amount equal to the depth of this undercut. Thus the necessity for accuracy in measuring the depth of the undercut is apparent. The undercut gauge should be placed against the tooth so that the tip of the gauge is in contact with the precise spot on the tooth surface that is to be occupied by the lower border of the clasp terminal, while at the same time, the shank of the gauge contacts the greatest convexity (the height of contour) of the tooth (Fig. 5.19). A mark should be made on the tooth at the exact point where the undercut gauge contacts the tooth surface (Fig. 5.20). The clasp is then outlined on the tooth with the lower border of the terminal precisely on the mark (Fig. 5.21).

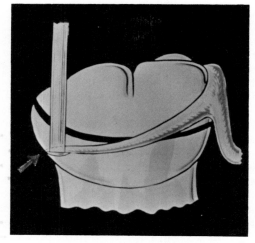

FIG. 5.20. To ensure that the retentive terminal of the clasp engages the exact amount of undercut that has been measured by the gauge, a mark is made with a pencil at the precise spot on the tooth that is contacted by the undercut gauge (*arrow*).

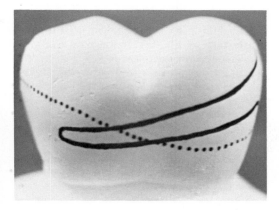

FIG. 5.21. The clasp is outlined so that the lower border of the terminal is precisely on the mark indicated by the gauge.

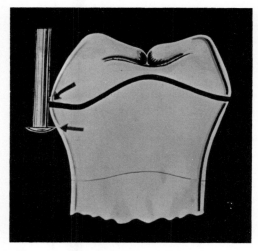

FIG. 5.19. The accurate measurement of the undercut on an abutment tooth is an exacting procedure. The shank of the undercut gauge should contact the height of contour of the tooth at the same time that the undercut gauge contacts the surface of the tooth in the undercut.

The Amount of Undercut to be Exploited

As a general rule of thumb, the retentive tip of a chromium-cobalt alloy clasp should engage no more than 0.010 inch of undercut for a bicuspid. As much as 0.015 inch might be engaged by a molar clasp terminal, while 0.020 inch would be approximately the proper amount for a clasp arm made of 18 gauge gold wrought wire.

Cast Tilting

If each abutment tooth on the cast is marked with a line with the graphite scriber around its greatest diameter, and the table is then tilted so that the cast is in a different horizontal plane after which each tooth is again marked, it is apparent that the position of the survey line on the crown can be thus modified. Altering the position of the cast in space by manipulating the cast table, or "tilting" as it is termed, changes the long axis of each tooth relative to the horizontal plane. The import of this to the designer is the fact that it changes the position of the survey line in relation to the horizontal plane and this, of course, changes the location of the undercut and non-undercut areas on each tooth. This might appear to provide an opportunity to create undercuts on areas of the tooth where no undercut existed prior to tilting the cast. Unfortunately, this is not precisely the case, however.

The Delusion of Creating a Retentive Undercut by Cast Tilting. It is delusive to consider an undercut created by tilting the cast on the surveyor as genuinely retentive because, unless an undercut is retentive relative to all paths of removal of the prosthesis, it will not provide the resistance to the clasp tip which enables it to resist the pull of a dislodging force. The reason for this is that dislodging forces which are generated against the prosthesis are operant primarily in a direction perpendicular, or at right angles, to the occlusal plane. In the maxilla, the occlusal plane is approximately parallel to the floor, and this relationship is comparatively constant as long as the patient is in an upright position. Thus, the forces of dislodgment exerted against the maxillary prosthesis are in an essentially vertical direction. In the functioning mandible the plane is not static, as it is in the maxilla, but moves on an arcuate path which is in an essentially vertical (upward and downward) plane. The point in space at which the greatest dislodging force is applied to the mandibular prosthesis (by a caramel candy, for example) is when the mandible is making its opening movement and is

traveling downward away from the maxilla. This is illustrated in the series of sketches in Figures 5.22A–D. If the path of escapement of the partial denture differs in significant degree from a direction that is at right angles to the occlusal plane, there will be some resistance to dislodgment of the prosthesis, by virtue of this fact, and it may be magnified by frictional contact of the prosthesis with well-formed guiding planes. However, this retention is operant in only a limited sense. *To be truly effective, the resistance of a clasp to dislodgment must be effective at right angles to the occlusal plane, regardless of the path of insertion.* Therefore, it follows that while the advantages of cast tilting do exist, they are extremely limited in terms of affecting the amount of retention. Simply stated, if there is no retentive undercut on a tooth with the cast in a horizontal plane, then tilting the cast to another horizontal plane will not create one that will be effective in retaining the prosthesis against dislodgment. In order to be genuinely retentive, an undercut must be operative in any possible path of escapement.

The Value of Cast Tilting. Is tilting of the cast, then, a totally illusory exercise? The answer is that under certain circumstances tilting can be employed to advantage. There are instances when it may be used to correlate the path of insertion with the axial walls of an anterior space, in order to make possible a more esthetic positioning of a replacement tooth or teeth. It can sometimes be used to advantage when a labial flange must be employed and the labial alveolar plate is severely undercut. The tilting technique may provide the resourceful designer with the means of discovering a compromise path of insertion that will allow the prosthesis to go smoothly into place, after which it is snugly resistant to dislodgment. Experimental tilting will disclose the varying effects of different paths of insertion and may point the way to the best possible compromise path from all standpoints. However, it should be borne in mind that undercut areas on a tooth, to be retentive, must resist escapement of

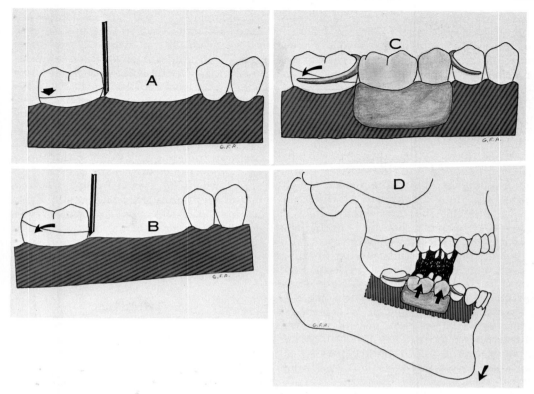

FIG. 5.22. These four sketches illustrate the fallacy of attempting to create retentive undercuts by tilting the cast on the surveyor. In *A* there is no usable retentive undercut on the buccal surface of the molar abutment with the cast in an essentially horizontal plane. At *B* the cast has been tilted posteriorly, which alters the survey line and creates a more substantial infrabulge area on the abutment tooth. If a clasp tip is designed to engage this undercut, as shown at *C*, and the denture is placed in the mouth, it becomes apparent at *D* that during mastication the retention created by cast tilting was in reality "false retention." A caramel candy, for example, exerts a dislodging force on the prosthesis that is in a direction essentially perpendicular to the occlusal plane, and since the false retention is not operant in this plane, the prosthesis is dislodged.

the clasp terminal in a direction at right angles to the plane of occlusion.

A Practical Approach to Establishing the Path of Insertion

Since the major dislodging forces acting upon the prosthesis are operant primarily in a direction at right angles to the occlusal plane, it would seem to be altogether logical to survey the cast in a horizontal plane. Unless usable undercuts can be demonstrated on the tooth surfaces with the cast in this plane, the clasps cannot be expected to be retentive. There are additional advantages to following this practice. (1) A prosthesis surveyed in this plane will be the least complicated for the patient to insert and remove (hence the least vulnerable to distortion or breakage). (2) Contouring the wax pattern for a surveyed crown is simplified, since the cast on which the crown is being waxed can be readily oriented on the surveyor at the same tilt as the one at which the master cast was surveyed. (3) It is somewhat easier to work in concert with a commercial dental laboratory when a standardized path of insertion has been mutually agreed upon.

Certainly, survey of the cast on a horizontal plane is not indicated in every instance. The mouth with an extreme labial undercut, which has already been mentioned, is a case where a compromise tilt of the cast may be advantageous. Generally, it is recommended for the routine partial denture, however, for the reasons enumerated.

The Definitive Design of the Prosthesis

When all of the mouth preparation has been completed and the master cast is available, the definitive design of the prosthesis may be drawn on the study cast. Drawing the framework design on the study cast and sending it to the laboratory, along with the master cast to supplement the written instructions, is to be recommended for several reasons. Foremost is the fact that it dispels any doubt as to the precise structuring that the dentist wishes the technician to incorporate into the metal skeleton. Second, it constitutes an accurate three-dimensional record of the desired framework, which can be used to compare with the metal framework when it has been fabricated. Finally, it helps the designer better to visualize the structure that he has conceived in his mind's eye and to focus his attention on each structural detail, thus minimizing the possibility that some facet of the design might be overlooked. The study cast should be reasonably current, although it is not essential that it be precisely accurate. If substantial changes have been effected in the mouth subsequent to making the initial study cast, a second cast should be made, either by making a "double pour" in the impression from which the master cast was obtained, or by duplicating it in agar type hydrocolloid. The design may then be drawn on this current study cast. Although this second cast cannot be relied on for complete fidelity in every dimension, it will be entirely adequate for the purpose of diagramming the outline of the partial denture framework which the dental laboratory technician is being authorized to fabricate.

The outline should be drawn on the study cast, rather than on the master cast, for two reasons: (1) drawing and erasing on the relatively soft surface of the cast renders it inaccurate in the precise areas where it should be completely accurate, and (2) it tends to complicate, unnecessarily, the technician's work in deciphering the various lines on the tooth and in integrating the marked master cast into the production routine of the laboratory. It is easier and more convenient for him to "read" the specifications on the study cast and then to apply them to the master cast, in accordance with the standard operating techniques used by his particular laboratory. The first laboratory step in the fabrication of the metal framework is the wax blockout prior to duplication, and an unmarked master cast is much preferred for this purpose.

Tripoding

In the survey, design, and fabrication of the removable partial denture, it frequently becomes necessary to remove a cast temporarily from the cast holder of the surveyor and subsequently to replace it in its original position. As an example, the laboratory technician routinely places the dentist's designed study cast on his (the technician's) own surveyor, in order to verify the path of insertion as well as the other details of the design. Tripoding enables him to do this. For another example, it is often desirable to verify or to remeasure an undercut on the master cast after wax-up of the framework has been started. This requires that the cast be returned to the same horizontal plane in which it was surveyed. The crux of the problem is to be able to remove a cast from the surveyor and then to relocate it in the same position in space, relative to the horizontal plane, at any time that it is necessary to do so. If all casts were identical in dimension, the problem could be solved by calibrating all movable parts of the surveyor. Then when a cast was surveyed the calibrations could be noted, and it could be returned to this position by adjusting the calibration at any time it was desired to do so. However, the base or capital portions of different casts vary in size and in contour, which would make the use of calibrations unreliable. Tripoding is a method of indexing the cast while it is on the surveyor, so that it can be removed and returned to its original position whenever it is desired to do so. There are two basic methods of accomplishing the tripoding procedure.

Tissue Surface Indexing

One method of tripoding is done by making three marks on the tissue surface of the cast, at three widely separated locations, with the lead marker in the surveyor spindle. The cast can then be removed from the cast holder and subsequently returned to its original position in space by tilting the table until the surveyor spindle again touches all three spots. If the vertical arm is locked in place after the tripod marks are made, the original position of the cast can be determined with relative ease, since it requires adjustment of only one variable, i.e., the cast in the horizontal plane. However, if it is necessary to change the position of the vertical marker after the tripod index marks have been made, the procedure is more complicated. The relative positions of two variables must be manipulated— the cast in the horizontal plane and the vertical marker.

Art Portion Indexing

A second method of tripoding is to scribe a line alongside the analyzing rod as it is held against the capital or art portion of the cast—one on the posterior or dorsal aspect, and one on each lateral surface. In employing this method, it is important that the spindle contacts the sides of the cast evenly throughout its length. If it cannot be made to do so because the cast is rough or uneven, the surface of the gypsum should be planed and smoothed until the spindle contacts it evenly. By means of these vertically scribed lines, the cast can be returned to its original position by tilting the table until the three lines on the cast are again parallel to the surveyor spindle. It is worth noting that

this latter method has the advantage that the scribed marks are transferred to the refractory cast during duplication, so that it (the refractory cast) can be placed on the surveyor at the original tilt if it should become desirable to do so at any time during the laboratory phase of fabrication.

A Summary of Uses of the Surveyor

The many uses of the dental surveyor in removable partial denture construction may be summarized by the following:

1. To analyze the planning cast during the preliminary phase of the planning. The analysis will consist of:
   a. Studying the contours of the axial surfaces of potential abutment teeth to assess their claspability.
   b. Locating tooth and soft tissue surfaces which may offer interference to easy insertion and removal of the contemplated prosthesis.
   c. Evaluating the cosmetic possibilities and problems associated with the placement of clasps, and teeth which will be visible in the mouth.
   d. Locating and analyzing existing and potential guiding plane surfaces.

When the above factors have been evaluated, a path of insertion can be selected which will represent the best possible compromise of all factors.

2. When the path of insertion has been determined, the surveyor can be used to:
   a. Mark the height of contour lines on the planning cast.
   b. Measure the exact amount of undercut to be engaged by the retentive clasp tips on each abutment.
   c. Mark the cast so that it can be removed from the surveyor and later returned to its original position relative to the horizontal plane (tripoded).
   d. Assist in contouring wax patterns for the abutment teeth so that retentive areas and guiding

planes can be properly related to the other teeth in the arch.

e. Assist in determining the most desirable contour of restorations that are needed in teeth located along the path of insertion.

Auxillary Uses of the Surveyor

Besides the functions enumerated above, the surveyor has additional uses.

3. The surveyor can be employed to
   a. Carve undercut wax during blockout of the master cast.
   b. Hold the dental handpiece in order to parallel frictional attachments in abutment teeth (requires a special handpiece holder).
   c. Aid in positioning precision and semiprecision attachments in abutment teeth.
   d. Analyze the abutment teeth prior to constructing a fixed prosthesis.

e. Determine parallelism in aligning teeth which are to be splinted together.

f. Determine the need for alveoloplasty for an edentulous area of the mouth.

Bibliography

Applegate, O. C.: *Essentials of Removable Partial Denture Prosthesis*, Ed. 3. W. B. Saunders Company, Philadelphia, 1965.

Craddock, F. W.: Clasp surveying and mysticism. Aust. J. Dent. *59:* 205–208, 1955.

Craddock, F. W., and Bottomley, G. A.: Second thoughts on clasp surveying. Brit. Dent. J. *96:* 134–136, 1954.

Dental Laboratory Technicians' Manual, AFM 160-29, Department of the Air Force. U. S. Government Printing Office, Washington, D.C., 1959.

McCall, J. O., and Hugel, I. M.: *Movable-Removable Bridgework*. The Dental Items of Interest Publishing Co., Brooklyn, 1950.

McCracken, W. L.: *Partial Denture Construction*. Ed. 3. The C. V. Mosby Company, St. Louis, 1964.

Chapter 6

TOOTH ALTERATION PROCEDURES

This chapter is concerned with the alterations, over and above those that are customarily accomplished with conventional types of restorations, which may be performed on the teeth for the purpose of improving the design, the function, and the prognosis of the removable partial prosthesis. It is organized under the subject headings which follow.

Introduction

The judicious employment of certain tooth altering procedures can bring about such a worthwhile improvement in the design and function of a removable partial denture that an understanding of these techniques should be a part of every prosthodontist's planning capability. One versed in the alterations that can be performed to improve the design of a prosthesis can exploit opportunities that may spell the difference between a highly successful prosthesis and one that is mediocre.

Tooth Alteration

The Responsibility for Tooth Alteration

Sometimes overlooked is the fact that the dental laboratory technician has an extremely limited control of the factors which play a pivotal role in the choice of structural details for the prosthesis. The technician can tilt the cast on the surveyor to effect a change in the path of insertion of the partial denture but, aside from this, his prerogatives are severely limited. In the last analysis he has no choice but to work with the cast which the dentist provides him. The dentist, on the other hand, enjoys a wide variety of options which he is free to exercise, in order to eliminate unfavorable factors and create favorable ones, being limited only by his breadth of knowledge, experience, and clinical skill. He can literally transform the entire structure of the mouth before making a cast and sending it to the technician for fabrication of a prosthesis. Well known is the fact that with surgical techniques he can ablate unfavorable bone or soft tissue undercuts, and that with restorative techniques he can completely transform the contour of the abutment teeth. Entirely apart from these clinical procedures, there are additional relatively simple techniques that can be employed which will improve the design of the prosthesis to a degree out of all proportion to the modest amount of time and energy required for their accomplishment.

Tooth Alteration as a Part of the Treatment Plane

Tooth alteration procedures should be accorded the same priority and receive the same meticulous attention to detail that any clinical procedure deserves. Whenever possible, they should be integrated into the treatment plan, so as to be accomplished at the same time that other clinical procedures are carried out in the same quadrant of the mouth. Thoughtful planning will serve to minimize the number of injections of local anesthetic required to accomplish the

119

treatment and may, in some instances, even reduce the number of appointments that must be scheduled. Moreover, it may contribute indirectly toward better mouth preparation, since an efficiently planned therapeutic sequence causes a minimum of discomfort, thus engendering optimal patient cooperation.

The Objectives of Tooth Alteration

One important objective in tooth alteration is to prepare the teeth that are to be clasped, so that the occlusal (lingual-incisal) rest directs stress along the long axis of the tooth. Another is to prepare the mouth so that the prosthesis can be inserted and removed by the patient without having it transmit wedging or torsional types of stress against the teeth with which it comes in contact. Still another is the recontouring of teeth when an altered contour will eliminate an interference or otherwise contribute to a better design. Finally, retention can be created, by a simple alteration procedure, in a tooth surface where none formerly existed. Techniques for accomplishing these objectives are discussed in the following paragraphs.

The Occlusal Rest

If it were possible for all partial dentures to be supported by natural teeth, there is little question but that the average removable partial denture would enjoy a much greater life expectancy than is presently the case, or that the clinical record of this type of prosthesis would be immeasurably improved. Indeed, it is difficult to overemphasize the important contribution that the natural teeth make to the support, retention, and stability of this type of oral prosthesis. Since the clasp is the connecting link which transmits the stresses borne by the prosthesis to the supporting teeth, it follows that proper design of the rest, as well as the configuration of its recess in the tooth, is of cardinal importance.

The Function of the Occlusal Rest

The occlusal rest has certain well defined functions that it must perform if it

is to contribute optimally to the biomechanics of the prosthesis. These are to:

1. Transmit stress along the long axis of the tooth.
2. Secure the clasp in its proper position on the tooth, so as to maintain a desired tooth-clasp and tooth-base relationship.
3. Prevent a spreading of the clasp arms, with subsequent displacement of the clasp and the prosthesis.
4. Assist in distributing the occlusal load among two or more teeth, so that each can bear a proportionate share of the masticatory load in concert with the residual ridges.
5. Prevent extrusion of the abutment tooth.
6. Prevent the ingress of food between the abutment tooth and the clasp, by deflecting it away from the immediate area.
7. Provide resistance to lateral displacement of the prosthesis.
8. Contribute indirect retention (in some instances).

Engineering the Rest Preparation

In order for tooth support to be optimally effective, it must be provided by sturdy rests, placed in properly engineered recesses, in the surfaces of the teeth. The planning and preparation of the recess should be carried out in consonance with well-established bioengineering principles. A fundamental fact is that the periodontal ligament is not designed by nature to provide a cushioning effect for the tooth but, on the contrary, is a suspensory ligament by means of which the tooth is suspended in its alveolus (Fig. 6.1). Thus, it may be seen that a horizontal stress applied against the tooth will be resisted by fewer than half of the periodontal membrane fibers, whereas a vertical stress will be resisted by all of the fibers with the exception of those at the apex. The forces which act on the tooth in a direction along its long axis are transferred by the periodontal ligament to the bone as tension, which is tolerated quite well. In contrast to this, the transverse or torsional stresses that are transmitted to the tooth are transferred to the periodontal ligament and to the bone as pressure, which is not well tolerated. Depending on the magnitude and the duration of the stress, the result may be

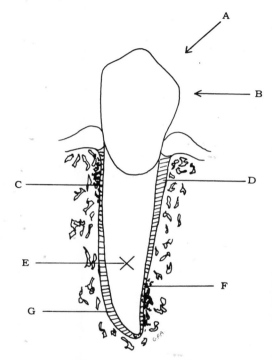

FIG. 6.1. When stress is directed against a tooth in a direction parallel to the long axis, it is resisted by all of the fibers of the periodontal ligament except those at the apex. However, when an oblique or horizontal force A or B is directed against the tooth, the resultant force is horizontal and the crown tends to move away from such a force in an essentially horizontal direction. Actually, the tooth rotates about an axis which is located, in a single-rooted tooth, at approximately the junction of the middle and apical thirds of the roots, E. As a horizontal force A or B is applied, the fibers of the periodontal ligament on the side of the tooth opposite to the force and above the rotation point offer no resistance to the force and are either compressed or crushed C, depending on the magnitude of the force and its duration. This is true also of the fibers below the rotation point on the opposite side of the tooth at F. Just the opposite is true of the fibers on the same side of the tooth as the applied force. Those above the rotation point at D, are stretched, as are those on the opposite side of the tooth below the rotation point, G.

crushing of the periodontal ligament, or even necrosis and bone resorption. Applying this principle to the foundation for the occlusal rest, it becomes apparent that the recess should be prepared within the confines of the greatest tooth mass, so that force directed against the tooth will be resisted by the greatest number of periodontal fibers. Of equal importance, the floor of the recess should be perpendicular to the long axis of the tooth, so that stress will be directed axially and so that torsional stresses are reduced to a minimum.

The General Configuration of the Recess. The occlusal rest must provide ample strength by being wide and comparatively thin, rather than narrow and thick. The ideal width for the occlusal recess is approximately one-half the measurement between the buccal and lingual cusp tips of the bicuspids (Fig. 6.2), and slightly less than this for the molars.

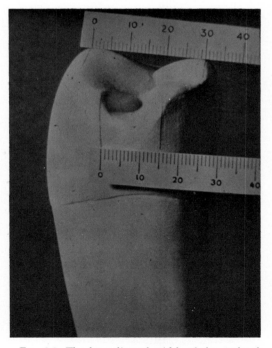

FIG. 6.2. The buccolingual width of the occlusal rest should be approximately one-half the distance between the cusp tips of bicuspids and slightly less for molars.

When the tooth is in normal alignment, the recess should be centered over the crest of the residual ridge (Fig. 6.3), although this is not always practical with teeth that are markedly rotated or tipped. It is important that the proximoocclusal line angle of the preparation not be sharp, but that it have the smoothly flowing contour of a waterfall. There are several reasons for this: (1) if the angle is left sharp, the rest may be too thin at this point, hence vulnerable to fracture (Fig. 6.4), (2) the resulting short, unprotected enamel rods are susceptible to breakage (Fig. 6.5), and (3) since the distal extension base will inevitably move to some extent in function, the entire bearing area of the recess should be formed so as to allow the clasp a slight degree of movement without transmitting a torsional stress to the tooth. *There is no place in a properly prepared recess for sharp angles* (Fig. 6.6 and 6.7).

Depth of the Recess. The recess in the tooth should be deep enough so that the occlusal rest can be made amply thick and sturdy enough to resist breakage, while at the same time not interfering with the opposing occlusion. However, the recess should not be made so deep as to create vertical walls against which the rest would be enabled to exert horizontal stress against the tooth. Further, if the recess is being prepared in an uncovered tooth surface, it should not be made so deep as to penetrate the enamel. If clearing the opposing occlusion will require a depth of the recess that risks penetration of the enamel into the underlying dentin, a gold restoration should be placed in the tooth. If the tooth cannot be restored with gold for one reason or another, it may be necessary to reduce the height of an opposing cusp in order to gain the needed interocclusal clearance (Fig. 6.8). In other circumstances, the solution to a lack of interocclusal space may be to locate the recess in another part of the tooth, the lingual groove of a lower molar, for example (Fig. 6.9). If penetration of the enamel does occur during the preparation of the recess despite due pre-

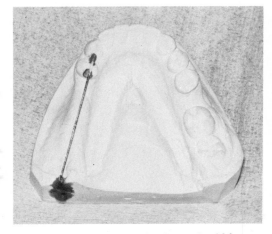

FIG. 6.3. Ideally, the occlusal rest should be centered over the crest of the residual ridge, although, when the tooth is rotated, this may not be feasible.

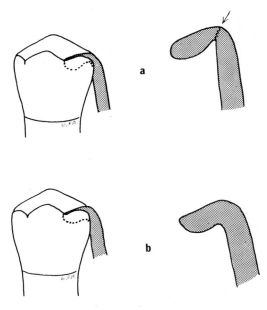

FIG. 6.4. The proximoocclusal angle of an occlusal rest should never be left sharp as at *a*, but rounded as in *b*.

cautions, a small cavity can be prepared in the dentin and filled with amalgam or gold foil. Fissures and grooves which lie adjacent to the boundaries of the recess should be made shallow and even, so as to

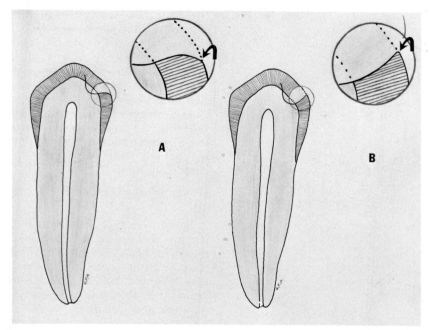

FIG. 6.5. Failure to round off the proximoocclusal line angle of an occlusal rest, as in *A*, will not only create a weak point in the occlusal rest as illustrated in Figure 6.4, but it may also leave short unprotected enamel rods as shown in *B*.

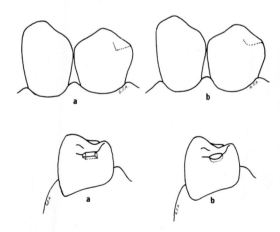

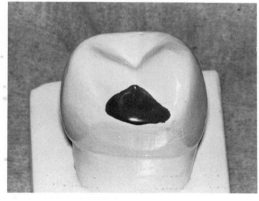

FIG. 6.6. The occlusal rest preparation should have no sharp angles as illustrated in *a-a* above, but should be rounded in all directions as shown in *b-b*, so that the denture has some freedom of movement without transmitting lateral stress to the abutment tooth.

FIG. 6.7. The occlusal recess, shown here in a mandibular molar, is rounded in all directions so that the metal rest can move to some degree, in a fashion similar to the movement in a ball-and-socket joint.

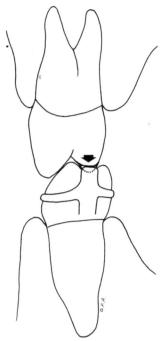

FIG. 6.8. When interocclusal space is very limited, it may be necessary to gain some access for the occlusal rest by reducing the height of the opposing cusp, rather than to attempt to secure all of the needed clearance at the expense of the abutment tooth. This is a frequent occurrence in the mandibular bicuspids when the lingual cusp of a maxillary bicuspid is in tight contact with the distal fossa of the lower tooth.

placed in the fossa of the abutment tooth adjacent to the edentulous space, although this is not an inviolable rule by any means. However, it is worthy of mention that placing the rest as far posteriorly in the mouth as possible in the distal extension base type of denture is advantageous from a standpoint of leverage control. By so doing, the lever arm is shortened while the indirect retainer may be made longer, anterior to the fulcrum line, hence mechanically more efficient.

Choice of Foundation Surface (See Table 6.1)

Tooth surfaces, upon which the recess for an occlusal rest must be prepared, differ in both contour and thickness of enamel from tooth to tooth, and from mouth to mouth. Thus, a measure of ingenuity and ability to improvise is often required in selecting the most suitable site for the recess, and in engineering its preparation to assure that the rest can be properly designed with ample strength while, at the same time, clearing the opposing occlusion.

The nearest thing to an ideal surface upon which to place an occlusal rest is gold alloy. Natural tooth enamel is next in order of suitability, followed by fused por-

blend smoothly with the margins of the preparation.

Site Selection and Preparation for the Occlusal Rest

Ofttimes the most suitable clasp design for a given clasping situation may hinge upon the availability of interocclusal space, and a proper site on the tooth for the rest recess. Thus, it follows that the selection of a particular clasp, for a given set of circumstances, presumes that space as well as a proper site are available for the occlusal (incisal, lingual) rest that is an integral part of that particular design of clasp. Generally, in the case of bicuspids and molars, the occlusal rest is

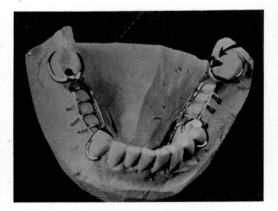

FIG. 6.9. The occlusal rest has been placed in the lingual groove of the mandibular molar shown here, because the occlusion was such that gaining sufficient space in the mesial fossa of the molar would have entailed an excessive amount of cutting of the abutment tooth, as well as its antagonist.

TABLE 6.1
Site Selection and Preferred Type of Surface for the Rest

Teeth	Enamel	Gold Alloy	Amalgam	Silicate or Acrylic Resin
Maxillary teeth				
Molars and premolars	Conventional preparations Usually in the mesial or distal fossae	Full crown, ¾ crown, inlay, or onlay	Replace with gold if minor connector contacts the proximal surface of the restoration	Replace with gold restorations
Canines	Cingulum. Inlay, full crown or ¾ crown often needed	Cingulum rest in gold provides the ideal surface	Might be employed under a cingulum rest in selected instances	Replace with gold restorations
Incisors	Cingulum rest (not feasible without a restoration)	Cingulum rest in inlay, full crown or ¾ crown	Replace with gold	Replace with gold restorations
Mandibular teeth				
Molars and premolars	Conventional preparations in the mesial or distal fossae	Full crown, ¾ crown, inlay, or onlay	Replace with gold if clasp connector contacts the proximal surface of the amalgam	Replace with gold restorations
Canines	Incisal (usually)	Cingulum rest in crown or inlay is ideal	Replace with gold	Replace with gold restorations
Incisors	Incisal rest sometimes used	Cingulum rest with two or more teeth splinted together	Replace with gold	Replace with gold restoration

celain and silver amalgam in that order. A rest should never be placed on a silicate cement restoration, nor on one of acrylic resin, because neither of these materials possesses the physical properties to sustain, for very long, the rigorous stresses to which it will be exposed under a partial denture clasp.

The Amalgam Restoration as a Rest Site. If a clasp is placed on a tooth containing a multisurface amalgam, in such a way that the clasp body and the minor connector must rest against the proximal surface of the restoration, scratching and abrasion of the amalgam will ensue. The reason for this is that the relative hardness of the partial denture alloy causes it to abrade the relatively softer surface of the amalgam as the prosthesis moves in function, and as it is inserted and removed from the mouth. If, on the other hand, the amalgam restoration is confined to the occlusal surface of the abutment tooth only, it can be depended upon to withstand the extra load of an occlusal rest, for many years of satisfactory service.

Clinical Steps in the Preparation of the Occlusal Rest

Prior to beginning the preparation of the recess in a natural tooth, it may be well to describe to the patient the procedure that is to be carried out, and to explain its purpose. The diagnostic casts are very useful in presenting an explanation that can be comprehended by the average lay person. If a study of the occlusion reveals that interocclusal space for the rest is extremely limited, it would be prudent to inform the patient at this time that some additional clearance will be required at the time of insertion of the prosthesis (or at the framework try-in), and that this will be accomplished by a slight alteration of a cusp of the opposing tooth. A straightforward explanation at this time will dispel the conclusion, which the patient might draw later, that the opposing tooth is being mutilated because of an oversight or mishap, or, to use a favored lay expression, "that the mouth is being altered to fit the prosthesis."

The clinical steps follow.

1. All disking should be accomplished first, for the purpose of creating guiding planes or for the elimination of unfavorable proximal undercuts.
2. A spoon- or saucer-shaped depression should then be prepared in the appropriate fossa. A round, diamond stone, approximately the size of a no. 8 bur, is the rotary instrument of choice for accomplishing this step. It

is advisable to establish the outline form of the recess with a larger stone, and then to deepen it with a smaller one. The rest should cover a width of approximately one-half the width of the distance between the buccal and lingual cusps of bicuspids, and slightly less for molars. It should be centered over the crest of the residual ridge, unless the tooth is rotated. The floor of the rest should be shallow and rounded in all directions.

3. The marginal ridge should be reduced and rounded, so that the angle formed between the floor of the rest and the axial surface of the tooth has a smoothly rounded contour. If the marginal ridge is left sharp and angular, a correspondingly sharp angle will be created in the metal on the side which contacts the tooth. This will weaken it and make it vulnerable to fracture. The angle formed between the floor of the recess and the axial surface of the tooth should ideally be less than 90°, but this is not always feasible because of the fact that a prominent triangular ridge of enamel is so often encountered. In such an instance, if the floor can be fashioned so that it is perpendicular to the long axis of the tooth, it will be perfectly adequate.

4. The depth of the prepared recess, with the teeth in occlusion (including excursive movements), should be observed, to ensure that the available space will permit an adequate bulk of metal for strength. Opposing cusps may be reduced if additional space is required, although it may be preferable to postpone this step until try-in of the metal framework, or even until final insertion of the prosthesis, to obviate the possibility of movement of the tooth or teeth subsequent to the alteration. Softened bite wax can be interposed between the occluded teeth as an aid in assessing the amount of available space which has been provided, or that still

needs to be created. If inspection of the wax reveals a very thin layer of wax between a marginal ridge and an opposing cusp, for example, it would indicate the need for additional clearance at this point.

5. When the rest preparation is complete, it should be smoothed with a rubber disk and polished with pumice. The application of a caries-inhibiting drug, to all recesses prepared in enamel, is a relatively simple procedure with much to recommend it.

The Rotated Tooth

When it is necessary to clasp a tooth which has rotated out of its normal position, the preferred treatment is to cover the crown with a restoration which realigns the surfaces of the tooth in a more conventional relationship to the other teeth in the arch. If the tooth is not to be restored, for one reason or another, it may be possible to alter its axial surfaces sufficiently to render it more suitable for clasping, and to place the occlusal rest in the mesial or distal fossae, even though these may be situated, as a result of the rotation, on the buccal or lingual side of the alveolar ridge. If it is not practical to site the rest in either fossae, it should be remembered that the occlusal rest may be placed anywhere on the surface of the tooth where a properly designed recess can be prepared to support it.

The Mandibular Bicuspid with a Rudimentary Cusp

The mandibular first bicuspid with a rudimentary lingual cusp presents a difficult surface upon which to fashion a conventional occlusal rest. All too often, an effort to prepare a recess in such a surface results in a preparation which falls short of meeting the minimum standards of a properly engineered rest seat. The most satisfactory solution is to cover such a crown with a gold restoration, building a quasi-cingulum rest into the wax pattern similar to the type employed for the mandibular cuspids.

The Indirect Retention Rest

The occlusal rest which is employed as an indirect retainer requires a recessed preparation in the surface of a tooth similar to that required for the conventional occlusal, lingual, or incisal rest for a clasp. A rest which is to be used for this purpose should be located as far anterior to the fulcrum line as mouth conditions permit. The reason for this is that, from a standpoint of mechanics, an indirect retainer positioned close to the fulcrum line will not be as effective as one placed farther from it. Other things being equal, the occlusal rest on a posterior tooth is preferred for an indirect retainer to the incisal or lingual rest on an anterior tooth, unless the lingual surface of the anterior tooth has been restored with gold so that an ideally contoured recess can be formed in it. Oftentimes the choices of a site for the indirect retainer rest may be narrowed down to the steeply inclined lingual surface of a cuspid, which is farthest from the fulcrum point and thus superior from a standpoint of leverage control, or the occlusal surface of a first bicuspid which, although closer to the fulcrum line, is much preferred as a foundation surface for the rest. One may take advantage of the best features of each tooth, in such an instance, by employing a rest which is supported by them both. The mesial fossa of the bicuspid is prepared in the conventional saucer shape. The rest for the indirect retainer is then designed to fit into the prepared recess on the bicuspid, and to extend over onto the lingual surface of the cuspid (Fig. 6.10). The lingual surface of the cuspid requires no preparation. Such a design exploits the excellent indirect retention which the cuspid is capable of supplying, and combines it with the equally excellent vertical support offered by the bicuspid.

The Rest Recess in the Abraded Tooth

The wisdom of preparing a rest recess in enamel which has already been worn thin may be questioned, and certainly, covering the tooth with a cast crown is the preferred treatment. Generally, however,

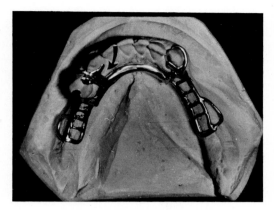

FIG. 6.10. When the choice of a site for a rest to house an indirect retainer narrows down to a bicuspid and a cuspid, one may take advantage of the best features of each tooth by preparing a recess in the mesial fossa of the bicuspid, in the conventional saucer shape, and extending the rest over onto the lingual surface of the cuspid. No preparation is necessary in the cuspid.

such a condition is found in a patient who is well beyond the age of high caries susceptibility, and whose dentin can usually be counted on to be extremely hard and caries resistant. The wear on the enamel which has already taken place may be prima facie evidence that the occlusion is exceedingly close and, if so, obtaining sufficient clearance to ensure adequate bulk for the rest, without excessive reduction of tooth structure, may require some ingenuity.

The Mesially Inclined Mandibular Molar

The severely tipped mandibular molar sometimes presents a problem for the placement of an occlusal rest because it is so difficult to engineer the recess in such a manner that stresses are directed along the long axis of the tooth (Fig. 6.11). Failure to direct the stress axially may permit the forces of occlusion to tilt the tooth farther mesially. One solution that may be effective is to place an additional occlusal rest in the distal fossa. In this location on the tooth, the floor of the recess may be more easily prepared to lie perpendicularly to the long axis than is the case in the mesial fossa. Moreover, a

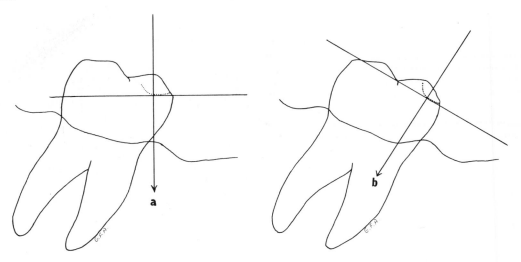

FIG. 6.11. The recess for a typical mesially inclined mandibular molar should be prepared with the floor perpendicular to the long axis of the tooth, so as to avoid tipping the tooth farther mesially. The recess shown at *a* will generate stresses which have a torsional component. The preparation shown at *b* will direct stress along the long axis, which will tend to stabilize the tooth.

rest so positioned will tend to counteract any tendency of the tooth to tip farther mesially.

The Embrasure Rest

The embrasure type clasp is, basically, two simple circlet clasps joined together, and the rest recesses should be fashioned on the two abutment teeth accordingly. Sufficient space must be created between the approximating teeth and the opposing cusps, to ensure that the rests and shoulders of the clasp can be of sufficient bulk and strength to withstand the rigors of mouth service (Figs. 6.12 and 6.13). Softened wax may be placed between the opposing teeth as a guide to assess better the amount of space that is available and the additional amount that will be required.

The Onlay Rest

It is sometimes advantageous to employ the onlay rest (Figs. 6.14 and 6.15) on the abutment tooth which has an occlusal surface that is partially below the plane of occlusion as a result of being tipped or rotated below its normal occlusal level. A properly contoured onlay rest may serve to restore the tooth so that it can contribute to more effective occlusal function while, at the same time, fulfilling its role as a vertical support for the prosthesis. Because of the imminent danger of enamel decalcification under this type of occlusal rest, it should be employed only in caries resistant mouths, unless the

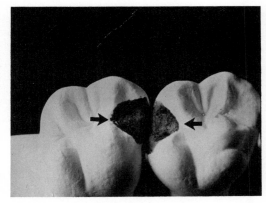

FIG. 6.12. The embrasure type of clasp is actually two simple circlet clasps joined together at the occlusal rest, and the recess for this clasp should be fashioned accordingly.

tooth is covered with a gold crown. It is essential that the patient's hygiene be maintained at a high level, and that a prosthesis with this type of an occlusal rest should be left out of the mouth for at least 8 of the 24 hours. When the occlusal surface of the abutment tooth is deeply fissured, the fissures should be widened and made more shallow before the framework is made, so as to render them as

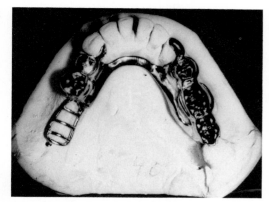

FIG. 6.15. The prosthesis shown here has elevated the occlusal surfaces of several teeth by means of onlay rests, thereby restoring the occlusal plane to its former position and making possible establishment of a more functional occlusion.

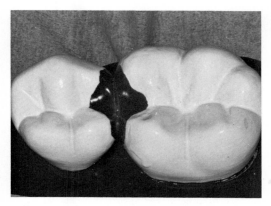

FIG. 6.13. It is important that sufficient space be provided in the interproximal embrasures to accommodate an adequate thickness of metal for the shoulders of the clasp.

self-cleansing as possible. An additional precaution, with much to recommend it, is to treat the tooth at each recall appointment with an anticariogenic drug.

The Rest Recess on Anterior Teeth

Anterior teeth do not naturally lend themselves to either clasping or to accommodation of a rest recess because of their morphology. Unfortunately, there often is no choice but to employ the cuspids as abutments and, at times, even the incisors. Employing the anterior teeth as abutments raises the problem of providing the clasp with support, so that it is prevented from exerting orthodontic movement against the tooth, or of the clasp arms spreading open, or of a combination of the two. If the clasp arms are permitted to spread so that the clasp slips downward on the abutment tooth, the result may be stripping of the gingival attachment, which is a grave sequela indeed (Fig. 6.16). Both incisal and lingual surfaces are used for the rest site, the choice depending on several variables.

The Cingulum Rest Preparation

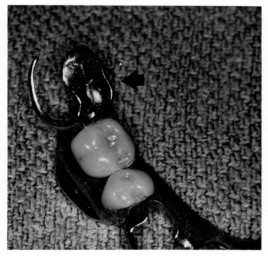

FIG. 6.14. The onlay rest may be employed to advantage when the plane of occlusion of the abutment tooth must be built up to improve the occlusion.

From a standpoint of mechanics, the cingulum rest on an anterior tooth has an important advantage over the incisal rest, in that it is closer to the center of rotation

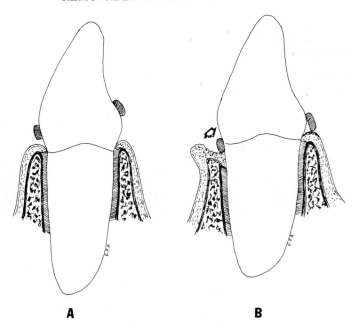

FIG. 6.16. Placing a rest on the inclined plane of an anterior tooth, without first preparing a recess for it, will result in either movement of the tooth or spreading of the clasp arms. If the clasp arms spread apart and slide down the steep lingual slope, irremediable damage may be incurred by the periodontal apparatus. The drawing shows the clasp in proper position at *A*, and after it has been permitted to slide down the steep lingual slope of the mandibular cuspid at *B*.

of the tooth and hence will exert less leverage (Fig. 6.17). It has, moreover, two additional advantages: (1) it can be discreetly hidden from view, and (2) it tends to be less bothersome to a curious tongue. It is preferred over the incisal rest for all three of these reasons, when it is feasible to employ it. However, all anterior teeth do not present lingual surfaces suitable for creation of a recess of sufficient depth, without penetration of the enamel. The maxillary cuspid is, in fact, the only one that does, by virtue of its prominent cingulum and a comparatively thick enamel cap. The lingual surface of the mandibular cuspid, on the other hand, is typically steep and precipitous with little or no cingulum (Fig. 6.18), and a relatively thin enamel covering. This is true also of the incisors. When the cingulum rest is employed with any anterior tooth other than the maxillary cuspid, the lingual surface

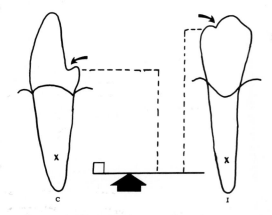

FIG. 6.17. The cingulum or lingual rest on an anterior tooth has an important advantage over the incisal rest, in that it is closer to the center of rotation of the tooth and the leverage factor is thereby reduced. In this sketch, *c* indicates the cingulum rest and *i* the incisal rest. The approximate location of the center of rotation for a single-rooted tooth is denoted at *x*.

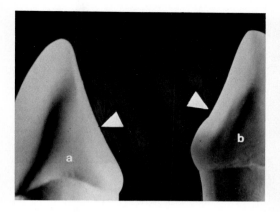

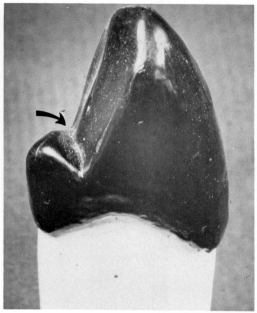

FIG. 6.18. The lingual surface of the mandibular cuspid, *a*, is typically precipitous, with little or no semblance of a cingulum. The maxillary cuspid, *b*, typically has a more prominent cingulum, which usually affords a more suitable site for a cingulum rest recess.

should first be covered with metal (Figs. 6.19 and 6.20). The cingulum rest should be of sufficient depth to afford a definite support for the lingual arm of the clasp. When used with a distal extension base partial denture, the floor of the recess should be semilunar in form from mesial to distal, to permit slight movement of the clasp in the recess as the base moves.

FIG. 6.19. When a lingual or cingulum rest is to be used on the mandibular cuspid, the lingual surface should be covered with metal, and the recess for the cingulum rest should be prepared in the wax pattern.

The Cingulum Rest on the Incisor Tooth

When mandibular incisors must be pressed into service as abutments, the method of choice is to splint two or three teeth together with crowns or pinledge inlays, so as to form a multirooted abutment. The metal coverings will also afford a surface upon which cingulum rests of ideal contour can be fashioned.

The Incisal Rest

The incisal rest may be employed on any anterior tooth, provided it will not interfere with the opposing occlusion, although it has some distinct disadvantages when compared with the cingulum rest. Perhaps the major disadvantage is its cosmetic shortcoming. Most individuals prefer to avoid a display of metal on an anterior tooth, if they have any choice in

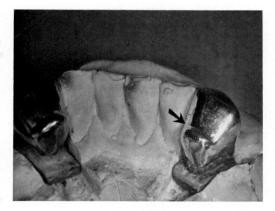

FIG. 6.20. The cingulum rest recess, prepared in metal in the mandibular cuspid is by any reckoning, the most satisfactory type of rest for this tooth. The recess should be made semilunar, mesiodistally, in configuration.

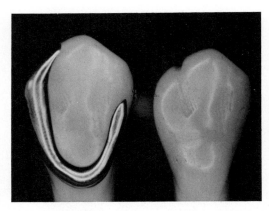

FIG. 6.21. The incisal rest, on the mandibular cuspid, is to be preferred to the lingual or cingulum rest if the recess for the latter is not properly prepared. Properly engineered, it can be a satisfactory rest both mechanically and esthetically in most mouths.

the matter. Because of its position in relation to the fulcrum point of the tooth, it permits the clasp to exert more leverage on the tooth; and because of greater tooth coverage, it is more apt to attract the notice of a curious tongue. Notwithstanding these weaknesses, however, the incisal rest is frequently used with success on mandibular canines, and certainly it is to be preferred to an improperly fashioned cingulum recess in enamel. Moreover, an incisal rest on the mandibular cuspid, situated as it is at the corner of the mouth, is ofttimes quite unobtrusive, and it may be acceptable to all but the most exacting type of patient (Fig. 6.21).

The Site for the Incisal Rest. Solely from a standpoint of mechanics, the incisal rest would best be sited on the mesial cusp arm of the cuspid, so that the clasp would not be as apt to be displaced by settling of the denture base as would be the case if it were placed on the distal cusp arm. However, unless the base is maintained well-fitted to the residual ridge, an incisal rest located on the mesial cusp arm has the potential of exerting more leverage on the tooth than would be the case with one on the distal cusp arm.

Oftentimes, the exact location on the incisal edge of the mandibular cuspid best

suited to support the rest will depend on the wear pattern of the individual tooth. Abrasion may have substantially altered the contour of the incisal edge, so that the sole criterion for siting the recess is simply where the opposing occlusion will best accommodate it. Another complicating factor may be the presence of synthetic restorations on the proximal surfaces of the tooth. Since it is not uncommon for the occlusion to be exceedingly close in this area, the preferred site may be dictated altogether by the availability of interincisal space. It should be borne in mind, too, that when assessing the amount of space between opposing teeth the occlusion is dynamic, not static, and hence, sight should not be lost of the space available during lateral and protrusive excursions.

Both the labial and lingual margins of the incisal rest preparation should be beveled.

The Internal Rest (The Milled Rest, The Semiprecision Attachment)

The internal rest consists of a narrow slot or keyway, built into a metal casting which has been constructed for an abutment tooth, and into which is fitted a male attachment that has been made a part of the removal partial denture framework. The advantages and disadvantages of this type of attachment are discussed in more detail in Chapter 18, Precision Attachments and Stressbreakers.

Guiding Planes

As the prosthesis is inserted and removed from the mouth, some portion of its rigid components, principally the truss arms must, perforce, contact various axial tooth surfaces that are situated along its path of insertion and removal. If these tooth surfaces are convex in contour, the prosthesis may wedge against them while the tooth makes a slight, momentarily accommodating movement in its alveolus. According to expectation, the effect on the periodontal apparatus of this whiplash stress, even though slight, may be damaging if continued over a long enough

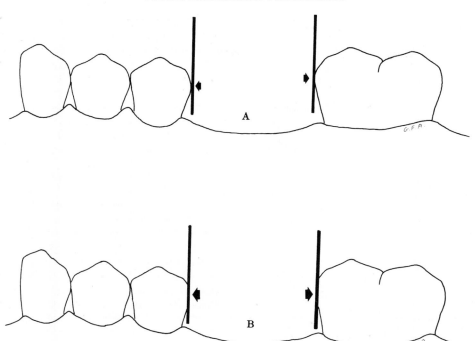

Fig. 6.22. Guiding planes are the prepared axial surfaces of the teeth, against which the prosthesis glides as it is inserted and removed from the mouth. *A* depicts the typical convex proximal surfaces of the teeth before preparation. *B* shows the same surfaces properly prepared to act as guiding planes for the partial denture.

time span. If, on the other hand, these convex tooth surfaces have been made flat, as well as parallel to the path of insertion (Fig. 6.22), the prosthesis will be enabled to glide smoothly into place against the flat planes, much as a desk drawer slides along its runners. A prosthesis so constructed will be easy for the patient to place and remove, and will transmit a minimum of stress to the teeth which support it. The prosthesis which is easily inserted and removed by the patient is much less vulnerable to breakage or distortion, particularly the latter, than is the case otherwise. Moreover, guiding planes contribute materially to the horizontal stability of the prosthesis and provide a measure of retention while, at the same time, assisting the reciprocal clasp arm to perform its intended function. Guiding planes are particularly effective when the edentulous spaces are tooth-

bounded. In addition, well prepared guiding planes tend to reduce undercuts between the proximal surface of the teeth and the minor connectors of the partial denture, thus making the prosthesis more hygienic. A further benefit which accrues from a properly prepared guiding plane is that lowering the height of contour of the proximal surface of the tooth permits the placement of some of the rigid portion of the clasp closer to the gingival margin of the tooth (Fig. 6.23). This makes possible a clasp design that is much less conspicuous, which is an undeniable advantage in an area of the mouth that is readily visible.

Creating Guiding Planes

Guiding planes may be present naturally on the axial surfaces of some teeth or, as is more often the case, there may be

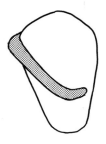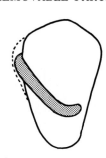

Fig. 6.23. Preparation of the guiding plane on the proximal surface of an anterior tooth may often lower the height of contour, so that some of the rigid part of the clasp (the body and shoulders) can be positioned farther gingivally on the tooth, thus greatly improving the esthetics.

a need to create them on tooth surfaces that are contacted by the rigid parts of the framework. The guiding planes on these tooth surfaces should be prepared parallel to the path of insertion, as well as parallel to one another. Ideally, each edentulous space should be bounded by parallel guiding planes, so as to direct the appliance along an interference-free pathway. Indeed, this is an important objective to be sought when planning the prosthesis. While a flat surface parallel to the path of insertion can be prepared on most teeth by judicious disking, teeth with short, conical shaped crowns which contact the surveyor spindle only at the cervix may have need of being restored with metal before they can provide the type of flat surface that is desired.

Tooth surfaces that are to be flattened, to create guiding plane surfaces, should be determined at the time of the initial analysis of the study cast on the surveyor, and the area to be reduced should be noted on the cast with a colored pencil. A recommended procedure is to prepare the guiding plane on the stone tooth, with the guidance of the analyzing rod in the spindle. The cast can then be used as a pattern at the time that the tooth alteration is accomplished intraorally.

Guiding Planes and the Distal Extension Base

In a discussion of the guiding plane principle, it is important that a distinc-tion be made between the guiding planes on abutment teeth that bound an edentulous space, and the one on the abutment tooth which supports a distal extension base. In the former instance, well engineered guiding planes are contacted by the truss arms of the framework as the prosthesis is inserted and removed, so that horizontal wedging is virtually eliminated. If the clasp has been properly engineered, all transverse stresses transmitted to the tooth are effectively neutralized, so that the whiplash effect is eliminated. In contrast to this, the creation of a flat distal surface on the abutment tooth next to an edentulous space has the effect of magnifying the stress which the denture base transmits to the abutment as the base moves in function. For this reason, a pronounced guiding plane is not recommended for the abutment tooth which supports a distal extension base (Fig. 6.24). The interface between tooth surface and clasp should be such that a slight degree of movement of the base and the clasp is permitted without, at the same time, transmitting torsional stress to the tooth. Enough flattening of the distal surface of the tooth should be accomplished to reduce the amount of the undercut between minor connector and abutment tooth, but the interface should not be formed to create a glove-like fit between the two surfaces.

A Summary of Functions of the Guiding Plane

The function of the guiding plane is to:
1. Minimize wedging stresses on the abutment teeth.
2. Make insertion and removal of the prosthesis easier for the patient.
3. Aid in stabilizing the prosthesis against horizontal stress.
4. Aid in stabilizing individual teeth.
5. Reduce the amount of blockout needed in areas of severe undercut, and thus minimize the amount of space between the denture and the tooth.
6. Contribute to the overall retention of the prosthesis.

Tooth Recontouring

The natural tooth surfaces which are contacted by the prosthesis are ofttimes not well contoured from a standpoint of ideal clasp design. Simple altering techniques performed with diamond stones and disks may serve to transform a tooth from an obstacle to a contributor to an improved design. As an example, the height of contour of the lingual surface of both maxillary and mandibular molars

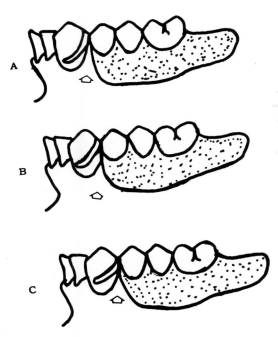

and bicuspids is usually higher than is the buccal surface. Because of this disparity in contour, the lingual or reciprocal arm of the clasp must be placed at a higher vertical level on the crown of the tooth than is the retentive arm. When the prosthesis is seated in the mouth, the retentive arm of the clasp will already have flexed into position in the infrabulge, before the reciprocal arm has even made contact with the tooth surface. The reciprocal action is most urgently needed, of course, at the exact fleeting instant that the retentive arm flexes, since it is at this juncture that the harmful transverse stress is directed against the tooth. This problem can be alleviated, if not completely eliminated, by lowering the height of contour on the lingual surface of the tooth so that the reciprocal arm of the clasp occupies a position at a vertical level opposite the retentive arm (Fig. 6.25).

Recontouring may be similarly helpful when a mandibular molar is employed as a distal abutment and the distobuccal surface presents a favorable undercut, except

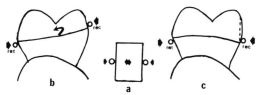

FIG. 6.24. In preparing guiding planes, it is important that a distinction be made between abutment teeth which adjoin an edentulous space, and the abutment which supports a distal extension base. If the guiding plane is too pronounced, it may increase the leverage-induced stress which is exerted by the distal extension base against the abutment tooth. In these sketches A shows the typical distal surface of a cuspid, unprepared and capable of offering very little guidance to the prosthesis. In B the distal surface of the tooth has been flattened to provide a good guiding plane, but such a surface will enable the distal extension base to exert a greatly magnified stress against the tooth. In C the surface has been modified to create an adequate guiding plane for the prosthesis, but the altered surface will still allow a moderate amount of movement of the base without creating a excessive stress against the tooth.

FIG. 6.25. Ideal balance between the two arms of the clasp is achieved when both arms contact the tooth surface simultaneously, so that stress exerted by the retentive arm is reciprocated by the bracing arm. This could be readily achieved if the tooth were cylindrically shaped, as shown at a. However, more often than not, the abutment teeth have contours like those shown at b, and the retentive arm will have flexed over the height of contour, inflicting its whiplash effect on the tooth, when the reciprocal arm has barely contacted the opposite tooth surface. If the height of contour is lowered on the lingual surface, as shown at c, the reciprocal arm can be positioned at the same vertical height as the retentive arm. Thus, all force directed against the tooth by the retentive arm is counteracted, at the same instant, by the reciprocal arm with an equal and opposite force.

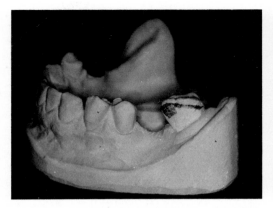

FIG. 6.26. The buccal surface of the mandibular molar frequently presents a very high height of contour, which complicates both the selection and the design of a clasp on this tooth. Note the survey line on the tooth pictured here, which is typical. The amount of reduction needed to lower the height of contour has been indicated with a colored pencil.

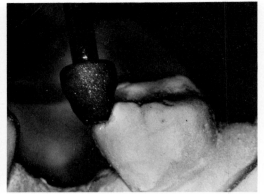

FIG. 6.27. This photograph depicts on the study cast the reduction in the height of contour of the tooth that will be accomplished in the mouth.

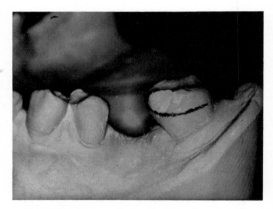

FIG. 6.28. The tooth has been reduced to lower the height of contour, so that advantage can be taken of the retentive undercut on the distal aspect of the buccal surface with a circumferential-type clasp. The clasp body and shoulder can now be more ideally positioned on the tooth.

that the survey line is extremely high on the mesiobuccal surface adjacent to the edentulous space (Fig. 6.26). A buccal surface so contoured would necessitate either positioning the shoulder of the clasp too high occlusally on the tooth for good clasp design or, as an alternative, choosing a different clasp design which might not be as suitable from other standpoints. Here again, the problem can be alleviated by reducing the tooth surface at its greatest convexity, so as to lower the survey line, thus making possible a lowering of the clasp shoulder (Figs. 6.27 and 6.28).

Other tooth surfaces which frequently require recontouring to reduce and lower the height of contour are the distal surfaces of cuspids, both maxillary and mandibular, the distobuccal line angle of maxillary bicuspids, the mesiolingual line angle of mandibular molars, and the mesiobuccal line angle of maxillary molars. It bears emphasis that tooth surfaces which require alteration should be recognized during the preliminary cast analysis. They can then be designated on the study cast and noted in the treatment plan, so that the required alteration can be accomplished at the most propitious time in the treatment sequence.

Paralleling Anterior Spaces

It is commonplace for the teeth adjacent to an anterior edentulous space to be bell shaped, thus creating an irregularly shaped space. To compound the problem, the teeth may be tipped or rotated (Fig. 6.29), which severely limits the opportunity of achieving a pleasingly natural appearance of the replacement teeth. The proximal surfaces of such teeth may be altered by disking, to make possible the fitting of a pleasing composition of re-

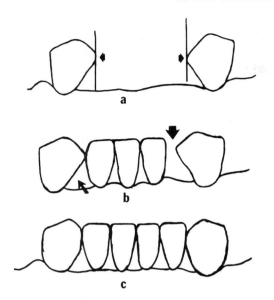

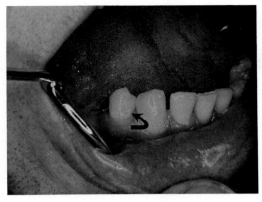

FIG. 6.31. The dimple is placed in the precise spot to be occupied by the clasp terminal.

FIG. 6.29. The teeth which border an anterior edentulous space are frequently so bell crowned that the mesiodistal width is markedly greater at the cervical border than it is at the incisal edge (*a*). This severely limits the esthetic opportunity and may be the root cause of food entrapment between the prosthesis and the teeth (*b*). The teeth can be altered by disking (*arrows*), so that the prosthetic teeth can be more pleasingly arranged while, at the same time, reducing the size of the embrasure between the teeth and the prosthesis (*c*).

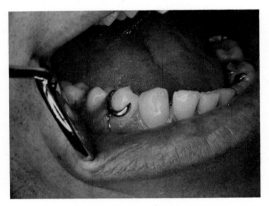

FIG. 6.32. A favored spot for this alteration is in the interproximal area where the enamel is comparatively thick and where the clasp terminal is customarily placed.

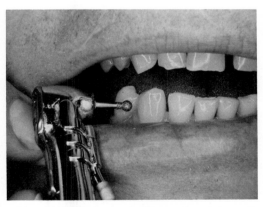

FIG. 6.30. When no retentive undercut is available on the surface of a tooth, and a crown or retentive restoration is contraindicated for one reason or another, a technique of dimpling the enamel may be employed. Dimpling consists in preparing a small, saucer shaped indentation in the enamel of the tooth with a round, diamond stone.

placement teeth into the space. The study cast can be used to determine the exact amount of disking required. If desired, the replacement tooth or teeth may be fitted into the space on the study cast, and the cast used as a blueprint in accomplishing the alteration when it is performed intraorally.

Dimpling

When there is a lack of sufficient retentive undercut on a surface of a tooth, which is of strategic importance as an abutment, and recontouring of the surface with a metal restoration is contraindicated for one reason or another, a technique known as "dimpling" may be employed. The dimpling technique consists in preparing a small indentation, or dimple, in the enamel of the tooth surface into which the retentive clasp can be placed (Fig. 6.30). When the clasp is cast, it will possess a small boss at its retentive tip, which fits the depression in the tooth. Most enamel surfaces will accommodate a 0.010 or 0.015 inch excavation without danger of penetration into the dentin, or otherwise damaging the tooth (Fig. 6.31). A favored site for this alteration is in the interproximal area where the enamel is thick, and where the retentive terminal of the clasp is customarily placed (Fig. 6.32). The prepared, dimpled surface should be smoothed and polished, and it is essential that the prosthesis be left out of the mouth at night. The dimpling procedure should be planned with the use of the study cast and the surveyor, so that the undercut can be precisely located at the most ideal site on the tooth surface. This technique may be employed to advantage on the mandibular cuspids, when no undercut exists and the patient does not wish, for cosmetic reasons, to have a metal restoration placed on the tooth. The dimple preparation should be treated with stannous fluoride following its completion, and the application should be repeated at subsequent recall appointments.

Bibliography

Gabel, A. B.: A new theory of the mechanics of tooth support. Dent. Cosmos 76: 677–683, 1934.

Hardy, I.: Partial dentures that function—partial dentures that fail. J. Amer. Dent. Ass. 25: 562–566, 1938.

McCracken, W. L.: Mouth preparations for partial dentures. J. Prosth. Dent. 6: 39–52, 1956.

Orban, B.: Tissue reactions encountered in partial denture construction. Illinois Dent. J. 10: 42–56, 1961.

Orban, B.: Orban's Periodontics, Ed. 2. The C. V. Mosby Company, St. Louis, 1963.

Perry, C. F., and Applegate, S. G.: Occlusal rest, an important part of a partial den. J. Michigan Dent. Soc. 29: 24–25, 1947.

Phillips, R. W., and Leonard, L. J.: A study of enamel abrasion as related to partial denture clasps. J. Prosth. Dent. 6: 657–671, 1956.

Schorr, L., and Clayman, L. H.: Reshaping abutment teeth for reception of partial denture clasps. J. Prosth. Dent. 4: 625–633, 1954.

Schuyler, C. H.: Planning the removable partial denture to restore function and maintain oral health. New York Dent. J. 13: 4–10, 1947.

Synge, J.: Phil. Trans. Roy. Soc. London, Series A231, 1933.

Chapter 7

PRINCIPLES OF PARTIAL
DENTURE DESIGN

This chapter is concerned with the biomechanical principles which form the basis for the design of the removable partial denture. The leverage factor, which is inherent in most removable partial dentures, is discussed, and various methods of controlling leverage-induced stresses are described and analyzed. The subject matter is organized in the following way.

Introduction

It is an axiom of prosthodontic practice that the fixed type of partial denture is the most nearly ideal of any oral prosthesis, and indeed, there is abundant evidence that it is well deserving of this eminent rank. Certainly, its record of clinical service is exemplary, and when compared with the removable type of partial denture the fixed type must be acknowledged superior in most respects. A critical analysis of the structural details and the similarities, as well as the points of difference between the two, serves to bring into focus the strengths and weaknesses of each. More to the point, the comparison provides insight which can be applied to the design of the removable type of denture, to improve its structure as well as its record of clinical service.

The Biomechanics of the Fixed Partial Denture

The typical fixed partial denture (Fig. 7.1A) is short in span (usually one or two teeth), and its architecture is such that the principal stresses are directed along the long axis of the abutments. Being supported and retained at both ends of the span, it is subject to no appreciable degree of movement in function, and for the same reason it is well stabilized in a mesiodistal plane. It is small in bulk, by virtue of which it enjoys almost instant acceptance by the patient. The fixed prosthesis seldom requires adjustment or repair, rarely needs refitting, and almost never becomes lost. Two of its shortcomings, besides the obvious limits in its applicability, are that it is not well stabilized in a buccolingual plane, and is not easily maintained in a thoroughly hygienic condition, because of its comparative inaccessibility. The latter fact is, perhaps, its major weakness.

The Biomechanics of the Removable Partial Denture

Unfortunately, the design of the typical removable partial denture must differ from its fixed counterpart in several respects and for a variety of reasons (Fig. 7.1B). The edentulous areas which it must restore are usually bilateral, the spans are

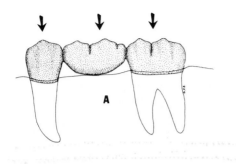

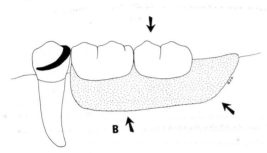

FIG. 7.1. The typical fixed partial denture, *A*, is short in span and supported at both ends by teeth, and the principle stresses are directed along the long axis of these abutment teeth. The typical removable partial denture, *B*, is usually longer in span and the support is provided by both abutment teeth and the residual ridge.

generally longer than one or two teeth, and even more important, the typical removable partial prosthesis must rely for a portion of its support on a resilient, displaceable foundation, the oral mucosa. This composite type of denture support means that the brunt of the masticatory stress must be shared between the relatively unyielding abutment teeth and the comparatively soft oral mucosa, undergirded though it is by a bony foundation. Because the support for the base is to some degree displaceable, it permits the distal extension base a degree of movement as occlusal loads are applied. Since the abutment tooth is capable of only a very limited amount of movement, a Class I lever is thus created, in which the abutment tooth plays the role of both ful-

crum and load (Fig. 7.2). Stress is transferred to the tooth by the clasp, and it is magnified by a leverage factor contributed by the denture base. Thus, it becomes increasingly apparent that a central concern in removable partial denture design must be the control, in one way or another, of such harmful, leverage-induced stresses. *Indeed, the evidence suggests that the nearer to complete neutralization of all leverages that a removable partial denture can be designed (like its fixed counterpart), the more favorable will be its prognosis.*

The Effect of Leverage-Induced Stress on the Partial Denture

The dental arch, with bilateral edentulous spaces which have terminal abutments at either end of the span, might, in a typical instance, be restored with either a fixed or a removable type of prosthesis. In this circumstance, the removable type of partial denture would have an extremely favorable prognosis, since it would be entirely supported by teeth and all leverages could thus be effectively neutralized (Fig. 7.3). It is worth noting that the removable prosthesis would be better stabilized in a buccolingual plane than would two fixed partial dentures, by

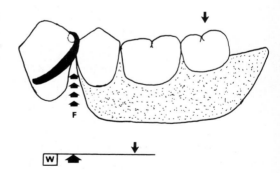

FIG. 7.2. Since the residual ridge is resilient, it permits the denture base a slight degree of movement as occlusal loads are applied. Hence, the abutment tooth becomes both the fulcrum, *F*, and the load, *W*, of a Class I lever. It is thus subjected to torsional types of stress transmitted through the clasp. To add to the gravity of the problem, the stress is magnified by the leverage of the base.

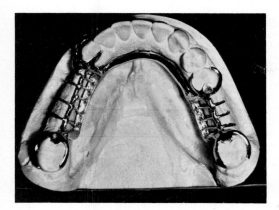

FIG. 7.3. The partially edentulous dental arch, which has bilateral spaces with an abutment tooth at both ends of both spans, has an extremely favorable prognosis, since it is entirely tooth-borne and all leverages are effectively neutralized.

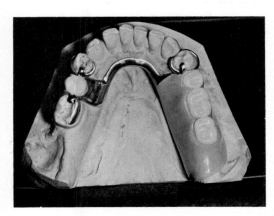

FIG. 7.4. When there are bilateral edentulous spans with a terminal abutment tooth on only one side, the prognosis is much less favorable than when abutment teeth are available on both sides, because movement of the distal extension base will generate torsional stress which will be transferred to the abutment teeth.

virtue of the cross-arch bracing which a rigid major connector would provide. However, when one of these terminal abutments is not available on one side of the arch for supporting and retaining the denture base (Fig. 7.4), the prognosis must be materially downgraded, because movement of the distal extension base will transmit torsional stress to all of the abutment teeth. The abutment tooth which

supports the distal extension base will, of course, bear the major share of the burden. Although the amount of movement of the distal extension base can be partially controlled by appropriate clinical techniques, so that the leverage factor is neutralized to some degree, some torsional stress on the abutment teeth is unavoidable.

When both terminal abutment teeth are missing, the prognosis becomes even less favorable (Fig. 7.5). In this circumstance, there will be some unavoidable movement of the denture bases on both sides of the arch, with a resulting transmission of torsional stresses to both abutments.

Allocating the Amount of Functional Load to be Borne by Each Structure

The vast majority of mouths that the prosthodontist is called on to treat will involve one or both distal extension bases, which means that the denture must rely for a portion of its support on the residual ridge. In the matter of allocating the proportionate share of stress that is to be sustained by each of these structures, i.e., the teeth and the residual ridges, there are differing schools of thought. The differences in viewpoints center basically around the question of whether the stresses should be borne principally by the

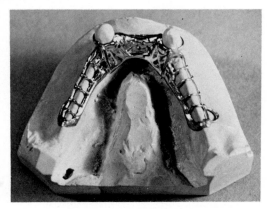

FIG. 7.5. When there are bilateral edentulous spaces and no terminal abutments, the prognosis must be downgraded, since both distal extension bases will transmit torsional stresses to the abutment teeth.

residual ridges or shared by both the natural teeth and the residual ridges, functioning in concert.

The Stressbreaker School. Those who advocate that the residual ridges bear the brunt of the burden, and that the teeth be spared all the stress possible, employ a flexible or a movable joint (a stressbreaker) between the teeth and the metal framework, so that the denture base can move independently of the clasp, thus theoretically, at least, sheltering the abutment teeth almost entirely from the stress created by movement of the base. (Stressbreakers are discussed in more detail in Chapter 18.)

The Wide-Distribution-of-Stress School. Opposed to this view is the opinion that while the support provided the prosthesis by a combination of abutment tooth and mucosa is far from ideal, it is a far better approach to the problem than permitting the residual ridges to bear virtually the entire load. Members of this school employ a variety of clinical techniques and design variations, in order to apportion functional stresses between soft tissue and remaining teeth in such a manner as to exploit the maximum load bearing capacity of each. This chapter will enumerate and analyze these approaches in some detail.

Factors Which Influence the Magnitude of the Stress That Is Transmitted to the Abutment Tooth

The amount of stress that is transmitted to the abutment tooth, by means of the clasp in a distal extension base type of partial denture, depends on an enormous array of factors, some of which are under the control of the prosthodontist, and others over which he has little or no control whatever.

The Length of the Span

The longer the edentulous span, the longer will be the denture base. The longer the base, the more will be the leverage factor, and hence the greater the stress that is transmitted to the abutment tooth. The base that begins next to the cuspid will have a greater degree of movement and will apply an increased amount of leverage, all else being equal, than will the one that begins distal to the second bicuspid.

The Quality of the Undergirding

The better the support provided by the stress-bearing soft tissues, the less will be the stress to be borne by the abutment tooth.

The Form of the Residual Ridges. Large, well-formed residual ridges will absorb more of the masticatory load, hence less stress will be transmitted to the abutment tooth. Well-shaped ridges permit the use of denture flanges that are contoured so as to contribute maximally to the stability of the prosthesis.

The Type of Mucosal Covering. Healthy mucosa, of normal thickness, is capable of bearing more of the functioning load than is thin, atrophic tissue. Unusually resilient tissue will permit more movement of the base in all directions, hence more stress on the abutment. Flabby tissue will contribute minimally to the support or to the stability, with the result that the abutment teeth will be required to bear a larger proportionate share of the stress.

The Clasp as a Factor in Stress

The type, design, and construction of the partial denture clasp can affect markedly the severity of the stress that is transmitted to the abutment tooth.

The Type of Clasp. The more resilient the retentive arm of the clasp, the less will be the stress transmitted to the abutment tooth. However, since stability, or resistance to horizontal stress, will likewise be reduced as the resiliency of the retentive clasp is increased, both the lateral and vertical stresses transmitted to the residual ridges will be increased.

The Design of the Clasp. A properly designed clasp can materially reduce the stress transmitted to the abutment. For example, a passive clasp will exert far less stress on the tooth than one that is not passive. A balanced clasp, i.e., one designed with effective reciprocal action, will eliminate the whiplash stress to which the tooth is exposed as the retentive terminal passes over the height of contour.

The Construction. A clasp made of chromium-cobalt alloy will exert more stress on the abutment tooth than will a gold clasp, all else being equal, because of the higher modulus of elasticity of the chromium-cobalt alloy. Similarly, a retentive clasp arm made of wrought alloy will be more resilient than one made of cast alloy, and so will transfer less stress to the abutment.

The Amount of Clasp Surface in Contact with the Tooth. The greater the area of tooth-to-metal contact between the clasp and the tooth, the more will be the stress exerted on the tooth.

The Type of Abutment Tooth Surface. A gold surface will offer more frictional resistance to movement of the clasp than will enamel, hence more stress will be exerted against the tooth which has been restored with a gold casting.

The Occlusion as a Factor

Several factors having to do with the quality and type of the occlusion have an important bearing on the stress that the prosthesis exerts on the abutment teeth.

The Harmony of the Occlusion or the Lack of It. A disharmonious occlusion will generate horizontal stresses which, when magnified by leverage, will be harmful to abutment tooth and residual ridge alike.

The Type of Opposing Occlusion. Individuals with natural teeth are able to exert a biting force of as much as 300 pounds. The wearer of an artificial denture may be reduced to a force as little as 30 pounds. Hence, the partial denture base which opposes an artificial denture will be subjected to a lessened amount of occlusal stress than will be the one which opposes healthy, natural teeth.

The Areas of the Base to Which the Load is Applied. There will be less movement of the base if the load is applied adjacent to the abutment tooth than if it is applied at the distal terminus of the base. Indeed, movement may be as much as fourfold greater at the distal extremity of the base than it is in the immediate vicinity of the clasp. It is worthy of mention, in this regard, that research studies have shown that the bulk of the masticatory load is normally applied to the dentition in the second bicuspid, first molar region.

Design Considerations in the Control of Stress

An understanding of the basic fundamentals of stress and its control will enable the partial denture planner to employ a combination of design and construction principles which will distribute the functional stresses equally between the hard and soft tissues, so that the effect of leverage is minimized and neither structure is stressed beyond its physiological tolerance.

Retention as a Means of Stress Control

Retention of the typical partial denture, which is, by definition, resistance to dislodgment by unseating forces, is provided principally by the clasps, but it is important to note that several other elements of the prosthesis contribute substantially to this objective. It should be clear that any retention supplied by units of the prosthesis, other than the clasps, has the salutary effect of reducing the amount of retention that the clasps are required to provide, which in turn diminishes the stress that must be borne by the abutment teeth. By exploiting retentive potential in various widely separated areas of the mouth, both support and stability may be enhanced at the same time that stress is effectively reduced. Factors other than the clasp which contribute significantly to the overall retention of the partial denture are discussed in succeeding paragraphs.

Adhesion. This is the affinity of the denture base, as well as the palatal connector, to the mucosa when an intervening layer of fluid (the saliva) is interposed between the two. The amount of retention contributed by this interfacial tension is in direct ratio to the amount of areal coverage, the accuracy of the adaptation of the base to the mucosa, and the character of the moisture film.

Atmospheric Pressure. This is not ordinarily a major factor in retention of a partial removable prosthesis, although in a large maxillary partial denture it may play an important role. Since gravity may be such a potent antiretentive force in the maxillary denture, any contribution to positive retention, from whatever source, may serve to relieve the abutment teeth of a portion of the leverage-induced stress which is threatened by a heavy prosthesis. The retentive potential of atmospheric pressure is exploited by sealing the peripheries of the denture, insofar as is possible, from the ingress of air between the denture base and the mucosa.

Frictional Contact. The retention created by a frictional contact between the teeth and the base, or other parts of the prosthesis, can be significant. Anterior replacement teeth, for example, often contact the proximal surfaces of the adjoining natural teeth, thus generating frictional resistance to vertical displacement of the denture. Properly planned and prepared guiding planes enable the truss arms to contribute substantially to the retention, as a result of frictional contact with adjacent tooth surfaces. Although not a consistently reliable source of retention, soft tissue undercuts can, under certain circumstances, assist materially in retaining the prosthesis in place. The mylohyoid ridge area and the tuberosities are prime examples of natural undercuts that can, under some circumstances, contribute to the retentive properties of the prosthesis.

Neuromuscular Control. The patient's ability to control the denture with the lips, cheeks, and tongue can be a major factor in the retentiveness of the denture, as witnessed by the large number of patients seen clinically who successfully "manage" dentures which have neither clasps nor other visible means of retention. Good neuromuscular control, coupled with properly contoured denture surfaces, is sufficient to transform a loose denture into one that is highly resistant to

dislodging forces. Contouring the base for maximum retention has been described as adding "handles" to the denture, a metaphor as apt as it is descriptive.

Strategic Clasp Positioning as a Means of Stress Control

Leverages can be controlled entirely by means of clasps, if there are sufficient abutment teeth and they are strategically distributed in the dental arch. However, even when the number and location of potential abutments is less than ideal, the harmful effects of leverage can often be reduced by the strategic placement of clasps.

Quadrilateral Configuration. When four abutment teeth are available for clasping, and the partial denture can be confined within these four clasps, all leverage is neutralized (Fig. 7.6). This quadrilateral pattern of clasping, with the prosthesis entirely confined within the four clasps, is ideal from a standpoint of both support and leverage control, and it should be employed whenever mouth conditions permit (Fig. 7.7).

Tripod Configuration. When the distal abutment on one side of the arch is missing, the inevitable lever is created by the distal extension base. In this circumstance, the leverage may be controlled, to some degree, by creating a triangular pat-

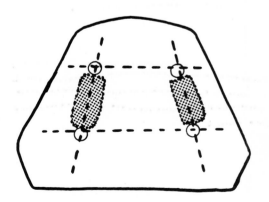

FIG. 7.6. When four abutment teeth are available for clasping and the partial denture can be designed within the confines of these four clasps, all leverages are neutralized.

tern of clasp placement (Fig. 7.8). When employing this pattern, the two clasps on the tooth-supported side should be placed on teeth as far separated as possible, consistent with acceptable esthetics (Fig. 7.9).

The Kennedy Class I. When two distal extension bases must be dealt with, the designer has little choice but to clasp the two distal abutments (Fig. 7.10 and 7.11). In this circumstance, the clasps exert little neutralizing effect on the leverage-induced stresses generated by the base, and they must be controlled by some other means.

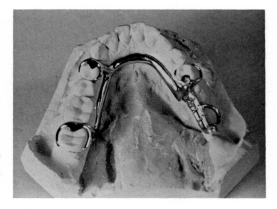

FIG. 7.9. The triangular, or tripod, pattern of clasp positioning. The clasps on the tooth-supported side should be placed as far apart as feasible, to neutralize the leverage of the distal extension base most effectively.

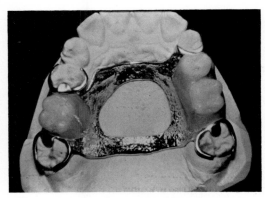

FIG. 7.7. A maxillary removable partial denture, in which all leverages are neutralized and stresses are directed along the long axis of the abutment teeth. This is an ideal method for neutralizing leverage and reducing stress.

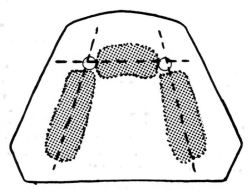

FIG. 7.10. When two distal extension bases must be dealt with, leverages must be controlled by other means. See also Figure 7.11.

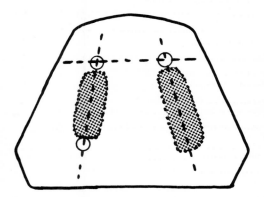

FIG. 7.8. When a distal terminal abutment is available on only one side, leverage may be partially controlled by employing a triangular pattern of clasp placement.

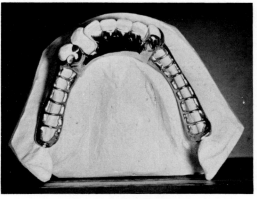

FIG. 7.11. See Figure 7.10.

The Unilateral Prosthesis. Leverage per se is not a problem with the unilateral type of edentulous span (Figs. 7.12 and 7.13). However, torsional stress on the abutments is generated by the prosthesis because of its tendency to rotate in a buc-colingual plane. The conventional solution is to cross the arch with a major connector and to clasp teeth on the contralateral side, thus making the prosthesis, in effect,

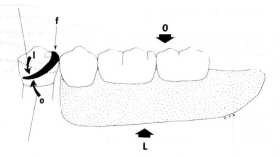

FIG. 7.14. This schematic shows the resultant stress transmitted to the abutment tooth by a circumferential-type clasp. When an occlusal force, O, is applied to the base, the terminal is moved upward as shown at o. When a lifting force, L, is applied, the terminal moves downward, l. The fulcrum is represented by f.

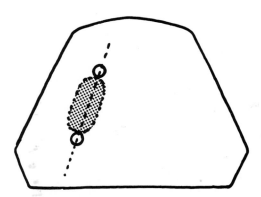

FIG. 7.12. Leverage, as such, is not a problem with the unilateral type of removable partial denture, although torsional stresses on the abutment teeth are operant because of the tendency of the prosthesis to rotate about a line which extends through the occlusal rests of the two clasps.

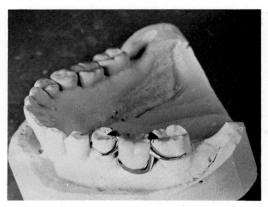

FIG. 7.13. A unilateral removable partial denture. Although the removable prosthesis is not usually the restoration of choice for such an edentulous space, the prosthesis shown in the photograph replaces one that the patient had worn successfully for 15 years. It was remade at the patient's request, because she had dropped and distorted the original prosthesis.

bilateral in design. Ordinarily this is the preferred approach to the problem. If the unilateral design must be used, all four clasp arms should be made retentive, to minimize the tendency of the prosthesis to rotate around a line which extends mesiodistally through the two abutment teeth.

Clasp Design as a Means of Stress Control

A comparison of the stress that is exerted on the abutment tooth by a circumferential clasp, as opposed to a bar type clasp, discloses the fact that the design of the clasp can affect markedly the type of stress that is transmitted to the abutment tooth. The clasp terminal of the circumferential type clasp, that engages the retentive undercut on the mesiobuccal surface of a bicuspid (Fig. 7.14), reacts to a tissue-ward displacement of the base by engaging the undercut. When a lifting force is applied to the base, the retentive terminal moves away from the undercut. Just the opposite is true of the bar type clasp, which engages an undercut on the distobuccal surface of the same tooth (Fig. 7.15). When an occlusal load is applied to the base, the retentive terminal of the bar type clasp moves away from the undercut. When the lifting force is applied, the terminal engages the undercut.

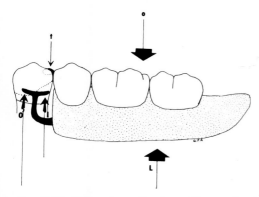

FIG. 7.15. This schematic shows the resultant stress from a distal extension base transmitted to the abutment tooth by a bar type clasp. A force, directed against the occlusal surfaces of the teeth at *o*, is transmitted to the abutment as an upward force at *O*. A lifting force at *L* is transmitted to the tooth as downward movement of the clasp at *l*. The fulcrum is at *f*.

Although this would seem to provide evidence that the circumferential clasp exerts more stress on the abutment than does the bar type clasp, such a conclusion is an over-simplification of an enormously complex problem.

The Combination Clasp as a Means of Stress Control

The combination clasp can be employed to reduce the stress that is transmitted to the abutment tooth by the distal extension base, because the wrought wire retentive arm of the combination clasp will absorb more stress than will the conventional cast clasp. The explanation for this is that, by virtue of its internal structure, the wrought wire is capable of flexing in any spatial plane (Fig. 7.16). This means that it can absorb the effect of a torsional stress as readily as one in a vertical or horizontal plane.

Indirect Retention as a Means of Stress Control

Indirect retention can be an effective retardant to movement of the distal extension base, thus reducing the stress to which the abutment teeth are exposed. An indirect retainer is an element of the re-

movable partial denture that is (usually) anterior to the fulcrum line, the function of which is to counteract the tipping forces which act on the prosthesis from the opposite side of the fulcrum line (Fig. 7.17). The fulcrum, or load, line is the imaginary line or lines which might be drawn through the abutment teeth, around which the partial denture would tend to rotate were it not prevented from doing so by other structural elements of the prosthesis. There might be one, two, or several fulcrum lines, depending upon the number and position of the remaining teeth and the location of the clasps. An embrasure rest, a lingual plate, a double lingual bar, an occlusal rest, or even a part of the denture base itself may perform the function of indirect retainer.

The principle of indirect retention is classically illustrated in the Kennedy Class I mandibular denture (Fig. 7.18). It enables the designer to exploit the mechanical advantage of leverage in the control of stress. The farther anterior to the fulcrum line that the indirect retainer can be positioned, the more effective will be its influence, since lengthening the counterbalance magnifies its neutralizing effect. Another advantage of an indirect retainer, such as a Kennedy bar or a lingual plate, is that the load is distributed to several teeth, thus minimizing the stress to be borne by any single tooth. Moreover, depending on the design, the indirect retainer may contribute a sub-

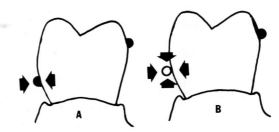

FIG. 7.16. The cast clasp, shown in cross section at *A*, is capable of flexing primarily in a mesiodistal direction, while the wrought wire clasp, shown at *B*, will flex in any spatial plane by virtue of its internal structure.

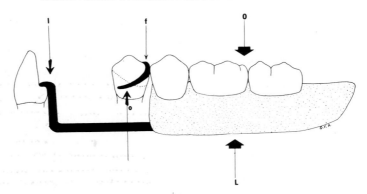

FIG. 7.17. The principle of indirect retention is depicted schematically here. The function of the indirect retainer, *I*, is to counteract lifting and tipping forces, *L*, which act on the prosthesis from the opposite side of the fulcrum line, *f*. When an occlusal force is applied at *O*, it is counteracted by the terminal of the circumferential clasp, *o*, engaging the undercut.

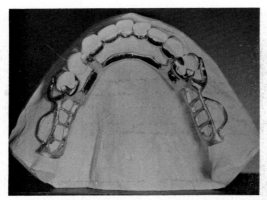

FIG. 7.18. A Kennedy bar, or double lingual bar, employed as an indirect retainer.

stantial measure of stability, as well as support, to the denture. Finally, the indirect retainer in the mandibular arch may serve a dual purpose by preventing rotation of a lingual bar of unusual length into contact with the underlying mucosa (Fig. 7.19).

The requirement for indirect retention is substantially less for the denture with only one distal extension base (the Kennedy Class II), because of the retention contributed by the two clasped teeth on the dentulous side of the arch. The indirect retainer should be placed as far anteriorly to the fulcrum line as is feasible, preferably on the contralateral side of the

midline from the distal extension base (Fig. 7.20).

The Kennedy Class III denture ordinarily requires no indirect retention, since there is no distal extension base to create a lever arm (Fig. 7.21). A fulcrum line may be created with the Kennedy Class IV denture, as for example, when embrasure type clasps are employed. In the photograph, Fig. 7.22, a fulcrum line extends

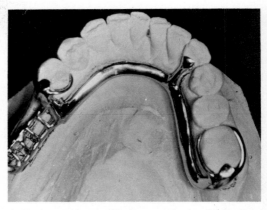

FIG. 7.19. A mandibular prosthesis which shows an application of indirect retention. The lingual rest on the right cuspid has been placed in a prepared recess in the tooth. This particular indirect retainer serves a dual purpose, in that it will also prevent the long lingual bar from rotating into contact with the underlying soft tissue should the denture base settle downward.

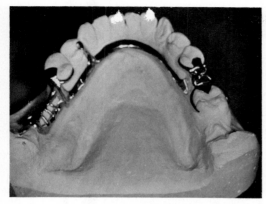

FIG. 7.20. The photograph shows an indirect retainer placed in the mesial fossa of the first bicuspid. The longer the edentulous span is, the greater the amount of leverage will be, and hence the greater the need for indirect retention.

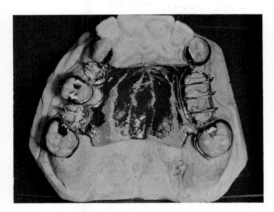

FIG. 7.21. The Kennedy Class III type of removable partial denture ordinarily requires no indirect retention, since there are no distal extension bases. The lingual rest, shown in the photograph on the right cuspid, is employed for support—rather than for indirect retention.

Functional Basing as a Means of Stress Control

As a result of the displaceable nature of the oral mucosa, the edentulous alveolar ridge is capable of assuming two markedly different contours. One, the resting or passive form, is registered when a soft impression material such as alginate or agar is used. The other is the supporting, or functioning, form which is the contour assumed when the denture base is subjected to an occlusal load. The theory underlying the technique of functional basing is that the residual ridge should be registered in its functioning form, instead of its resting form, so that when subjected to occlusal loading it will not be displaced to any appreciable extent. Hence, the magnitude of the stress transmitted to the abutment will be substantially reduced.

The Occlusion as a Means of Stress Control

The type of occlusion can contribute materially to the stability of the denture thus taking a load off the supporting structures, or it can add to the load to which they are subjected. Several factors govern the quality of the occlusion of the removable partial denture.

Harmonious Intercuspation. A smoothly functioning intercuspation will

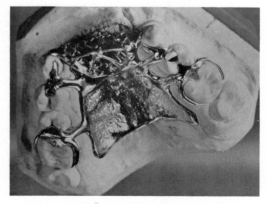

FIG. 7.22. In the photograph shown here, the fulcrum line extends through the occlusal rests of the molars clasps. Indirect retention is supplied by the occlusal-lingual rests on the bicuspids and cuspids.

through the occlusal rests of the molar clasps. Indirect retention is supplied by the occlusal-lingual rests on the bicuspids and cuspids on either side of the arch. The prime purpose of the rests shown here, however, is for support of the anterior segment of the denture rather than for retention of the denture by indirect means.

create a minimum of tipping forces, hence will transmit a minimum amount of stress to abutment teeth and residual ridges.

The Size of the Food Table. A large food table has the potential of transmitting considerably more pressure on both the residual ridges and the abutment teeth than does a small one. This factor would be negligible with a small morsel of food between the teeth, but would become substantial when the teeth were forced to penetrate a mass of fibrous food resistant to comminution.

The Occlusal Pattern of the Posterior Teeth. The occlusal pattern of the posterior teeth may influence the amount of stress. Cuspless teeth will generate more load on the denture base than will sharp cusp teeth, because of the increased power needed to force them through the bolus. The steep inclines of cusp teeth, on the other hand, may introduce horizontal forces which generate torsional stresses.

The Denture Base as a Means of Stress Control

A properly designed denture base can add materially to the stability, support, and retention of the prosthesis.

The Size and Configuration of the Base. Coverage of a large area of soft tissue by the base will distribute the functional stresses over a greater area of support, thus reducing the burden that must be borne by each supporting structure. The greater the number of teeth missing, the more urgent is the need for the stabilizing effect of having the denture flanges extend into the vestibules, in accordance with the principles of complete denture coverage. Flanges should provide a seal with the border tissues whenever it is possible to do so.

The Accuracy of the Adaptation of the Base to the Tissue. The more intimately the base fits the mucosa, the greater will be its adhesion, the less will be its tendency to movement, and the smaller will be the magnitude of the stress that is transmitted to the abutment.

The Form of the Polished Surfaces. Proper contour of the polished surfaces of the denture base will enable the adjacent musculature to exert a substantial degree of control over the base, thus diminishing the movement, hence the load that is transferred to the supporting units.

The Maxillary Connector as a Means of Stress Control

The major connector of the maxillary partial denture can contribute enormously to the support, stability, and retention of the prosthesis, thereby relieving the abutment teeth of a substantial amount of stress to which they would otherwise be exposed. This factor is dealt with in more detail in Chapter 9, The Design of Structural Units—Major Connectors.

A Summary of Basic Design Principles

The following paragraphs summarize an approach to partial denture design, based on a philosophy of wide stress distribution between the hard and soft tissues, which exploits the maximum supportive properties of each structure. The essence of the concept is the employment of multiple clasps and rests, broad tissue coverage, and harmonious occlusion.

1. Retention of the prosthesis should not be considered the prime objective of design. Instead, efficiency, esthetics, comfort, and preservation of oral health are the attributes which should be considered paramount.

2. The simplest type of clasp that will accomplish the design objectives should be employed. Clasps should be designed so as to have good stabilizing qualities, remain passive until activated by functional stress, and to accommodate a minor amount of movement of the base without transmitting a torque to the abutment tooth. Clasps should be strategically positioned in the arch to achieve the greatest possible control of stress.

3. Tooth support should be exploited to the extent that it is available. Abutment teeth should be prepared with rest seats which direct stress along the long axis of the tooth.

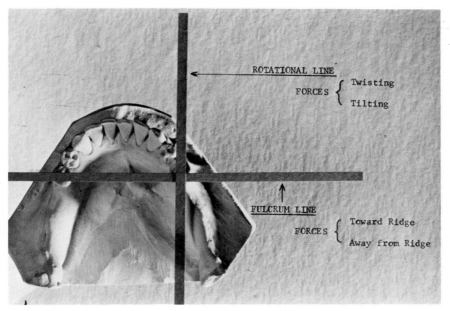

FIG. 7.23. The photograph shows a cast for a Kennedy Class I removable partial denture. Unseating and dislodging forces act around two principle fulcrums. One runs through the two abutment teeth—the *fulcrum line*. The second runs through each abutment in a mesio-distal direction—the *rotational line*.

Type of Force	Resultant Stress	Controls
	An Analysis of Forces Which Act Around the Fulcrum Line	
Occlusal loading	Towards the ridge Torsional stress on abutments	1. Occlusal rests 2. Base design (wide coverage) 3. Connector design (maxillary only) 4. Selection of proper tooth 5. Fewer teeth 6. Narrower teeth
Lifting force	Torsional stress on abutments	1. The clasps 2. Indirect retention 3. Base design 4. Tooth arrangement 5. Gravity (mandible only)
	An Analysis of Forces Which Act Around the Rotational Line	
Occlusal loading	Vertical and torsional stress on ridges Torsional stress on abutments	1. Harmonious occlusion 2. Good base design 3. Rigid connectors 4. Indirect retention 5. Clasp design
Lifting force	Torsional stress on abutments	

FIG. 7.24.

4. The simplest connector that will accomplish the objectives should be selected. Maxillary connectors should be chosen that will contribute to the support of the prosthesis commensurate with the requirements.

5. No part of the prosthesis should be permitted to impinge on the free gingival margin.

6. All connectors, major and minor, must be rigid.

7. The principle of indirect retention should be employed, when feasible, to neutralize unseating leverages.

8. A harmonious occlusion should be developed, to minimize the destructive types of stress on the residual ridges and the abutment teeth. This is accomplished by:
   a. Establishing true centric relation. Ideally centric occlusion and centric relation will coincide.
   b. Positioning the teeth in relation to the residual ridges, so as to be as mechanically advantageous as possible. Lower posterior teeth should be positioned over the crest of the mandibular ridge.
   c. Using smaller and/or fewer replacement teeth, and ones that are narrower buccolingually than the natural teeth.
   d. Ensuring that the replacement teeth will function efficiently, by providing sharp cutting edges and ample escape-ways.
   e. Providing a free-running, harmonious occlusion, and eliminating all interceptive contacts.

9. The base for the partial denture should be constructed on a cast of the mouth which has captured the soft tissue in its functional form.
   a. The base should be designed with broad coverage so as to enable the residual ridges to bear a substantial share of the load, and so that this load is distributed over as wide an area of support as the patient can comfortably tolerate.

The base must be intimately adapted to the underlying mucosa.
   b. The polished surfaces of the base should be contoured so as to enable the patient to exercise maximum neuromuscular control.

A Summary of Stress and Its Control

Functional pressures and forces that act on the denture base are operant around two principle fulcrums. One extends through the two abutment teeth and is termed the fulcrum line. The other, termed the rotational line, extends through the abutment tooth from mesial to distal (Fig. 7.23). The chart (Fig. 7.24) shows an analysis of the different types of functional stresses which are operant around each fulcrum, points out the resultant stress that is transmitted to the supporting structures, and gives an enumeration of the design factors which may be employed to counteract the harmful effects of these stresses.

Bibliography

Akers, P. E.: A new and simplified method of partial denture prosthesis. J Amer. Dent. Ass. *12:* 711–717, 1925.

Applegate, O. C.: Keeping the partial denture in harmony with biologic limitations. J. Amer. Dent. Ass. *43:* 409–419, 1951.

Augsburger, R. H.: Evaluating removable partial dentures by mathematical equations. J. Prosth. Dent. *22:* 528–543, 1969.

Elliott, F. C.: Partial denture prosthesis as a health service. J. Michigan Dent. Soc. *20:* 163–169, 1938.

Frechette, A. R.: The influence of partial denture design on distribution of force to abutment teeth. J. Prosth. Dent. *6:* 195–212, 1956.

Girardot, R. I.: History and development of partial denture design. J. Amer. Dent. Ass. *28:* 1399–1408, 1941.

Glickman, I.: The periodontal structures and removable partial denture prosthesis. J. Amer. Dent. Ass. *37:* 311–316, 1968.

Granger, E. R.: Mechanical principles applied to partial denture construction. J. Amer. Dent. Ass. *28:* 1943–1951, 1941.

Hickey, J. C.: Responsibility of the dentist in removable partial dentures. J. Kentucky Dent. Ass. *17:* 70–87, 1965.

Hughes, G. A.: Review of basic principles of removable partial denture prosthesis. Fortn. Rev. Chicago Dent. Soc. *13:* 9–13, 23, 1947.

Kaires, A. K.: Effect of partial denture design on bilateral force distribution. J. Prosth. Dent. *6:* 363–385, 1956.

Kaires, A. K.: Effect of partial denture design on unilateral force distribution. J. Prosth. Dent. *6:* 526–533, 1956.

Kelley, E. K.: The physiologic approach to partial denture design. J. Prosth. Dent. *3:* 699–710, 1953.

Perry, C.: Philosophy of partial denture design. J. Prosth. Dent. *6:* 775–784, 1956.

Potter, R. B., Appleby, R. C., and Adams, C. D.: Removable partial denture design: A review and a challenge, J. Prosth. Dent. *17:* 63–68, 1967.

Schuyler, C. H.: Stress distribution as a prime requisite to the success of a partial denture, J. Amer. Dent. Ass. *20:* 2148–2154, 1933.

Steffel, V. L.: Fundamental principles involved in partial denture design. J. Amer. Dent. Ass. *42:* 534–544, 1951.

Trapozzano, V. R., and Winter, G. R.: Periodontal aspects of partial denture design. J. Prosth. Dent. *2:*101–107, 1952.

Weinberg, L. A.: Lateral force in relation to the denture base and clasp design. J. Prosth. Dent. *6:* 785–800, 1956.

Chapter 8

THE DESIGN OF STRUCTURAL UNITS—THE PARTIAL DENTURE CLASP

This chapter deals with the makeup and function of the clasp and with the various types of clasps which are commonly employed in construction of the removable partial denture. Basic principles of clasp design are discussed as they relate to the clasp's intended function; the various criteria employed in selecting the most suitable clasp to satisfy a variety of clasping requirements are set forth, and the structural designs of seven basic clasps are described. Indications for the use of each clasp are presented. The chapter is organized into the sections which follow.

Introduction

The typical removable partial denture is made up of five structural elements, each of which plays a role in restoring function and preserving the remaining oral structures. These five structural units are: (1) the clasp, (2) the major connector, (3) the minor connector(s), (4) the base, and (5) the teeth. This chapter will be confined to a discussion of the clasp.

The clasp is often described as having a structure roughly analogous to man, being composed of a body, shoulders, and arms.

Actually, this is quite a fitting metaphor when applied to the circumferential clasp, although it is much less applicable to the bar type clasp. The components of the individual clasp have been given names, for convenience in discussion. In addition to the body, shoulder, and arms, other parts are the terminal, strut, and approach arm (Fig. 8.1).

The Functional Elements of the Clasp

Although it is customary to think of the clasp as being the working unit of the partial denture that retains the prosthesis in place, the reality is that, in addition to providing retention, the clasp has other equally important functions to perform. From a standpoint of function, the clasp has two arms (a retentive and a reciprocal arm), an occlusal rest, and a minor connector. Each of these elements fulfills as essential requirement of the prosthesis.

The Retentive Arm

The function of the retentive arm is to resist displacement on the tooth, thus maintaining the prosthesis in its proper position in the mouth. The retentive arm is structured so that the terminal third is flexible, the middle third has a limited flexibility, and the third which joins the body (the shoulders) has no flexibility whatever (Fig. 8.2).

The Reciprocal Arm

The reciprocal arm of the clasp is placed on the surface of the tooth opposite

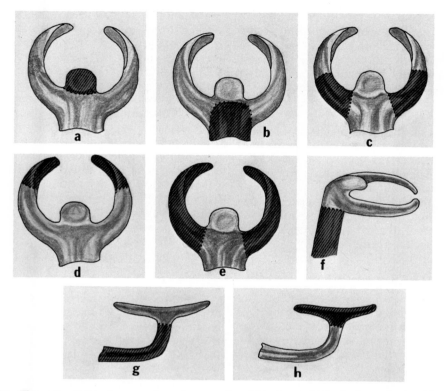

FIG. 8.1. The parts of the clasp are shown here: *a*, the occlusal rest; *b*, the body, *c*, the shoulders; *d*, the terminals; *e*, the clasp arms; *f*, the strut; *g*, the approach arm; and *h*, the terminal.

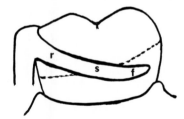

FIG. 8.2. The retentive arm of the clasp is made up of a retentive terminal which has a flexible portion, *f*, a part that has a limited flexibility, *s*, and a rigid part, *r*. Only the portion of the clasp with flexibility should be placed below the survey line.

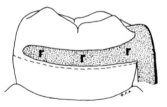

FIG. 8.3. The reciprocal arm of the clasp is rigid (*r*) throughout its length, and should always be positioned above the survey line.

the retentive arm. Its function is to counterbalance any stress generated against the tooth by the retentive arm. The reciprocal arm is rigid throughout its length. It contributes substantially to horizontal stability, and gives some support and a limited amount of retention, by virtue of its contact with the tooth surface (Fig. 8.3).

The Occlusal Rest, (lingual or incisal)

The occlusal rest is positioned in a prepared recess on the tooth surface, and resists displacement of the clasp in a gingival direction. In fulfilling this function it also prevents the clasp arms from spreading apart, which might occur if the clasp were permitted to slip gingivally on

occlusal rests - gingival & horizontal

the tooth. This applies, in particular, to the cingulum rest which has been placed on the steeply inclined lingual surface of the typical mandibular canine. The rest also contributes a substantial amount of resistance to horizontal movement.

The Minor Connector

This part of the clasp unites the body and arms to the remainder of the framework. Other terms by which it is frequently designated are truss arm, standard, tail, tang, and upright.

The Approach Arm. The approach arm is the minor connector which unites the clasp terminal of a bar type clasp with the remainder of the framework.

The Kinds of Clasps

Partial denture clasps are fabricated of several different alloys and combinations of alloys, and in a wide variety of shapes and forms, to meet a diverse array of requirements as well as to satisfy different design philosophies.

Clasps Classified on a Basis of Construction

Partial denture clasps may be classified on a basis of construction into (1) the cast clasp, (2) the wrought wire clasp, and (3) the combination clasp.

The Cast Clasp. The cast clasp is cast (with either gold or chromium-cobalt alloy) into a mold which has been formed by a wax or plastic pattern. The cast clasp is employed in perhaps 95% of removable partial dentures fabricated in the United States, a fact which would certainly attest to its wide acceptance by the profession, and would appear to speak for its merits as well.

The Wrought Clasp. The wrought wire clasp is usually made of gold alloy wire to which an occlusal rest is added by means of gold solder. The clasp is attached to the framework by means of a minor connector, or the minor connector may be simply processed into an acrylic resin base. The wrought form of any alloy is different in its internal structure from the cast form, as a result of the process by which it is

made. Gold wrought wire is made by the refiner from gold alloy which has been rolled, swaged, and drawn through progressively smaller die plates into a desired shape and gauge. The fabricating process imparts to the wire a fibrous structure which accounts for its toughness and resiliency. This unique difference in internal structure can be verified by examination and comparison of the two forms of the alloy under magnification. When observed under the lens of a microscope, the cast gold appears to be crystalline in structure, whereas the wrought wire is seen to be fibrous-like—not unlike the intertwined strands of a steel cable. As might be expected, the wrought wire form of the gold is extremely resilient. However, for this very reason, it possesses poor stabilizing properties.

The wrought wire clasp is not in widespread use today, mainly because the casting process has been so improved, and the cast type of partial denture so perfected, that it has been largely supplanted by the cast clasp.

The Combination Clasp. The combination clasp is essentially a cast clasp in which wrought wire has been substituted for the usual cast retentive arm. The combination clasp is customarily made by either of two methods. (1) The wrought wire arm can be attached to the body of the cast clasp with solder, or (2) the wrought wire can be embedded in position in the wax pattern of the clasp, the assembly invested, and the melted metal cast into the mold to envelope the wrought wire. The combination clasp may be constructed of several combinations of materials. These are: (1) gold wrought wire with cast gold alloy, (2) gold wrought wire with cast chromium-cobalt alloy, and (3) chromium-cobalt alloy wrought wire with cast chromium-cobalt alloy. The prime advantage of the combination clasp is the fact that the most worthwhile features of both types of clasp can be exploited: the resiliency of the wrought wire in the retentive arm, and the less resilient but better stabilizing features of the cast gold for the body, rest, and reciprocal arm.

Advantages of the Combination Clasp. Not only is the wrought wire retentive arm more resilient than its cast counterpart, but it has, in addition, the capability of flexing in all spatial planes (Fig. 8.4). This is a profoundly important advantage, because it enables the clasp to neutralize better the torsional type of stress to which the abutment tooth may be subjected in service. The retentive arm of the cast clasp is also capable of flexing, but the flexure will be principally in a horizontal plane, albeit some degree of edgewise movement is possible. However, if this be true, then it is equally true that the extreme flexibility of the wrought wire arm reduces the horizontal stability of the combination clasp, and it may be fairly contended that the increased movement of the base which this permits will subject the residual ridges to a proportionately greater degree of lateral stress.

Clasps Classified on a Basis of Design

Cast clasps are designed in a wide variety of shapes, in order to engage the multitude of different configurations of tooth surfaces where usable retentive undercut areas happen to be located, as well as to cope with an almost infinite variety of tooth size, long axis inclination, and retention requirements. Clasps are often classified on a basis of design into (1) the circumferential type clasp (also Akers, suprabulge), and (2) the bar type clasp (also vertical projection, Roach, infrabulge).

The Circumferential Type Clasp. The circumferential type clasp is characterized by the fact that the retentive terminal approaches the undercut of the tooth from above the survey line (Fig. 8.5a). This type of retention is sometimes described as a "pull" type of retention.

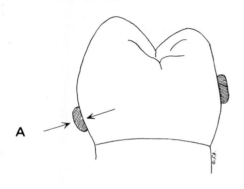

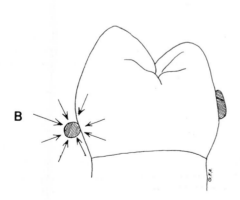

Fig. 8.4. The wrought wire arm of the combination clasp is capable of flexing in all planes, as depicted by the arrows in *B*. The cast clasp arm, shown in *A*, will flex readily in a horizontal plane (*arrows*), but has a severely limited capability of flexing in any other plane.

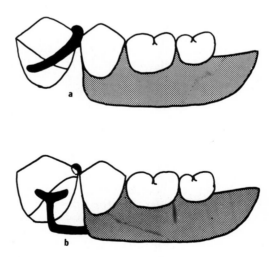

Fig. 8.5. The retentive arm of the circumferential type clasp approaches the undercut from an occlusal direction (*a*). The retentive arm of the bar type clasp approaches the undercut from a cervical direction (*b*).

The Bar Type Clasp. The bar type clasp is characterized by the fact that the retentive terminal approaches the undercut on the tooth from below the survey line (Fig. 8.5b). The bar type clasp is said to have a "push" type of retention.

The Six Attributes of a Properly Designed Clasp

The function of a properly designed clasp is to contribute retention, stability, and support to the prosthesis. The clasp should also possess the attributes of encirclement, reciprocity, and passivity.

Retention

Retention is the property which enables the clasp to resist dislodgment from the tooth in an occlusal direction. A dislodging force may be activated by speech, muscle action, mastication, deglutition, sticky foods, or gravity. The clasp arm is retentive, by virtue of the fact that it is positioned on a surface of the tooth that is cervical to its greatest circumference, and the alloy resists the distortion (flexion) which is required for the clasp arm to escape from this area beneath the bulge of the tooth. Thus, a measure of its flexibility is its capability of distorting momentarily as it is forced over the greatest diameter of the tooth. Another, although far less effective, factor in retention is friction. The degree of frictional resistance is dependent on the type of interface which exists between the tooth and the clasp. Gold offers more resistance to the clasp arm that does enamel, for example. Other factors are the amount of tooth surface covered, the intimacy of tooth clasp contact, the type of alloy (the cast form of the alloy is more retentive than is the wrought wire form), and the direction of approach of the retentive terminal. The prime factor influencing the degree of retention possessed by the clasp is, of course, the amount of horizontal undercut engaged by the retentive tip, coupled with the resiliency of the clasp arm. The degree of resiliency possessed by the clasp arm is dependent on the following factors:

1. The length of the clasp arm. The greater the length, the greater the resiliency.

2. The diameter of the retentive arm. The smaller the diameter, the greater the resiliency.
3. The cross-sectional form. A round clasp arm is more resilient than one that is half round or oval in shape.
4. The taper. Proper taper can increase flexibility as much as fourfold. Taper makes possible the thin, highly flexible fishing rod, and allows the archer's bow to bend without breaking. The retentive arm of the clasp should taper evenly and uniformly from its origin at the body of the clasp to its terminal extremity. In the case of a circumferential clasp arm, the arm should measure approximately one-half the diameter at the tip that it measures at its origin. A clasp so tapered will have approximately four times the degree of flexibility of one which has not been properly tapered. Similarly, the approach arm of the bar type clasp should be tapered uniformly from its origin at the framework to the terminal.
5. The kind of alloy. The chromium-cobalt alloys have a higher modulus of elasticity, hence are not as resilient as gold alloys of the same diameter.
6. The type of alloy. An alloy in wrought form is more resilient than the same alloy of identical diameter in cast form, because of its internal structure.
7. Heat treatment of the alloy. Proper heat treatment, of gold in particular, will increase the resilience substantially, whereas improper heat treatment may render it brittle and with no resilience whatever.

Stabilization

Stabilization, or bracing, is the resistance which the clasp contributes to displacement of the prosthesis in a horizontal plane. All of the clasp components, with the exception of the retentive terminal, contribute this property in varying degrees. It is worthy of note that the cast circumferential clasp is a better stabilizing clasp than is either the bar clasp or the combination clasp, by virtue of having two rigid clasp shoulders, and also because the retentive elements of those two clasps are more resilient.

Support

Support is the property of the clasp which enables it to resist displacement in a gingival direction. The occlusal (lingual or incisal) rest is the prime support unit of the clasp, although the body and the shoulder of the clasp, positioned as they are above the greatest diameter of the tooth, also contribute a substantial amount of support.

Encirclement

The clasp should be so designed that it encircles at least 180 degrees of the crown of the tooth, to preclude movement of the tooth out of the confines of the clasp arms as stresses are applied.

Reciprocity

Reciprocation may be defined as "the means by which one part of the appliance is made to counter the effect created by another part." Applying this to the partial denture clasp, reciprocity may be defined as "the means by which the effect of the retentive clasp arm on the abutment tooth is countered by the action of the nonretentive clasp arm" (Fig. 8.6). Reciprocation is needed most when the retentive terminal flexes over the bulge of the crown during insertion and removal of the prosthesis. Unless the clasp is properly designed, this reciprocating force is not operant at the precise instant that it is most needed. Many clasps do not fulfill

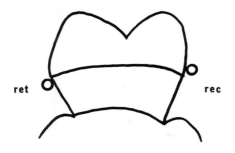

FIG. 8.6. The reciprocal arm of the clasp (rec) acts on the tooth surface opposite the retentive arm (ret) to counteract any stress which the retentive arm exerts against the tooth.

this important requirement because the contour of the abutment tooth is such that the reciprocal arm of the clasp must be placed much higher occlusally on the surface of the tooth than is the retentive arm. When this is true, the reciprocal arm may barely have come into contact with the tooth surface at the instant that the retentive arm flexes over the height of contour and arrives at its terminal position in the infrabulge. As a result, the retentive arm exerts a fleeting, unreciprocated thrust (whiplash) against the tooth each time that the prosthesis is inserted or removed from the mouth. Whether the clasp arm flexes or the tooth shifts momentarily, or a combination of the two occurs, is dependent upon the relative mobility of the tooth and the flexibility of the clasp. Whichever occurs, the periodontal ligament may be stretched or pinched, or both, depending on the magnitude of the force and the direction of movement. The periodontal apparatus may have the capacity to withstand this relatively minor stress over a prolonged period of time, depending on the host resistance factor, but there is little question that the prognosis for the abutment tooth would be materially improved if it were not permitted to occur. From a standpoint of abutment longevity, *all clasps should be planned and designed so that the two arms of the clasp are in balance, i.e., with the two arms positioned on their respective tooth surfaces at the same horizontal level. Thus any thrust exerted by the retentive arm is simultaneously counteracted by the reciprocal arm.* Careful surveying, when the treatment plan is being formulated, coupled with judicious alteration of the tooth surface, may serve to spare the tooth from this damaging overload. The principle of reciprocity should also be operant in stabilizing the prosthesis against the horizontal types of stress which are generated by functional movement of the prosthesis.

Passivity

When the clasp is in place on the tooth, it should be passive. This means that it should exert no pressure against the tooth until it is activated either by movement of the prosthesis in function, or in being removed from the mouth. Since some slight movement of the denture base in function is inevitable, because of the inherent displacability of the soft tissue foundation, passivity is an important requirement of a properly designed clasp. A clasp so designed will permit a slight degree of movement of the base without transmitting any appreciable amount of stress to the abutment tooth.

Miscellaneous Considerations in Clasp Design

The Retentive Undercut

The term "retentive undercut" is ofttimes misunderstood, because there is a tendency to confuse the three spatial planes which are involved. The dimension of pivotal importance, which critically affects the degree of retention possessed by the clasp, is the one in a buccolingual direction in the horizontal plane. This is the dimension (A-B) in Figure 8.7. This is the plane in which the retentive tip of the clasp flexes as it passes over the bulge of greatest circumference of the tooth and into the undercut. The dimensions of the clasp, relative to the other spatial planes, are of much less significance as depicted in the sketch.

Buccal versus Lingual Retention

The question of whether or not it is permissible to place the retentive clasp arm on the lingual surface of the tooth is sometimes raised. When the most favorable retentive undercut is on the lingual surface of the abutment, there is no logical reason for not placing the retentive arm on this surface and the reciprocal arm on the buccal surface. The one drawback to this procedure is that it may be more difficult for the patient to remove the clasp from the tooth when the retentive terminal is on the lingual surface. A question closely related to the foregoing is: When lingual retention is employed on one side of the arch, is it imperative that lingual retention be employed on the other side of the arch also? Since the clasps are passive until activated, and are united by a rigid connector, there is no valid reason why this need be done. Buccal retention on one side of the arch, opposed to lingual retention on the other side, is perfectly permissible and may be employed with no fear of ill effects.

How Much Undercut?

Oftentimes the retentive properties of a removable partial denture will be extolled because it "snapped into place" when it was inserted. The reality is that, far from denoting a virtue, this indicates an excessive amount of retention. Assuming proper diameter and taper of the clasp arm, it indicates that the resilient clasp tip is required to flex over too great a

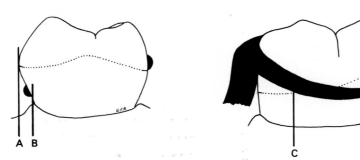

FIG. 8.7. Retentive undercut is measured by the amount that the clasp terminal must flex in a horizontal plane, as dipicted by the dimension AB. The dimension indicated by CD is much less significant, while the dimension EF plays a very minor role in the amount of retention possessed by the clasp.

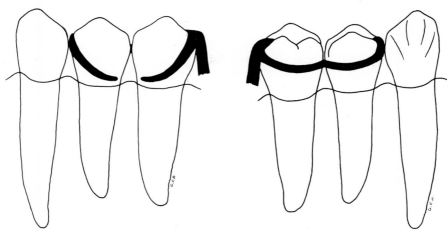

Fig. 8.8. Clasps can be employed to splint two or more teeth together, in instances when a fixed splint cannot be used. Two teeth united by two connected circlet clasps to form a multiple circlet clasp are shown on the left in a buccal view and on the right in a lingual view.

diameter of the tooth in order to enter an excessively severe undercut on the tooth surface. Unless the retentive clasp arm is perfectly balanced by the reciprocal arm, this is very apt to overstress the tooth over a period of time. It must be clear from the foregoing that a properly designed clasp should require only a moderate amount of pressure to seat on the tooth, and there should be no sensation of snapping or clicking as the clasp arms glide into the infrabulge.

The degree of retention supplied by a clasp relates directly to the flexibility of the retentive arm, and to the depth of the tooth undercut into which the terminal is placed. Therefore, when designing the clasp, the factors of (1) type of alloy to be used (gold is more flexible than chromium-cobalt), and (2) tooth to be clasped (a molar clasp arm is longer, hence more flexible than a bicuspid or a cuspid clasp arm), must be borne in mind so that an amount of undercut commensurate with these factors can be employed. As a general rule of thumb, a clasp made of chromium-cobalt alloy for a bicuspid should engage approximately 0.010 inch of undercut, while 0.015 inch of undercut is approximately the right amount for a molar clasp arm. An undercut of 0.020 inch would normally be excessive for a chromium-cobalt

clasp because of its relatively low resilience (high modulus of elasticity), but this amount of undercut might be used for a gold wrought wire retentive clasp arm on a molar tooth.

How Many Clasps?

This question cannot be decided by any formula but, from a standpoint of ideal design, a sufficient number of clasps should be employed, so that the stress which is borne by each abutment tooth is safely below its physiological tolerance level. Obviously, this entails taking into account the retention, support, and stability contributed by all of the other components of the prosthesis, and weighing them in the balance against the dislodging forces which the prosthesis may reasonably be expected to withstand.

Splinting with Clasps

Properly designed clasps can be employed to splint two or several teeth together for the same reasons that fixed splinting is done (Figs. 8.8 and 8.9). The procedure is, in fact, an excellent means of accomplishing a wide distribution of masticatory loads, and it has the advantage over the typical unilateral fixed splint of being stabilized against hori-

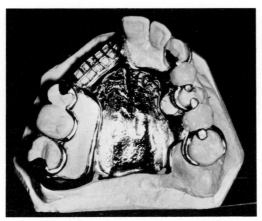

FIG. 8.9. All of the maxillary teeth shown here are, in effect, splinted together, with the exception of the central and lateral incisors. Stress is divided among six teeth, thus reducing the amount of stress that must be borne by any one tooth.

zontal stress by teeth on the other side of the arch. However, since the prosthesis should be left out of the mouth for an interval of sleep, the benefits of splinting are lost during this period.

Retention of Bar versus Circumferential Type Clasps

The retentive properties of the bar type clasp and the circumferential type clasp are often compared. The bar type clasp is said to have a "push" type retention, while the circumferential clasp is described as a "pull" type retention. In comparing the effectiveness of the two clasps from a standpoint of retention, the analogy is sometimes used of the force required to push a wheelbarrow over a curb, as compared to the force required to pull it over the curb. The analogy highlights the fact that the bar type clasp is more retentive, all else being equal. It might be expected, therefore, that the push type clasp is easier to seat on the tooth but more difficult to remove from it, while the pull type clasp requires more force to seat it and less to remove it. This could be an important consideration in an instance where the abutment tooth offered a less-than-ideal amount of retentive undercut.

Leverage and Esthetics in Clasp Design

A fundamental of clasp design is that the arms should be placed as low on the crown, within limits, as the survey line will permit, so as to reduce the effect of leverage. It should not be placed so close to the marginal gingiva that this area is not self-cleansing, however (Fig. 8.10).

The Basis for Clasp Selection

If there were such an entity as an ideal clasp it would first of all, be applicable in any clasping situation. Besides providing adequate retention, support, and stability, it would encircle more than 180 degrees of the tooth, possess balanced reciprocation and, when in place on the tooth, it would remain passive until activated. The clasp arms would make minimal contact with the tooth surface and would not increase the circumference of the crown. Finally, it would be neither complicated nor expensive to construct, relatively simple to adjust or repair, and completely acceptable from a viewpoint of esthetics. Although it is obvious that no such paragon of claspdom exists, the simple circlet clasp, when considered from all aspects, manages to come closer to meeting these specifications than any other. While it cannot be employed universally, and is not always the most esthetic, it is the most versatile by any standard, and fulfills the

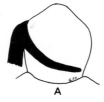
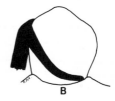

A   B

FIG. 8.10. Clasp arms should be placed low on the crown of the tooth, to minimize the effect of leverage and to be less obtrusive esthetically, as shown in A. However, the retentive arm should not be placed so low as to interfere with self-cleansing of the tooth surface, or the natural stimulation of the gingival margin. The clasp arm shown in B may harbor debris, because it is too close to the gingival margin.

requirements of retention, stabilization, support, encirclement, passivity, and reciprocity as well as any, and better than most, other clasps.

Factors in Clasp Selection

Factors which govern the selection of a particular clasp for a given clasping situation are (1) the tooth to be clasped (whether molar, bicuspid, or cuspid), (2) the tooth surface (lingual, labial or buccal), (3) the area on the tooth where the most favorable retentive undercut is to be found (mesial or distal), and (4) the esthetic requirement (will it be visible?). Additional factors of no less importance are the requirements for interocclusal space in the case of the embrasure clasp, for example, and the need for sufficient tooth surface for a double width of clasp in the case of the hairpin clasp. Not to be overlooked is the requirement for a suitable site on the tooth surface to accommodate a rest recess. A cardinal principle of partial denture design is to select the simplest clasp that will fulfill the requirements.

The surfaces of an abutment tooth suitable for clasping, i.e., the buccal or lingual, can usually be divided by the survey line roughly into quadrants (Fig. 8.11). These quadrants may be designated mesioocclusal, and distoocclusal, mesiogingival, and distogingival. The two occlusal quadrants of either tooth surface may be ignored for purposes of tooth clasping, because there is rarely a usable undercut in this region of the tooth, and if one were present it would be esthetically poor, as well as mechanically unsound, to place a retentive clasp tip on this area of the tooth. Thus, for all practical purposes, the designer may consider either of the four gingival quadrants as suitable zones into which to place the clasp tip. These zones are depicted in the drawings (Fig. 8.12) as shaded areas which indicate the quadrants where undercuts are typically present, and the manner in which four types of clasps might be adapted to exploit each undercut. A variety of clasp designs, applied to undercuts on different areas of the tooth, are shown in the sketches (Fig. 8.13).

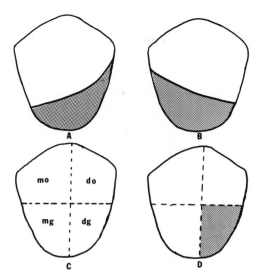

FIG. 8.11. The surfaces of the abutment tooth, both buccal and lingual, may be roughly divided by the survey line, A, and B, into four quadrants—mesio- and distoocclusal, and mesio- and distogingival—as depicted in C. The shaded quadrant in D indicates the location of a typical retentive undercut.

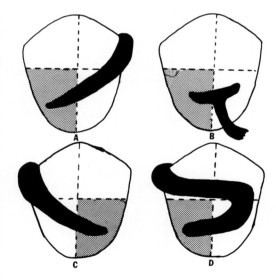

FIG. 8.12. The gingival quadrants of either the buccal or lingual surfaces are ideal sites for the clasp terminal, provided they possess a retentive undercut. This sketch depicts four different clasp designs, engaging retentive undercuts in different quadrants (*shaded areas*).

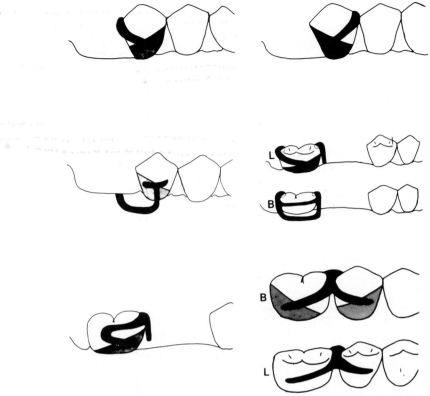

FIG. 8.13. Depicted schematically are six clasp designs designs showing appropriate undercuts. *Upper left*, simple circlet clasp; *upper right*, reverse approach circlet; *middle left*, "T" bar; *middle right*, ring clasp; *lower left*, reverse loop clasp; *lower right*, embrasure clasp.

Seven Basic Clasp Designs

When the simple circlet clasp is supplemented by six additional clasps of varied design but similar attributes, the designer is prepared for most of the clasping problems commonly encountered in practice. The following seven clasps will collectively meet the demands of all but the most extraordinary clasping requirement.

The Simple Circlet Clasp

The most universally employed of all clasp designs, the simple circlet clasp is highly versatile and lends itself to use on any tooth, maxillary or mandibular, when a retentive undercut exists in a favorable location. Generally, this is on the surface of the abutment remote from the edentulous space (Fig. 8.14). It is customary to design the buccal arm into a retentive undercut, but it is perfectly acceptable to place the lingual arm into a lingual undercut when it is the more favorable one. When the lingual arm is made retentive, the buccal arm should be made the reciprocal element, by making it inflexible and positioning it on or above the guide line.

The properties of retention, support, reciprocity, stability, encirclement, and passivity are readily designed into the simple circlet clasp, and it is not only easily adjusted, but comparatively simple to repair, as well. With all its merit, however, it does possess some disadvantages. It increases the circumference of the crown and tends to deflect food off and away from the tooth, thus depriving the pericoronal gingiva of needed physiological stimulation. Another negative attribute is the fact that the circumferential clasp is sometimes not as acceptable,

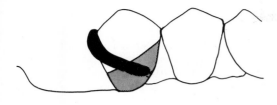

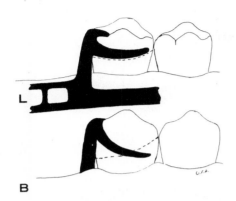

B

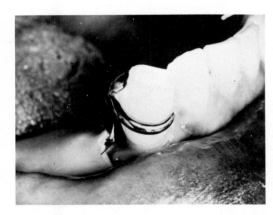

FIG. 8.14. The simple circlet is the most commonly used clasp when the undercut is in the mesiogingival quadrant of either the buccal or lingual surfaces of an abutment which is adjacent to an edentulous space.

from a cosmetic standpoint, on teeth in the anterior part of the mouth that are frequently on display. Finally, the retentive undercuts on some teeth are difficult to reach with the retentive terminal of this clasp.

The Reverse Approach Circlet (Fig. 8.15)

This clasp is most often employed on mandibular bicuspids, when the most fa-

vorable retentive undercut is on the distobuccal surface adjacent to the edentulous area. It is particularly useful when the bar type clasp is contraindicated because the approach arm must bridge over a soft tissue undercut, or when a hairpin clasp is not suitable because the crown of the abutment tooth is too short to accommodate the double width of clasp. An advantage of this clasp, from a biomechanical standpoint, is the fact that the occlusal

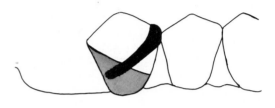

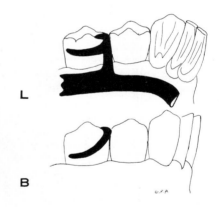

L

B

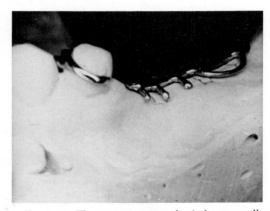

FIG. 8.15. The reverse approach circlet generally is used to engage an undercut in the distogingival quadrant adjacent to an edentulous space.

rest, located in the mesial fossa, exerts a mesially directed force on the abutment where it is reciprocated by an adjacent tooth, as opposed to a distally directed force exerted by the simple circlet clasp. Another advantage is that the stresses transmitted to the abutment by this clasp may be less stressful than those of a simple circlet clasp, because when the base is depressed the retentive tip swings away from the retentive bulge, and thus does not exert a torsional stress on the abutment tooth. When the base is dislodged by sticky food, the retentive tip engages the bulge and the base is stabilized. Because of this stabilizing influence, the reverse approach circumferential clasp may sometimes be employed to advantage, in lieu of an indirect retainer. It is particularly suitable when a distal extension base partial denture is opposed by a complete denture, so that securing adequate interocclusal clearance for the shoulders and rest poses no problem. One disadvantage of the reverse approach circlet clasp is that the gingival mucosa at the distal of the abutment tooth may not be as well sheltered as would be the case with the conventional circlet clasp.

Because of its position on the mesial surface of the tooth, it may be poor esthetically, and so it is not usually the clasp of choice for the maxillary bicuspids. The reverse approach circlet clasp may be contraindicated when the opposing occlusion is extremely tight, so that creating the needed space for the rest and shoulders would require a prohibitive amount of cutting of the abutment tooth and/or its antagonist.

The Bar Clasp (Fig. 8.16)

The "T" bar clasp, or one of its modifications, best exemplifies the type of clasp which is characterized by the fact that the retentive terminal approaches the undercut from a gingival direction. One of the most frequent applications of this clasp is to retain the distal extension base type of denture by engaging an undercut on the distobuccal surface of the abutment

tooth. It may be employed with either cuspids or bicuspids, and even molars, although much less often. It is used often on the distolabial surface of mandibular cuspids and the distobuccal surface of bicuspids, because the retentive tip can normally be discreetly hidden from view in this location. It is rarely indicated on

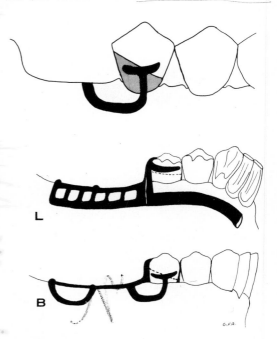

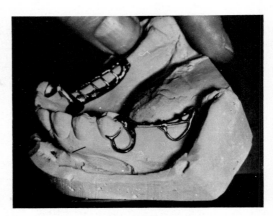

FIG. 8.16. The "T" bar clasp, or one of its variations, is the most commonly employed bar type clasp. It is frequently employed, as portrayed here, to engage an undercut on the distobuccal surface of a mandibular bicuspid adjacent to a distal extension base.

the tooth surface with an unusually high survey line, and it should not be employed in situations where the approach arm must bridge over a soft tissue undercut, because of the hazard of fibrous food retention. While the bar clasp is esthetically superior to the circumferential type clasp in some circumstances, it does not contribute stability to the degree that the circumferential clasp does, because of the flexibility of its retentive element.

As a general rule, only half of the terminal should be placed in the infrabulge.

The Ring Clasp (Fig. 8.17)

This clasp is most often used on mandibular molars which are tipped out of normal alignment so that the most favorable undercut is typically on the mesiolin-gual surface. It is employed, although less frequently, on maxillary molars which typically tip mesiobuccally. When used on a maxillary molar, the clasp encircles the tooth beginning on the mesiolingual surface and terminates in an infrabulge on the mesiobuccal surface. The ring clasp should not be designed without an auxiliary bracing arm, because without this rigid element the clasp does not possess reciprocity and contributes little to horizontal stability, since such a large portion of the clasp is flexible. A further disadvantage of the ring clasp without an auxiliary brace is the fact that it is prone to get out of adjustment and is difficult to readjust. Such a clasp is also difficult to repair. The ring clasp is contraindicated when there is a soft tissue undercut in the buccal area adjacent to a mandibular

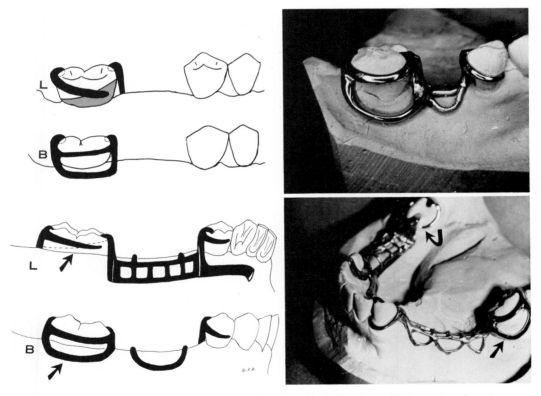

FIG. 8.17. The ring clasp is especially suited for the lingually inclined mandibular molar when the retentive undercut is on the mesiolingual surface. Note the auxiliary bracing arm on the buccal side. The ring clasp requires adequate space in the buccal vestibule for the auxiliary brace, which is essential in providing a rigid reciprocal arm on the buccal surface of the tooth.

molar, which must be occupied by the auxiliary reinforcing arm. Similarly, it is not a good choice when the buccinator muscle attachment is so close to the crown of the tooth that there is danger that the auxiliary brace might encroach upon it.

Occlusal rests in both mesial and distal fossae are preferred when this clasp design is used.

The Reverse Loop Clasp (The Hairpin Clasp) (Fig. 8.18)

This clasp design can be employed when the usable undercut is on the buccal surface of the tooth adjacent to the edentulous space. Its most common use is on mesially inclined mandibular molars when the most favorable retentive area is on the mesiobuccal surface. It may be employed on mandibular bicuspids when the reverse approach circlet or bar clasp are not suitable for one reason or another. However the crown of the abutment must be of at least average height, to provide sufficient surface for the double width of clasp arm. Only the lower arm of this clasp should enter the undercut.

This clasp is far from ideal from a cosmetic standpoint, and for this reason its use is confined primarily to abutments that are not readily observable from the front of the mouth. It is seldom the choice on maxillary bicuspids because of their prominence, although it is often used with success on mandibular bicuspids.

The Embrasure Clasp (Fig. 8.19)

This clasp is essentially two simple circlet clasps joined at the bodies, hence the

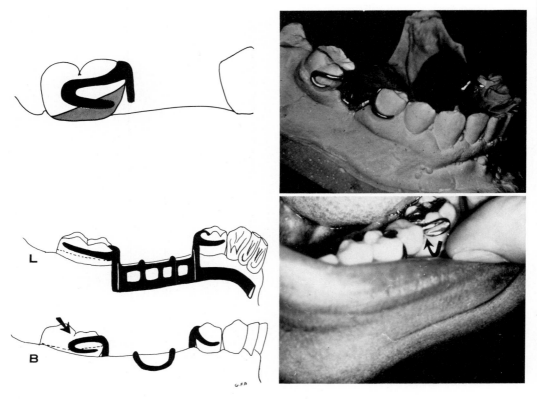

FIG. 8.18. The reverse loop clasp lends itself well for use when the usable retentive undercut is in the mesiogingival quadrant of the buccal surface of a mandibular molar. The reverse loop requires that the crown of the abutment tooth have sufficient vertical height to accommodate the double width of the retentive clasp arm.

commonly used synonyms of "double Akers" and "back to back" clasp. The embrasure clasp is indispensable in a quadrant of the mouth where retention must be obtained and there is no edentu-

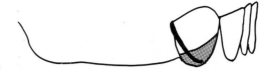

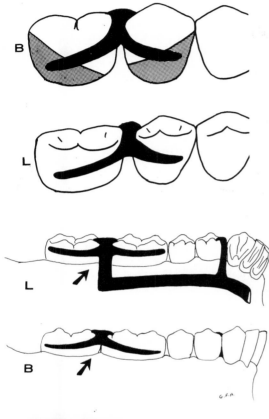

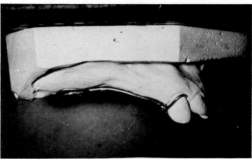

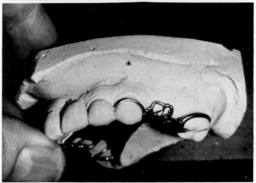

FIG. 8.20. The combination clasp may be indicated when the undercut on the abutment tooth is unusually severe, as a result of an anomalous contour or of tipping of the tooth. The exceptional flexibility of the wrought wire allows the retentive arm to flex sufficiently to pass over the bulge and into the undercut without overstressing the tooth. Because the wrought arm of the combination clasp reflects light differently from the cast arm, it may be more acceptable, cosmetically, on an anterior tooth when placed near the gingival margin.

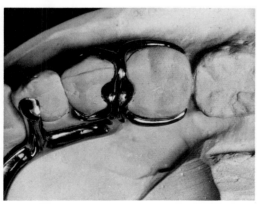

FIG. 8.19. The embrasure clasp is usually indicated when the retention must be secured in a quadrant of the mouth that is completely dentulous.

lous space to provide ingress for a simpler design of clasp. Its application in the Kennedy Class III typ of partial denture is a typical example. Since the embrasure clasp must cross the occlusal surfaces and occupy the occlusal embrasures of two adjoining teeth, it is essential that ample space be provided for the clasp shoulders so that they do not interfere with the opposing occlusion, and that definite recesses are provided for the occlusal rests to preclude any wedging effect that the clasp might otherwise exert on the teeth. The ideal approach, when this clasp is to be employed, is to crown the two abutments and in the fabrication of the crowns to provide ample clearance in the wax patterns. If crowns cannot be used for valid reasons, and a prohibitive amount of grinding is needed to create interocclusal space, it is sometimes preferable to extract a bicuspid on the dentulous side of the arch, thereby making possible the clasping of the two teeth adjacent to the edentulous space.

The Combination Clasp (Fig. 8.20)

The prime application for the combination clasp is for the abutment tooth that must be sheltered from all but a minimal amount of stress. Thus it is indicated for the abutment tooth that has been weakened by bone loss from periodontal disease. Similarly, it may be a boon to any abutment tooth that supports a distal extension base when indirect retention is not obtainable. By virtue of its extreme resiliency it can be used on a tooth when the undercut is exceptionally severe, thus requiring that the retentive arm distort an inordinate amount in order to enter the undercut.

The combination clasp is sometimes superior to any other clasp from a cosmetic viewpoint. Because of the manner in which light is reflected from the spherical surface of the wrought wire, and due to the fact that the wire can be positioned close to the gum line, it may be so unobtrusive as to escape notice completely in some mouths.

The end of the wrought wire arm should always be rounded and smoothed before the denture is placed in service, since damage to the tooth surface or injury to the gingiva is likely to result if the end of the wire is left sharp from being cut by the edge of the pliers.

Bibliography

Craddock, F. W., and Bottomley, G. A.: Second thoughts on clasping. Brit. Dent. J. *46:* 134–137, 1954.

DeVan, M. M.: Embrasure saddle clasp—its principles and design. J. Amer. Dent. Ass. *22:* 1352–1362, 1935.

Kratochvil, F. J.: Influence of occlusal rest position and clasp design on movement of abutment teeth. J. Prosth. Dent. *13:* 114–123, 1963.

Roach, F. E.: Mouth survey and design of partial dentures. J. Amer. Dent. Ass. *21:* 1166–1176, 1934.

Sayre, L. D.: Partial denture work. Dent. Cosmos *73:* 383–390, 1931.

Schuyler, C. H.: The partial denture as a means of stabilizing abutment teeth. J. Amer. Dent. Ass. *28:* 1121–1125, 1941.

Stone, E. R.: The tripping action of clasps. Dent. Cosmos *74:* 960–967, 1932.

Tench, R. W.: Fundamentals of partial denture design. J. Amer. Dent. Ass. *23:* 1087–1092, 1936.

Chapter 9

THE DESIGN OF STRUCTURAL
UNITS—MAJOR CONNECTORS

This chapter is concerned with the selection of major connectors for the removable partial denture. The various criteria which are applied to the selection process are discussed, and the structural details of proper design of the different connectors are described. Subject matter is organized according to the following format.

Introduction

Major connectors for both the mandible and maxilla have in common the fact that the primary function of each is to unite the various structural elements of the prosthesis. Aside from this one point of commonality, however, there are more differences than similarities between the two. The maxillary connector, for example, in addition to its function of unification, contributes substantially to the support of the prosthesis, while the mandibular connector has a very limited capability in this regard. The mandibular connector, for its part, may contribute indirect retention, a function which the maxillary connector does not ordinarily perform. Because of the inherent differences of these two structural elements, they will be discussed separately in this chapter.

The Types of Major Connectors

The maxillary connectors customarily employed in the design of the removable partial denture are the palatal strap, the double palatal bar, the horseshoe, and the full palatal connector. Selection of the most suitable one in a given instance will be based on the need for support, the number and location of the teeth to be replaced, and the number of clasps, as well as certain anatomical imperatives peculiar to the maxilla.

Commonly employed mandibular connectors are the lingual bar, the double lingual bar, and the lingual plate. The labial bar, although not often indicated, deserves mention since it may be the only connector that can be employed in some circumstances. Selection of the proper mandibular connector will depend on the need for indirect retention or for horizontal stabilization, as well as on certain anatomical imperatives peculiar to the mandible.

Criteria for Selection of the Maxillary Connector

Although there are several criteria for selecting the most suitable maxillary connector, certainly the requirement for support is a major one. If a dental arch that is to be fitted with a prosthesis has four abutment teeth situated in each of the four quadrants of the arch, the need for support from the palatal tissue and the residual ridges is minimal. In contrast, if there are only two abutment teeth remaining, the palatal tissues should contribute maximally to the support of the prosthesis, so as to reduce to a minimum the stresses which are transmitted to these teeth. Many times there is a reluctance to employ a maxillary connector which covers more than a minimum amount of palatal area, because of the patient's presumed resistance to the greater areal coverage and because of the resultant increase in bulk. This attitude is, in part, a holdover from an era of dentistry when palatal coverage was accomplished with either acrylic resin or gold alloy. It must be conceded that palatal coverage with acrylic resin, that meets the requirement for strength, must be relatively bulky, whereas wide coverage with gold alloy increases the weight of the prosthesis substantially. However, as a result of the improved physical properties and advanced techniques of fabrication of the chromium-cobalt dental alloys, it is possible to cover the palate with a very thin though extremely strong, rigid covering which adds little to either the bulk or the weight. Moreover, the patient's individual palatal topography can be reproduced in the metal. Since the chromium-cobalt alloys are polished by a deplating process, which eliminates the areas of uneven thickness so often present in the gold alloy casting as a result of hand polishing, problems due to excessive bulk are infrequent and phonetic difficulties are a rarity. When one considers the obvious benefits to the abutment teeth of employing the palatal tissues for support, and their eminent suitability for providing it, there should be no hesitancy in using the connector which results in minimal stress on the abutment teeth. It should be remembered, too, that in addition to providing unification and support, a properly designed maxillary connector can contribute materially to both stability and retention of the prosthesis, the latter by virtue of the interfacial tension which is operant between the metal and the mucosa. The amount of retention, stability, and support contributed will be directly proportional to the amount of areal coverage.

Additional factors in selection of the most suitable palatal connector are: (1) the presence of palatal tori, (2) the need for anterior tooth replacement, (3) the requirement for indirect retention, (4) the need for stabilization of infirm teeth, (5) phonetic considerations, and (6) the mental attitude of the patient.

The Presence of Palatal Tori. The presence of a torus palatinus may alter the requirements for the major connector, depending on the size, position, and configuration of the anomaly. A small torus can usually be covered with the connector, provided it is not lobulated or undercut. If it is, however, it will be necessary to circumvent it by designing the connector to pass either anteriorly to it (a horseshoe) or both anteriorly and posteriorly to it (an A-P bar).

The Need for Anterior Tooth Replacement. The prosthesis that must supply replacements for missing anterior teeth will require a maxillary connector of different configuration from the prosthesis that replaces only posterior teeth.

The Requirement for Indirect Retention. The requirement for indirect retention is normally not a major item of concern in the maxillary arch. Moreover, it is not often feasible to employ the conventional form of indirect retention, because the sites customarily used as support areas are located where interocclusal space is stringently limited. Furthermore, the denture which has an axis of rotation through the abutment teeth can often be satisfactorily stabilized by a posterior seal, which contributes greatly to the retention and stability of the prosthesis.

The Need to Stabilize Weakened Teeth. The need for the stabilization of periodontally weakened teeth will influence the choice of the major connector, in some instances. Teeth which have a marginal crown/root ratio may be reinforced against lateral stress by contact with the major connector, thus upgrading the prognosis for their longevity.

Phonetic Considerations. Although the problem of difficulty in articulation of speech sounds, stemming from wear of a maxillary partial denture, is not often encountered, there is no escaping the fact that a certain few individuals are abnormally sensitive to any alteration, however slight, in the anterior third of the palate, the so-called speech zone. Unless anterior teeth must be replaced, this area can be avoided altogether by proper connector selection, provided the patient has given some sign of his idiosyncrasy prior to design of the prosthesis. It is hard to escape the conclusion, however, that such complaints have a spurious air of untruth when coming from an individual who cannot adapt to a thin, lightweight metal covering in which the natural rugae have been reproduced.

The Mental Attitude of the Patient. An occasional individual will be accepted for treatment who objects to anything but minimal coverage of the roof of the mouth. Typically, this occurs with the patient who has previously worn a small prosthesis, such as a single palatal bar, for whom full palatal coverage is now prescribed, perhaps because of the loss of additional natural teeth. The usual explanation to such a patient of the need for increased palatal support, for the pupose of protracting the useful life of the remaining teeth, will generally suffice to gain his acquiescence and cooperation. Moreover, there is ofttimes presumptive evidence, at least, that the prime reason the prosthesis is being remade is that the previous one was designed with a connector which failed to provide adequate support.

The Palatal Strap

The palatal strap is the most versatile maxillary connector, and for this reason it is the most widely employed. It can be made relatively narrow, for the small tooth-supported prosthesis (Fig. 9.1), or much wider when the edentulous spaces are longer and the requirement for support correspondingly greater. It is rarely annoying to the patient, and there is minimal interference with phonetics. The palatal strap is an especially suitable connector when (1) only one or two teeth are being replaced on each side of the arch, (2) the edentulous spaces are tooth-bounded, and (3) the need for palatal support is minimal. It is frequently employed with only three supporting teeth, in which case the areal coverage of the strap should be increased so as to improve its load-bearing potential (Fig. 9.2). No sharp dividing line can be drawn between the wide palatal strap and the full palatal coverage connector. The one portrayed in Figure 9.3, for example, might be referred to as either type of connector.

Structural Details

The palatal strap should be made wide and thin, rather than narrow and thick, to achieve the required rigidity and to be as innocuous as possible to the tongue. The areal coverage should be governed by the

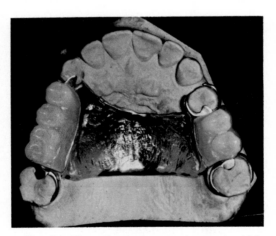

FIG. 9.1. The palatal strap is the most widely used maxillary connector.

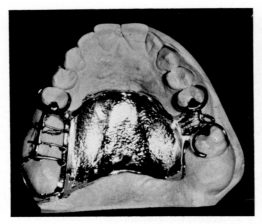

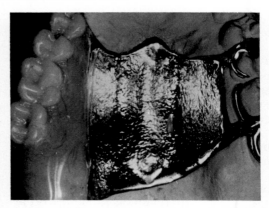

FIG. 9.2. The palatal strap can be made relatively narrow for the all tooth-supported denture, or wider when more palatal support is required.

FIG. 9.4. The width of the palatal strap should be based on the length of the edentulous span(s), and the amount of support that the connector will be expected to contribute in supporting the prosthesis.

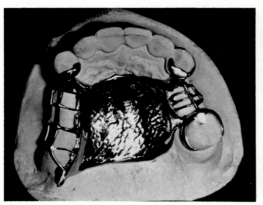

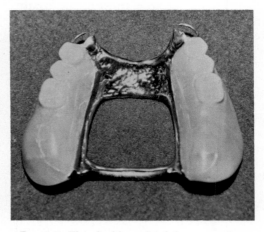

FIG. 9.3. No sharp dividing line can be drawn between a large palatal strap and the full palatal coverage connector. The connector shown here might be designated by either term.

FIG. 9.5. The double palatal bar cannot contribute the amount of support to the prosthesis that either the palatal strap or the full palatal coverage connector can give.

length of the edentulous span(s) and the amount of support that it will be required to contribute (Fig. 9.4). The anterior and posterior borders of the strap should be lightly beaded to ensure intimate contact with the mucosa, except over hard structures such as a prominent median raphe or a torus palatinus.

The Double Palatal Bar (the A-P Bar)

The double palatal bar is often used when the anterior and posterior abut-

ments are widely separated and the full palatal connector is not to be used for one reason or another. The two bars may be made wider or thinner, as dictated by the needs and the available space, in a particular case.

The Maxillary Arch with a Torus Palatinus. The A-P bar (Figs. 9.5 and 9.6) may be the connector of choice for the maxillary arch which has a torus palatinus that is either undercut, lobulated, or too massive to be covered with a full coverage

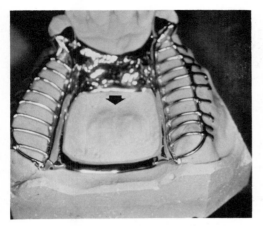

FIG. 9.6. A common use of the double palatal bar is to circumvent a torus palatinus (*arrow*) when it is not desirable to cover it.

connector or a strap. Sometimes the maxillary torus extends so far anteriorly that a horseshoe connector cannot be made wide enough for rigidity without impinging on it, and the A-P bar may be a solution. However, when the torus extends so far posteriorly that it preempts space that would normally be occupied by the posterior bar, the horseshoe connector is probably a better choice.

The Patient's Mental Attitude. The A-P bar may be used as a compromise for the patient who strongly objects to the greater bulk or areal coverage of the full palatal connector. Although the double palatal bar may serve adequately, to all intents and purposes, in such a circumstance, it cannot equal the full palatal connector from a standpoint of support, and hence the probable service expectancy of the abutment teeth must be rated somewhat less than favorable. Then too, there is presumptive evidence, at least, that the multiple metal margins of the two bars have the potential of being more annoying, to a patient with a restless tongue, than any other maxillary connector.

Structural Details

The anterior bar should be wide and flat, with its borders positioned in the depressions and slopes of the rugae rather

than on the crests (Fig. 9.7). Occasionally, however, a crest will have to be crossed almost at right angles. When this is the case, there is no alternative to doing so, although this fact may tip the balance for selection of another type of connector. Both borders should be gently curved and beveled to elude notice by the tongue, and the borders of the posterior bar should be lightly beaded on the tissue surface. The posterior bar should be located well back in the palate, just anterior to the vibrating line.

The Palatal Horseshoe Connector

The palatal horseshoe connector has two principle applications, when (1) several anterior teeth are to be replaced, and (2) a palatal torus that cannot be covered extends so far posteriorly that a posterior bar cannot be properly positioned without impinging on it. A third indication, which arises much less frequently, is when periodontally weakened anterior teeth require some stabilizing support.

Replacing Anterior Teeth. When one or several anterior teeth are to be replaced by the partial denture, the horseshoe connector often lends itself better than any other for this purpose (Figs. 9.8 and 9.9).

The Troublesome Torus Palatinus. A torus which cannot be crossed, because of

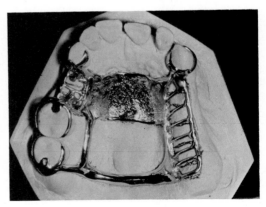

FIG. 9.7. The anterior bar of the A-P bar connector should be wide and flat. The anterior border should be positioned in the valleys between the rugae.

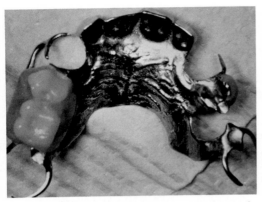

FIG. 9.8. When several anterior teeth are to be replaced by the prosthesis, the horseshoe connector often lends itself better for the purpose than does any other maxillary connector.

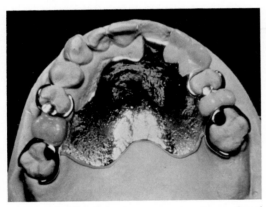

FIG. 9.9. The horseshoe connector is employed here to replace two anterior teeth, in addition to restoring the posterior edentulous spaces.

ciprocated thrust in a labial direction is avoided (Fig. 9.10), and the free gingival margins that are bridged by the connector should be liberally relieved to avoid their impingement.

Structural Details

The horseshoe connector should be made as thin as possible, consistent with strength and rigidity, and the natural rugae should be reproduced in the metal, to minimize the possibility of phonetic difficulties. The posterior borders of the connector should be lightly beaded, except over an unusually prominent median raphe.

The Full Palate Connector

The full palate connector covers a wider area of the palate than any other maxillary connector and, by virtue of this fact, contributes maximum support to the prosthesis. The extensive areal coverage makes possible a wide distribution of the functional load, so that the amount of stress to be borne by any single unit of area is minimal. Also of importance is the fact that, as a result of the increased areal coverage, there will be very little movement of the base during function. This has relevance because movement of the prosthesis in function is what creates the torsional and horizontal stresses which are so

its size or because it is undercut, may extend so far posteriorly that it preempts the space that a posterior palatal bar would normally occupy. In this instance, employment of the horseshoe palatal connector may be the most feasible solution to the problem.

Stabilizing Anterior Teeth. When periodontally weakened anterior teeth require support from the connector, the horseshoe may be designed to contribute to this need by partially engaging the lingual surfaces. When the connector is employed for this purpose, vertical stops should be provided on the anterior teeth, so that unre-

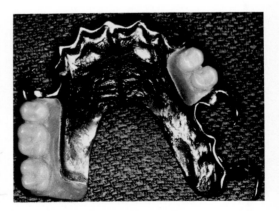

FIG. 9.10. When periodontally weakened teeth require some stabilizing support from the connector, the horseshoe may lend itself well for the purpose.

destructive to the abutment teeth. It must be emphasized once more, that a cardinal objective of design is to control movement of the prosthesis, thus minimizing the stresses that movement generates.

Two Distal Extension Bases. In most instances of bilateral distal extension bases, the need for support will be a major requirement. Increasing the amount of palatal coverage will assist in relieving the abutment teeth of some of the load to which they would otherwise be subjected (Fig. 9.11). When the denture flanges are extended well into the vestibules, and the posterior border is in intimate contact with the post dam seal area of the palate, the patient will generally feel as comfortable and secure as with any type of maxillary connector.

Six Remaining Anterior Teeth. When only six natural anterior teeth remain in the maxilla, the mechanical problems created by a partial prosthesis are so formidable that full palatal coverage may be considered essential in all but exceptional instances. Since the unfavorable effect of gravity, magnified by a leverage factor, poses such a grave threat to the well-being of the teeth that are clasped, every possible effort should be directed towards relieving the few remaining teeth of all stress possible. A major step in this direction is to ensure that palatal coverage of the edentulous areas is identical to that which would be employed for a complete denture, thereby exploiting to the fullest possible extent the factors of cohesion, adhesion, and atmospheric pressure. This is sometimes best accomplished by forming the posterior border of the prosthesis with acrylic resin, so as to make possible an accurate, though modifiable, post dam seal (Fig. 9.12). The denture flanges should be extended into the vestibules, to obtain all possible peripheral seal, in a similar manner to that employed for a complete denture.

Structural Details

The full palate connector should be thin, with the natural anatomy of the palate reproduced in the metal (Fig. 9.13).

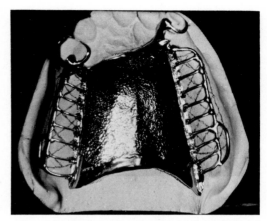

FIG. 9.11. In most instances of bilateral distal extension bases, the need for maximum support from the palatal structures makes the full coverage connector the one of choice.

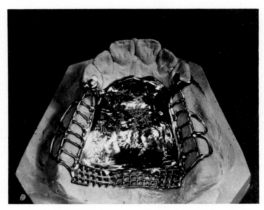

FIG. 9.12. When the prognosis for the remaining teeth is less than favorable, it may be prudent to employ the full palatal coverage connector, and to design it very much like a complete denture. Such a denture may play the role of a transitional prosthesis.

The material which covers the residual ridges should be one that can be refitted easily (acrylic resin), since this is the area of the mouth that is most susceptible to atrophic change. The posterior border can be fabricated of either metal or acrylic resin.

If it is made of metal, the border must be precisely established, because if overextended it will quickly induce soreness, and the metal is difficult to alter satisfac-

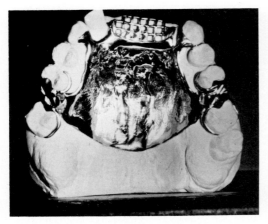

FIG. 9.13. The full palate connector should be thin, and the natural anatomy of the palate should be reproduced in the metal.

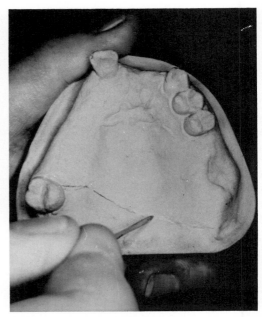

FIG. 9.14. A slight bead should be provided in the metal by lightly scraping the refractory cast prior to forming the wax pattern for the framework.

torily. A slight bead should be provided in the metal by lightly scraping the refractory cast, prior to forming the wax pattern for the framework (Fig. 9.14).

The acrylic resin border is preferred when maximum adhesion and atmospheric seal is needed, and it has the advantage of being easily altered. The post dam seal should be located in the zone of the palate where the mucosa is resilient but not movable (Fig. 9.15). This will be found at, or very near, a line drawn from one hamular notch to the other, through the fovea palatinae. It may be located quite precisely in the mouth by observing the region of the fovea palatinae while the patient says "aH." Articulation of the "aH" sound raises the palatal curtain, thus disclosing the junction of movable and nonmovable tissue.

Normally the full palate connector requires no relief unless there is a prominent palatal raphe or a large torus palatinus.

Criteria for Selection of the Mandibular Connector

Although the maxillary connector is able to contribute substantially to the support of the prosthesis, the mandibular connector has a very limited capability for doing so, because of the differences in the

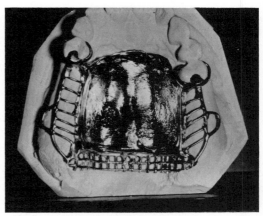

FIG. 9.15. The post dam seal should be located in the zone of the palate where the mucosa is resilient but not movable.

anatomy of the two jaws. Since the residual ridges of the mandible provide so much less support, indirect retention is sorely needed to help stabilize the mandibular partial denture, and fortunately two of the mandibular connectors are well suited for the purpose. Hence, the need for indirect retention is a major criterion used in the selection of the mandibular connector.

A basic tenet of partial denture design is that neither mucosa nor teeth should be covered with the prosthesis unless there is a valid reason for doing so. The reason for this is that when a lingual plate, for example, covers the free gingival margins of the mandibular teeth, as well as a portion of the teeth themselves, it deprives the teeth of the cleansing action of the saliva and the sweeping action of the tongue. Similarly, it deprives the marginal mucosa of the benefits of the gentle stimulation which it normally receives from the passage of food over it during mastication. Thus it follows that, all else being equal, the double lingual bar would be a better choice of mandibular connector than would be a lingual plate. It must be emphasized, however, that the lingual plate is oftentimes the connector of choice, notwithstanding this drawback.

In addition to the requirement of indirect retention, other criteria for selection of the mandibular connector are: (1) the need to stabilize infirm teeth, (2) anatom-ical considerations, (3) esthetics, (4) contingency planning, and (5) patient preference.

The Requirement for Indirect Retention. When an axis of rotation has been created through the principal abutments by the design of the partial denture, a properly selected and designed mandibular connector can contribute by indirect means a substantial amount of needed retention and stability to the prosthesis (Fig. 9.16).

Horizontal Stability and Stress Distribution. Well known is the fact that both the lingual plate and the double lingual bar contribute materially to the horizontal stability of the mandibular partial denture. Sometimes overlooked, however, is the fact that these connectors perform a very valuable auxiliary function by distributing masticatory stresses to all of the teeth with which they come in contact. This, of course, relieves the abutment teeth of a substantial amount of the stress to which they would otherwise be subjected.

Anatomical Considerations. The presence of inoperable lingual tori may influ-

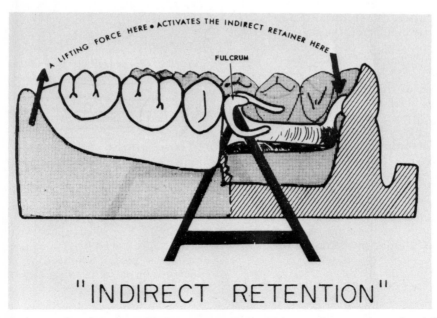

FIG. 9.16. A properly selected mandibular connector may supplement the retention and stability of the prosthesis by indirect means thus helping to counteract dislodging forces.

ence the type of mandibular connnector that can best serve. In similar manner, a different connector may be required, for a mouth in which the lingual frenum is attached abnormally close to the crest of the residual ridge, from the one that is more normally structured. Finally, the contour of the mucosa around the lower anterior teeth may influence the selection of the mandibular connector. For example, if the teeth have been treated for periodontal disease, and the interproximal embrasures are large, there may be a problem of either food retention or esthetics, or of both. The problem may be either alleviated or aggravated by the choice of mandibular connector.

Esthetics. When there are diastemas or abnormally large interproximal spaces between the teeth a connector should be selected which is least observable from a conversational distance.

Contingency Planning. Planning for the possible future loss of natural teeth, by anticipating their method of replacement, may dictate the use of one mandibular connector over another, since artificial teeth can be more conveniently attached to some connectors than to others.

The Patient Preference Factor. The mandibular connector, because of its location in the tongue's playground, can be a distracting source of annoyance to some individuals. Therefore as a general rule, the design of the major connector should not be changed for a patient who has successfully worn a previous removable partial denture. The double lingual bar should not ordinarily be used for the patient who has previously worn a lingual plate with comfort and satisfaction, unless there is a compelling reason for doing so. The converse is also true. When a change in connector design is contemplated for a good reason, the reason should be explained to the patient beforehand.

The Lingual Bar

The lingual bar (Fig. 9.17), is the simplest of the mandibular connectors and should be employed when there are no extraordinary requirements other than

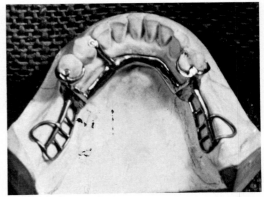

FIG. 9.17. The lingual bar is the simplest mandibular connector, and is the one of choice for the routine prosthesis which has no unusual requirements.

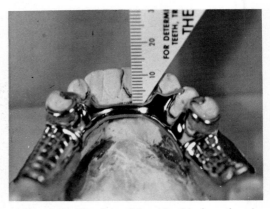

FIG. 9.18. The lingual bar should clear the gingival margin of the mandibular anterior teeth by a minimum 2 to 3 mm.

unification of the various elements of the prosthesis.

The Routine Mandibular Partial Denture. When there is no requirement that the connector supply indirect retention or stabilization of weakened teeth, and there are no obstacles to placement of the bar in its proper position, it is the mandibular connector par excellence. Because of its simplicity and limited coverage, it is better tolerated, by a broader spectrum of patients, than any other type of mandibular connector.

Structural Details

The most nearly ideal configuration for the lingual bar is one-half pear shape in cross section, with the thicker part making up the inferior border. The superior border of the bar should clear the gingival margins of the lower anterior teeth by a minimum of 2 to 3 mm. (Fig. 9.18). This distance is not as critical in the mandible as it is with the maxillary connector, because the mandibular connector does not contact the underlying mucosa. The inferior border must not interfere with the lingual frenum (Fig. 9.19), or the genioglossus muscle when the floor of the mouth is at high level, i.e., with the tongue in the roof of the mouth. The bar should follow closely the contour of the lingual surface of the mandible, just barely short of contact with the mucosa.

The Double Lingual Bar (the Kennedy Bar), the Split Bar

This connector is often referred to as a "continuous lingual clasp" since it is, in some ways, suggestive of a series of clasp arms connected on the lingual surfaces of the lower anterior teeth (Fig. 9.20). In addition to being an excellent indirect retainer, it makes a major contribution to the horizontal stability of the prosthesis, as well as giving a minor amount of support. A feature of the Kennedy bar, sometimes overlooked, is that it distributes stress to all of the teeth with which it comes in contact, thereby reducing the stress to be borne by each supporting unit.

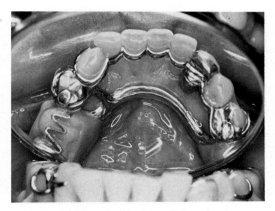

FIG. 9.20. The double lingual bar is, in some ways, suggestive of a series of lingual clasp arms on the incisors, and for this reason it is sometimes referred to as a "a continuous lingual clasp."

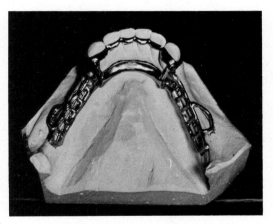

FIG. 9.21. When indirect retention must be supplied by the major connector, the double lingual bar is capable of fulfilling this function admirably.

Indirect Retention with Periodontally Treated Teeth

The double lingual bar is without peer when the connector must supply indirect retention in a mouth where periodontal disease and its treatment have created large interproximal embrasures between the lower anterior teeth (Fig. 9.21). A lingual plate may create dead-end tunnels between the teeth in such a way that food tends to enter from the labial side, and is unable to escape lingually, because of the lingual plate. Not unexpectedly, this is very annoying to the patient. In contrast, the double lingual bar allows the free flow

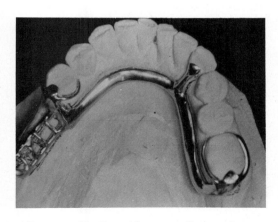

FIG. 9.19. The lingual bar must allow ample room for functional movement of the lingual frenum and the floor of the mouth.

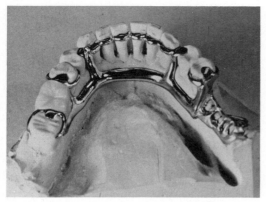

Fig. 9.22. When periodontal disease and its treatment have left in their wake large interproximal spaces between the mandibular incisors, the double lingual bar is usually the most self-cleansing type of connector.

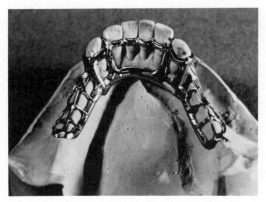

Fig. 9.23. The double lingual bar permits the free flow of saliva around and through the interproximal embrasures.

of food and saliva through the interproximal embrasures (Figs. 9.22 and 9.23). For this reason, it is a better connector from the standpoint of periodontal health than is the lingual plate. It should be employed with circumspection in the case of markedly crowded lower anterior teeth, because of the numerous undercuts so often created by the overlapping teeth, which make it difficult to fit the bar closely to the lingual surface of each tooth.

Structural Details

The lower border of the upper bar

should rest on the top edge of the cingula, where it will be optimally effective and minimally obtrusive. When it is so located, the area between the two bars will usually be self-cleansing. If the two bars cannot be separated enough to ensure a self-cleansing area between them because of anatomical anomalies (short teeth and a high lingual frenulum attachment, for example), the lingual plate may be a better choice of connector. The two bars must be attached to each other by means of minor connectors at either side of the span. The minor connectors should be positioned opposite embrasures, so as to be as innocuous as possible. It is absolutely essential that positive vertical stops (occlusal, incisal, or lingual) be provided at either terminus of the bar, to prevent its settling downward or exerting orthodontic pressure against the anterior teeth. The lower lingual bar should have the same design as a single lingual bar, i.e., one-half pear shape in cross section.

The Interrupted Double Lingual Bar

When the Kennedy bar is indicated for use, but its presence will be cosmetically distracting because of a prominent diastema, a modification in the conventional Kennedy bar design may be resorted to (Fig. 9.24). When so designed, the upper bar is virtually indiscernible from a conversational distance (Fig. 9.25), yet the connector loses none of its functional effectiveness.

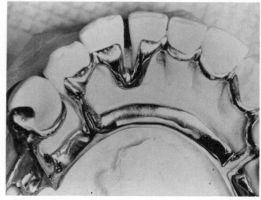

Fig. 9.24. The double lingual bar may be modified in design to circumvent a diastema.

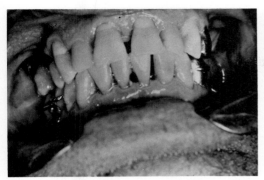

FIG. 9.25. The interrupted double lingual bar shown here is indiscernible from a conversational distance.

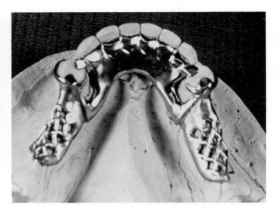

FIG. 9.26. The lingual plate is an excellent indirect retainer.

The Lingual Plate

(Linguoplate, Lingual Strap, Lingual Apron, Lingual Shield)

The lingual plate (Fig. 9.26) is by all odds the most controversial of the mandibular connectors. Criticism usually centers around the fact that coverage by the metal prevents the customary physiological stimulation of the lingual gingival tissues, and the self-cleansing by the saliva and tongue of the lingual surfaces of the mandibular anterior teeth. It must be conceded that instances of erosion of the lingual surfaces of teeth are not unknown when the prosthesis has been worn continuously, in the absence of adequate oral hygiene. Certainly, when this connector is prescribed, the prosthesis must be left out of the mouth for at least 8 of the 24 hours, and the mouth must be maintained in a state of scrupulous cleanliness.

Notwithstanding this drawback, the lingual plate has considerable merit, and when employed where indicated, properly designed, and adequately maintained by the patient, no mandibular connector can take its place. It is an excellent indirect retainer and stabilizer.

The Presence of Lingual Tori. When large lingual tori (Fig. 9.27) are inoperable for reasons of the patient's health, the proper placement of a conventional lingual bar may not be possible. The lingual plate may be the most feasible alternative in such a circumstance. Usually, this connector can be designed to avoid con-

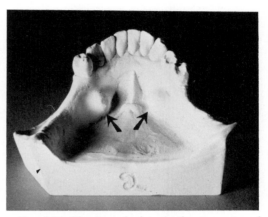

FIG. 9.27. The lingual plate is the connector of choice when a large lingual torus, or tori, occupies space that would normally be occupied by a lingual bar and cannot be removed for one reason or another.

tact with the tori, while still being wide enough to satisfy the requirement of rigidity.

The Abnormally High Lingual Frenum. A lingual frenum attached near the crest of the mandibular ridge (Figs. 9.28 and 9.29) may sometimes interefere with placement of the conventional lingual bar, and the lingual plate (Fig. 9.30) may provide a practical answer to the problem. The lingual plate can be designed to avoid the frenum, while still retaining the required rigidity and without being made overly thick.

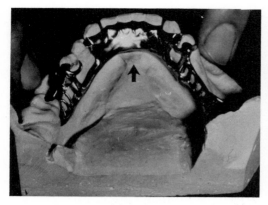

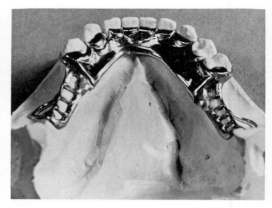

FIG. 9.28. The lingual plate may be employed when an aberrant lingual frenum attaches so high on the lingual surface of the mandible that it interferes with proper positioning of a lingual bar.

FIG. 9.30. The lingual plate can usually be designed to avoid interfering with the aberrant lingual frenum, while still being wide enough to possess the required rigidity without undue thickness and bulk. This is the same mouth shown in Figure 9.29.

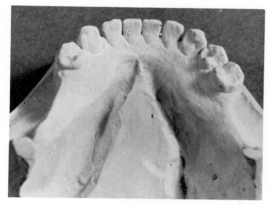

FIG. 9.29. The lingual frenum shown here was not operated because of the patient's age and poor health status. A lingual plate was employed as a connector for a removable partial denture as shown in Figure 9.30.

Heavy Calculus Formation. The lingual plate may be the connector of choice for the patient who deposits calculus very rapidly on the lingual surfaces of the anterior teeth. The metal plate will act as a repository for the calculus, so that the periodontium escapes its deleterious effects and, of course, it can be more easily removed from the surface of the metal than from the natural teeth.

The Need for Indirect Retention. When the mandibular connector must supply some of the retention by indirect means, this connector may be the best solution from all viewpoints. As with the double lingual bar, it also distributes lateral stress to many teeth, thereby contributing substantially to the overall stability of the prosthesis. It should be noted, however, that it is not a suitable connector for the mouth in which periodontal disease and its treatment have created large interproximal embrasures, because it may be distractingly visible between the teeth (Fig. 9.31).

A Stabilizer. The lingual plate may be a very effective stabilizer for anterior teeth which have been weakened from periodontal disease. It is particularly suited for stabilizing extruded mandibular anterior teeth after they have been reduced in height to harmonize with the occlusal plane (Fig. 9.32). It should be noted, too, that lingual plating can be extended onto the mandibular bicuspids, for the purpose of stabilizing the prosthesis and/or covering interproximal spaces that would otherwise act as food traps (Fig. 9.33).

Contingency Planning. If the loss of additional anterior teeth is recognized as a distinct possibility for the future, the

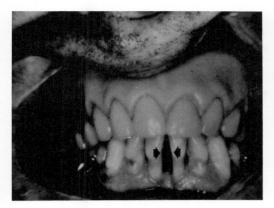

FIG. 9.31. The lingual plate is ordinarily not the connector of choice for the mouth in which periodontal disease and its treatment have created large interproximal embrasures, as it may be visible and hence cosmetically detracting. In this photograph the patient had a large diastema in addition to a large interproximal embrasure. The lingual plate which he wore was plainly visible, although he seemed to be unaware of its unsightly appearance.

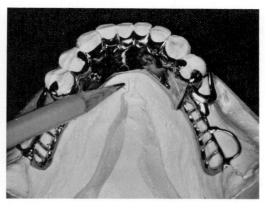

FIG. 9.33. "Plating," or extending the metal of the connector up onto the lingual surfaces of the teeth, is done to provide indirect retention, to contribute splinting support, to avoid creating a dead-end aperture, and to strengthen the connector without thickening it. In this photograph the plate has been extended to cover the interproximal spaces of the bicuspids in order to avoid food traps. The pencil calls attention to the high lingual frenum attachment, which is a common reason for employing the lingual plate connector.

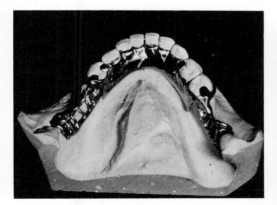

FIG. 9.32. The lingual plate is particularly suited for stabilizing extruded mandibular anterior teeth after they have been reduced in height to harmonize with the occlusal plane.

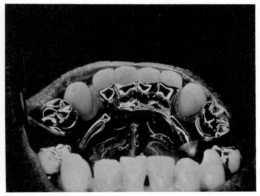

FIG. 9.34. The superior border of the lingual plate should be located in the middle third of the lingual surfaces of the mandibular anterior teeth, and it should fit the tooth surface intimately.

lingual plate may be employed as the connector of choice because of the ease with which retentive loops may be attached to the lingual plate and a prosthetic tooth added to it.

Structural Details

The upper border of the apron should be placed in the middle third of the lingual surface of the mandibular anterior teeth (Fig. 9.34). It is important to good patient acceptance that the metal be contoured to simulate the lingual surfaces of the anterior teeth, and that its superior margins be intimately adapted to the lingual surface of the teeth. Like all connectors, it must be absolutely rigid, and it is essential that it be supported at either terminus, by prepared recesses in the natural teeth, to preclude any settling tissue-ward (Fig. 9.35).

The Interrupted Lingual Plate

When the lingual plate connector is indicated for use, but its presence will be unsightly because of large interdental spaces, a modification of the conventional design may be employed. When this variation in design is used, the lingual plate is divided into units which are extended onto the lingual surfaces of each individual tooth (Fig. 9.36). When properly executed, this configuration is virtually indiscernible from a labial view, yet loses none of its effectiveness as a connector.

The Labial Bar

The labial bar has a limited application but, in the rare instances when it is indicated, there is no feasible alternative. The lower anteriors and bicuspids may be so severely inclined lingually as to prevent proper positioning of a conventional lingual bar (Fig. 9.37). The favored solutions are to modify the offending teeth by recontouring, if the change is not major, or to place on them protective coverings which restore them to a more normal alignment in the arch, if substantial change is needed. However, in instances

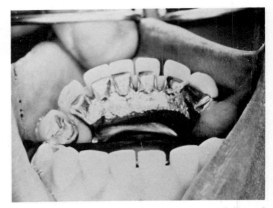

FIG. 9.36. Shown here is the interrupted lingual plate, which lends itself well for use with spaced anterior teeth.

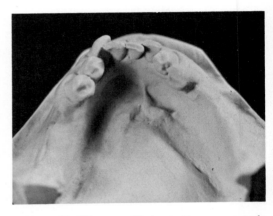

FIG. 9.37. When mandibular teeth are so severely inclined lingually as to interfere with proper placement of a conventional mandibular connector, the favored treatment is the realignment of the teeth with restorations. When this cannot be accomplished, recourse may be made to the labial bar.

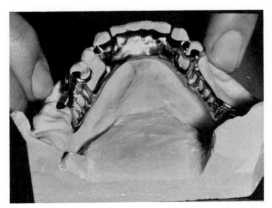

FIG. 9.35. The lingual plate must be supported at either end of its span by occlusal, incisal, or lingual rests.

where these teeth are inoperable for one reason or another, the labial bar may be the connector of choice, although it must be conceded that there is little to commend it architecturally (Fig. 9.38).

Structural Details Which Apply to All Major Connectors

Certain design fundamentals apply to all connectors, and these are discussed in the next few paragraphs.

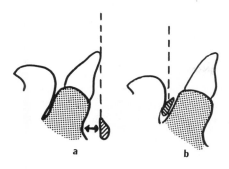
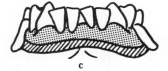

FIG. 9.38. This schematic shows at *a* the position of a lingual bar necessitated by the lingual inclination of the mandibular teeth. Shown at *b* is the customary position of the labial bar and at *c* an anterior view of the bar, showing its position labial to the anterior teeth.

Rigidity

Connectors should be completely rigid, so that all stress is transmitted throughout the area of coverage of the prosthesis, thus distributing it among the largest possible number of stabilizing elements. A connector which lacks rigidity will allow rotation and flexion within the structure of the connector itself. This will result in the transmission of horizontal and torsional stresses, which are damaging to the abutment teeth as well as to the residual ridges. The use of rigid major connectors is an inviolate rule of design.

Impingement of the Free Gingival Margin

The connector should never be permitted to impinge on the free gingival margin of any of the remaining teeth, since this structure is highly vascular, hence extremely susceptible to injury from pressure. Ideally, the maxillary connector should by-pass the gingival margin altogether by a distance of 4 to 6 mm. (Fig. 9.39 and 9.40). However, the distribution of the remaining teeth may be such that this is not always feasible. When crossing the gingival margin with the connector cannot be avoided, it should never be terminated on this delicate structure, but instead, extended up onto the lingual surfaces of the teeth (Figs. 9.41 and 9.42), and the gingival margin should be liberally relieved, so that the metal bridges over it. This is true also of the gingival margins of the mandibular ante-

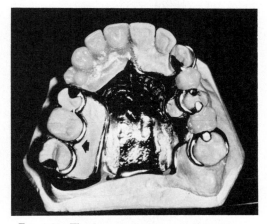

FIG. 9.39. The free gingival margin is highly vascular and extremely susceptible to injury from pressure. For this reason, the maxillary connector should never be permitted to impinge upon this delicate structure.

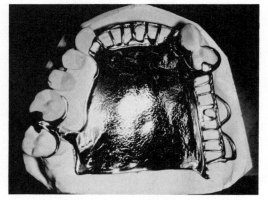

FIG. 9.40. Ideally, the connector should by-pass the gingival margin by a distance of 4 to 6 mm.

rior teeth which are covered by a lingual plate. Failure to take this precaution will result in inflammation and edema.

The Avoidance of Dead-End Apertures

The creation of dead-end apertures (Fig. 9.43) with the connector, or any part of

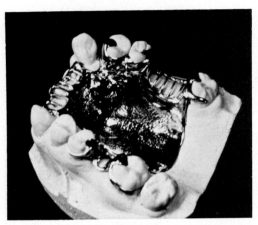

FIG. 9.41. If by-passing the free gingival margin is not feasible, the connector should be extended up onto the lingual surfaces of the teeth, as it has been between the left bicuspids in this photograph.

the framework, should be avoided. Besides being annoying to most patients, they are difficult to maintain in a state of cleanliness and, when debris is permitted to stagnate in such a shelter, the result will be inflammation of the mucosa. The recommended solution is to cover the area with a thin metal plate (Fig. 9.44).

Border Contour

All long borders of the maxillary connector should be gently curved—never sharp or angular—and the edges of all connectors should be beveled so as not to arouse the notice of a curious tongue. The ideal connector is one that earns the patient's acceptance by being so contoured that shortly following its insertion he is no longer conscious of its presence.

Beading the Borders

The borders of the maxillary bars and straps that contact soft resilient tissue should be lightly beaded on the refractory cast to ensure intimate contact between the metal and the palatal mucosa. This

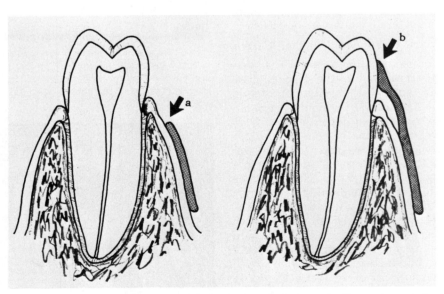

FIG. 9.42. In areas where the connector must cover the free gingival margin, the master cast should be liberally relieved prior to duplication, so that the metal does not impinge on this delicate structure. At *a* is shown the connector, in cross section, clearing the gingiva. Depicted at *b* is the connector crossing the gingiva. It is not in contact with the gingiva because the master cast was relieved in this area.

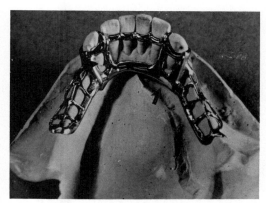

FIG. 9.43. The creation of dead-end apertures with the framework should be avoided. The areas around the cuspids (*arrows*) shown here will invite food entrapment. Covering of this area with a thin plate would be preferable.

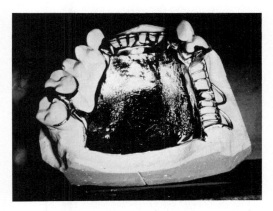

FIG. 9.44. Creation of a dead-end aperture has been avoided between the left cuspid and bicuspid by extending the connector onto the lingual surface of both teeth (plating).

is true also of the posterior border of the full palatal coverage connector. The reason for this is that when the molten alloy passes from a semiliquid stage to a solid state, during the casting procedure, there is a slight dimensional change in the

casting. Although actually miniscule in amount, it can affect, however slightly, the intimacy of contact between the soft tissue and the metal, and the purpose of the beading is to compensate for this discrepancy. The beading should not extend onto relatively hard, unyielding areas such as the median raphe or a torus palatinus, nor is it indicated over the rugae. Since this procedure is performed on the refractory cast, it is normally a laboratory procedure and can be performed in a perfectly satisfactory manner by a competent technician. If there is any room for doubt as to which of the areas should be beaded, or if there are anomalous soft or hard areas in the palatal region to be covered, this fact should be made known to the technician, who otherwise has access only to the information which he can glean from inspection of the stone cast. This communication is best accomplished by indicating on the study cast the areas that are to be either relieved or beaded, in addition to making a brief note on the laboratory authorization form.

Bibliography

Blatterfein, L.: A systematic method of designing upper partial denture bases. J. Amer. Dent. Ass. *46:* 510–525, 1953.

Chappelle, W.: Partial denture design. Dent. Cosmos *76:* 183–193, 1934.

Dirksen, L. C., and Campagna, S. J.: Mat surface and rugae reproduction for upper partial denture castings. J. Prosth. Dent. *4:* 67–72, 1954.

Hardy, I.: Partial lower denture design. Dent. Dig. *44:* 57–61, 1938.

Kelley, E. K.: The physiologic approach to partial denture design. J. Prosth. Dent., *3:* 699–709, 1953.

Kennedy, E.: *Partial Denture Construction*, Ed. 2. Dental Items of Interest Publishing Company, New York, 1951.

McClean, D. W.: Fundamental principles of partial denture construction. J. Tennessee State Dent. Ass. *19:* 109–118, 1938.

Chapter 10

DESIGN OF THE MINOR CONNECTOR AND MISCELLANEOUS DESIGN CONSIDERATIONS

This chapter deals with the design of the minor connector and with proper structuring of the retention latticework for the removable partial denture. The advisability of creating a distal extension base with a single tooth is considered, and the proper design of the unilateral type of removable prosthesis is discussed. Finally, a systematized method for drawing the design of the framework on the study cast is described. The subject matter is organized in the following way.
Design of the Minor Connector
Design of the Retention Latticework
The One-Tooth Extension Base
The Unilateral Removable Prosthesis
Drawing the Design on the Study Cast

Design of the Minor Connector

The minor connector, like the other components of the framework (with the exception of the terminal third of the retentive clasp arm), should be rigid so that all forces directed against it are distributed among all of the structures which support and stabilize the prosthesis. Notwithstanding the requirement for strength and rigidity, the minor connector should not be bulky. When it is employed to unite the major connector with a clasp on a terminal abutment adjacent to a distal extension base, it should be made wide buccolingually for strength, but it should be kept thin mesiodistally. This configuration is desirable so that the connector will interfere minimally with placement of the substitute tooth, which must be adapted closely to the clasp in order to achieve the best esthetic effect. (Fig. 10.1). The minor connector shown in Figure 10.2 is far too bulky, and will interfere with proper positioning of the prosthetic tooth.

When the minor connector is placed in an embrasure between two teeth, as in the case of an embrasure clasp, for example, or of an occlusal rest which is employed as an indirect retainer, it should be triangular in form, so as to fit into the embrasure between the teeth and to occupy a minimum of space consistent with strength and rigidity (Fig. 10.3). The junction of the minor connector and the major connector should be rounded rather than angular, and the surface of the metal which is exposed to the tongue should be beveled and smooth, so as to be as innocuous as possible. The marginal gingiva must always be relieved at the point where it is crossed by the minor connector.

Design of the Retention Latticework

The prime purpose of the retention latticework of the partial denture framework is to provide secure anchorage for the acrylic resin base. It should be designed so as to (1) retain the acrylic resin of the

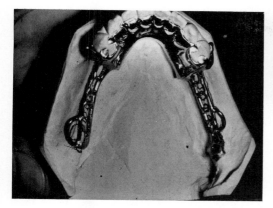

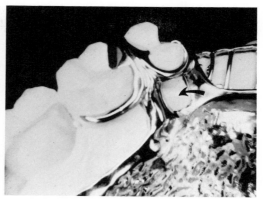

FIG. 10.1. The minor connector that unites the clasp with the major connector which is adjacent to an edentulous space should be made small enough in bulk to allow for proper positioning of the prosthetic tooth while, at the same time, being strong and rigid. It should be made wide buccolingually for strength rather than thick mesiodistally.

FIG. 10.3. The minor connector which is placed in an interproximal embrasure should be roughly triangular in cross section. It must be strong and rigid without being bulky. The outer surface should be smoothly beveled to be minimally obtrusive to the tongue.

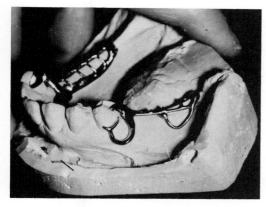

FIG. 10.2. The minor connector which connects the "T" bar clasp to the framework in this photograph is extremely bulky and will interfere with proper positioning of the prosthetic tooth.

base securely, (2) be strong enough for rigidity and to resist breakage or distortion, and (3) be small enough in bulk so as to interfere minimally with proper positioning of the substitute teeth. A common mistake in design is to place the main brace of the latticework along the crest of the alveolar ridge. When placed in this position it occupies interridge space often critically needed for proper positioning of the artificial teeth. Since interridge space

is typically at a premium in this region, the presence of the brace on the ridge crest necessitates drastic reduction in size of the prosthetic teeth, and thinning of the acrylic resin base. This may so weaken the base that fracture of the teeth, the base, or both occurs after a short period of mouth service.

The Form of the Latticework

The form of the retention latticework is not important, provided it satisfies the requirements enumerated in the paragraph above. The mesh type (Fig. 10.4) is exceptionally strong but requires more space than does the open type of latticework (Fig. 10.5), which is amply strong, light in weight, and not overly bulky. The open type is the more versatile and is recommended for routine use.

Tissue Stops

The retention latticework for the distal extension base should include a tissue stop which contacts the residual ridge of the cast (Fig. 10.6). The purpose of this stop, or "foot," is to preclude the possibility of the framework being sprung downward as the acrylic resin dough is being packed into the mold. It is apparent that unreciprocated pressure on the

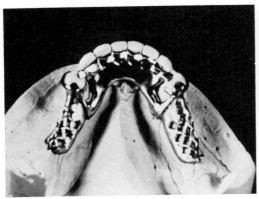

FIG. 10.4. The mesh type of retention shown here is very strong but is more bulky than the open type; hence, it should be employed only when there is abundant interridge space.

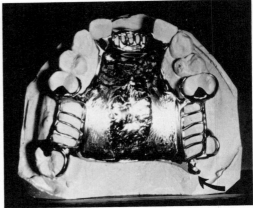

FIG. 10.6. The retention latticework should include a tissue stop (*arrow*), the purpose of which is to avert the possibility of the metal framework being distorted as the acrylic resin dough is packed into the denture mold. The stop is created in the metal by forming a small opening, approximately 2 x 2 mm., in the saddle relief wax on the crest of the ridge prior to duplication of the master cast.

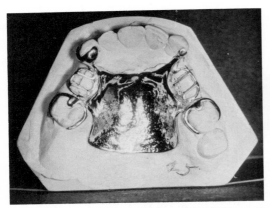

FIG. 10.5. The open type of retention latticework shown here can be adequately strong without undue bulk or weight, and provides a maximum space for the prosthetic teeth.

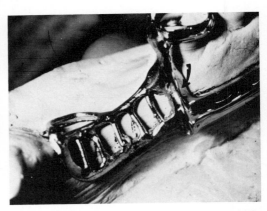

FIG. 10.7. A sharp, definite finish line should be provided in the metal at any point where it is joined with acrylic resin (*arrow*). This area of the framework is sometimes inadvertently thinned to a point that it is dangerously weak and vulnerable to breakage in service.

framework at this point could result in distortion of the metal.

Finish Lines

Sharp, definite finish lines should be incorporated into the metal at any point where the acrylic resin joins the metal. This will ensure a neat junction of the two materials and will preclude the creation of a thin feather edge of acrylic resin overlapping the metal, which is unsightly in addition to being unhygienic. A rather common error, which should be avoided, is to place too deep a finish line at the junction of the lingual bar and the retention latticework. This causes a dangerous thin-ning of the metal at a point that is vulnerable to breakage in service.

External finish lines should be formed in the wax pattern in a way that provides ample thickness of both metal and resin, to preclude fracture of the former and an overlapping feather edge of the latter (Fig. 10.7).

Internal finish lines are formed by the

edge of the saddle relief wax, which is placed on the master cast by the laboratory technician prior to duplication (Fig. 10.8). As is true of the external finish line, it is important that the internal finish line be formed so as to provide a definite, even junction between metal and resin.

The Metal-Framed Base

When the edentulous space is tooth bounded, the acrylic resin base may be framed in metal to create a neat, easily maintained denture base (Fig. 10.9). The method is not recommended for the distal extension base because of the likelihood that the border of the finished denture will need alteration. Moreover, the distal extension base denture is much more apt to require refitting at some future date, which would be complicated by the metal border.

The One-Tooth Extension Base

The question frequently arises, in design of the denture, as to the advisability of replacing a single posterior tooth (usually a second molar) on one side of the arch by adding a small distal extension base. As a general rule, the potential harm that this cantilevered appendage can create far outweighs any possible benefit that it might contribute to the restoration of occlusal function. Although the small amount of leverage-induced stress created by such a free-end segment is probably inconsequential, of far greater importance is the difficulty of maintaining the distal surface of the terminal tooth in a hygienic state (Fig. 10.10). Unless the patient's oral

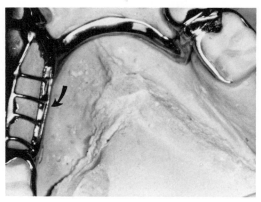

FIG. 10.9. When the edentulous space is tooth-bounded, the acrylic resin base can be framed in metal as shown here.

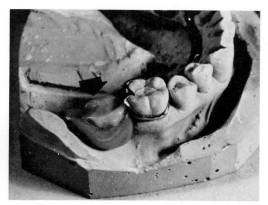

FIG. 10.10. Adding a base to one side of a removable partial denture for the purpose of supplying a single tooth is generally a poor practice. Besides adding a lever arm, which will generate stress, it also creates a bacterial sanctuary on the distal surface of the abutment tooth that may be very difficult for the patient to maintain in a state of cleanliness. The molar abutment shown here had been attacked with root caries on the distal surface and was saved and restored only as a result of heroic effort. The patient's oral hygiene was considered excellent except that she apparently was not able to scrub the distal surface of this one tooth with dental floss. The tooth would have been in large measure self-cleansing were it not for the prosthetic appendage that "sheltered" its distal surface.

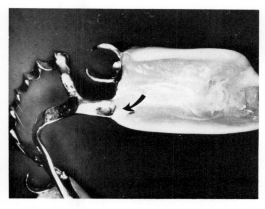

FIG. 10.8. Internal finish lines are formed by the saddle relief wax that is placed on the master cast prior to its duplication to obtain the refractory cast. Unless the junction of the metal and acrylic resin is sharp and definite, the acrylic resin will form a feather edge that overlaps the metal as shown here. Such a thin overlay of acrylic resin is unhygienic.

hygiene is faultless, bacterial plaque retention with its usual sequelae is virtually inevitable in the area of tooth and periodontium sheltered by the base. There is one circumstance, however, wherein the one-tooth base may be justified and that is when its presence will prevent a tooth in the opposing arch from extruding into the space. Even this obvious benefit must be weighed against the fact that the distal surface of the abutment tooth is rendered much more vulnerable to both carious attack and periodontal disease by the presence of the base, which in effect creates a bacterial sanctuary. An alternate solution, when a tooth opposes the edentulous space and has no surface against which to occlude, is to cantilever a small pontic off a restoration in the distal abutment, for the sole purpose of preventing its extrusion. This solution, of course, may pose its own problem of hygienic maintenance.

The Unilateral Removable Prosthesis

It is sometimes desirable to restore the small, unilateral (one- or two-tooth) edentulous space with a removable prosthesis. The favored design for this type of partial denture is to cross the mouth with a rigid connector, and to clasp a tooth or teeth on the contralateral side, so that in effect,

the design is conventionally bilateral. However, the unilateral design is sometimes preferred, and when it is, the clasps should be designed so that they are retentive on all four tooth surfaces. Such clasps will probably not possess reciprocity, and stress distribution is far from ideal. Finally, the possibility of the patient swallowing or aspirating a small unilateral prosthesis should not be overlooked.

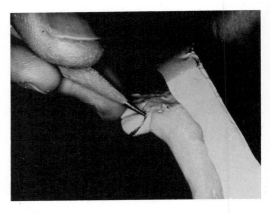

FIG. 10.12. The desired amount of undercut is measured with the undercut gauge and marked on the infrabulge area of the abutment tooth. The clasp is drawn so that it curves gracefully into the infrabulge area, with the lower border of the terminal precisely on this mark.

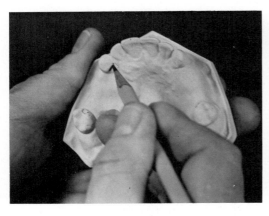

FIG. 10.11. If proper finger rests and reasonably sharp pencils are used, the task of drawing the design on the planning cast can be accomplished quickly and easily.

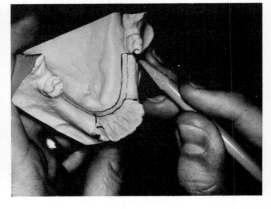

FIG. 10.13. The major connector may be sketched in first or it may be added after the clasps have been outlined.

Drawing the Design on the Study Cast

The outline of the proposed partial denture should be drawn on the study cast, and the study cast should accompany *the unmarked master cast* to the laboratory. If there has been substantial change in the

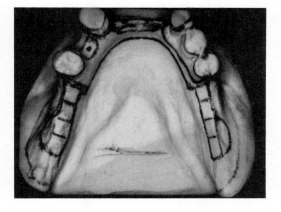

FIG. 10.14. This photograph shows the finished sketch on the planning cast.

abutment teeth, as a result of placing restorations and/or tooth alteration, the master cast should be duplicated to produce a currently accurate study cast. The use of several pencils of different colors is recommended for sketching the various units of the prosthesis. For example, if pencil "lead" (graphite) is used to mark the survey line, then the framework might be drawn in red and the outline to be occupied by the base in blue. If the same colors are employed consistently to designate the same structural elements, the procedure should contribute in worthwhile measure to a good working rapport between dentist and laboratory technician.

The exact sequence to be followed in sketching the various components is immaterial, but a standardized routine is recommended. If proper finger rests and reasonably sharp pencils are employed, the task can be accomplished quickly and easily (Fig. 10.11). The following is a suggested routine.

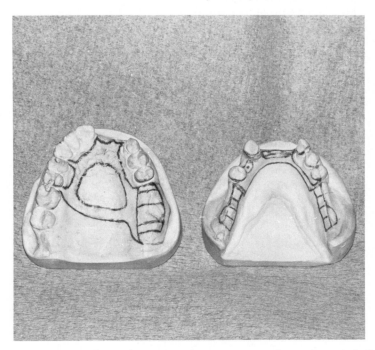

FIG. 10.15. The planning casts shown above are ready to accompany the master casts to the laboratory, as a supplement to a properly prepared work authorization.

Marking the Height of Contour. The study cast should be positioned on the surveyor in the same horizontal plane which was selected at the time of the preliminary analysis and planning, and the survey line should be marked on each abutment tooth.

Measuring Undercut. An undercut gauge of the proper size should be placed in the spindle. The gauge should be positioned on the surface of each of the abutment teeth so that the foot of the gauge contacts the tooth surface in the precise spot that will be contacted by the retentive clasp terminals, at the same time that the shank of the gauge contacts the height of contour. A small mark should be placed at the point at which the gauge contacts the surface of the tooth.

Drawing the Clasps. The clasp should be drawn so that the retentive terminal descends gracefully into the infrabulge area of the tooth (Fig. 10.12), *with the lower border of the clasp terminal precisely on the mark which indicates the desired degree of undercut to be engaged.* The reciprocal arm is drawn, being careful to maintain the inferior border on or above the survey line. The occlusal, incisal, or cingulum rest should be drawn in next, by delineating the outline of the prepared recess.

Drawing the Connectors. The major connector is drawn, including the retention latticework (Fig. 10.13). The minor connectors are added to unite the clasps with the major connector. The area to be occupied by the base may be drawn last, if the laboratory is to accomplish this phase of the construction (Fig. 10.14).

Miscellaneous Notations. Notations that will clarify other structural details such as the type of replacement tooth, e.g., "T" (for the tube tooth), "M" (for metal tooth), and "F" (for facing), may be placed on the capital portion of the cast opposite the appropriate edentulous space. Areas that are to be relieved, as well as borders that are meant to be beaded, should be indicated by a mutually understood code.

The diagram should represent a blueprint of the structural details of the framework that is to be fabricated (Fig. 10.15).

Bibliography

The Dental Laboratory Technician's Manual, AFM 160-29, Department of the Air Force. U.S. Government Printing Office, Washington, 1959.

Chapter 11

TRIAL FITTING OF THE FRAMEWORK

This chapter deals with the procedures which are followed in fitting the metal framework to the mouth. It is organized in the following way.

Introduction
Checking the Framework
Fitting the Framework to the Teeth
Adjusting the Framework to the Opposing Occlusion

Introduction

The metal framework should be tried in the mouth as soon after it is returned from the laboratory as is practicable. If there has been any error in technique, either in the dental office or in the laboratory, it should be discovered at this juncture, in order to determine the extent of the discrepancy and to make a judgment as to its effect on the prosthesis. Proper steps can then be taken, either to accomplish the appropriate adjustment or to begin anew by obtaining an impression.

Checking the Framework

The framework will typically fit the stone cast very tightly and may, in fact, be quite difficult to remove from it (Fig. 11.1). This should not be construed as conclusive evidence that it will exhibit the same degree of retention in the mouth, because a portion of this resistance to removal is due to the friction between the rough surface of the stone and the clasp. Typically, the clasps will not fit as tightly in the mouth. The framework which is moderately tight on the cast will generally

fit the mouth with the precise degree of tightness desired.

The Framework Fits the Cast but Not the Mouth

When a framework fits the master cast, but does not fit the mouth, it is prima facie evidence that the cast is not an exact replica of the mouth. This would indicate either an inaccurate impression or an improperly poured cast, provided one can be certain that (1) the cast has not been altered, or (2) the natural teeth have not changed position during the interval between obtaining the impression and fitting the framework. In the first instance, alteration of the cast can occur if an inexperienced laboratory technician forces the framework on and off the cast as he accomplishes the finishing operation on the metal. Each time that the frame is forced onto the cast, some of the stone is rubbed off the surface. The areas of the cast that become abraded and inaccurate are the precise areas where the framework does not fit the mouth. A discrepancy thus created can usually be recognized by close scrutiny of the cast surface in the areas where it is contacted by the metal. The second possibility, migration of the teeth, is not likely to occur unless there has been an unusually long time lag between the time the impression was obtained and the time of fitting the framework. However, migration may take place if a tooth adjacent to an abutment tooth has recently been extracted, and the opposing occlusion has been permitted to exert a tor-

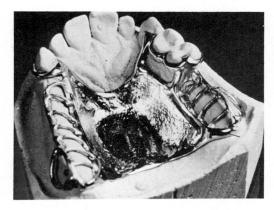

FIG. 11.1. The metal framework typically fits the stone master cast very tightly and may be difficult to remove.

sional stress on the abutment during the interval between the impression and fitting the framework. The latter contingency may be averted by reasonable precautions in planning the treatment sequence and in scheduling the required appointments so that they can be most expeditiously carried out. In either case, it may be possible to deal successfully with the discrepancy by knowledgeable adjustment of the framework, provided it is relatively minor in extent.

Examining the Tissue Side of the Casting

Prior to beginning the fitting operation, the tissue side of the framework should be examined carefully, under magnification and with adequate lighting, for the presence of blebs, bubbles, or other artifacts on the metal that might act as an impediment to smooth insertion of the framework onto the teeth. If there are any present, they should be removed with suitable abrasives before the framework is taken to the mouth for fitting. Gold alloy may be altered with ordinary carborundum stones, mounted in either the dental handpiece or the conventional bench lathe. The chromium-cobalt alloys, because of their hardness, require harder abrasives especially manufactured for the purpose, with rotating speeds of at least 20,000 rpm.

Although the metal framework will usually go into place and fit reasonably well with little need for adjustment, it is almost always possible to improve the fit to some degree by judicious machining operations on the metal. Fitting the metal framework to the mouth logically divides itself into two phases: (1) fitting the framework to the abutment teeth, and (2) adjusting it to the opposing occlusion. They are best accomplished in that order.

Fitting the Framework to the Teeth

Fitting the framework to the teeth is begun by positioning it over the abutments, placing the balls of the fingers on all (if possible) of the rests, and applying pressure in a direction parallel to the path of insertion. Practice instills a kind of sixth sense or "feel," so that any unusual resistance to seating is felt immediately upon being encountered, and the probable area of obstruction is usually known intuitively. If more than moderate pressure is required to seat the framework completely, one may confidently suspect an obstruction caused by a minor connector being forced against the proximal surface of an abutment tooth or, less commonly, a clasp arm which has become distorted.

Adjusting the Clasp

If a clasp arm is causing an obstruction, the contouring pliers can be employed to correct the problem, so that the frame can be seated. Pliers with smooth beaks should be used to effect the needed bend, so as not to scratch, nick, or otherwise weaken the metal of the clasp arm. While it must be conceded that the chromium-cobalt alloys are not as pliant as the gold alloys and do not lend themselves to adjustment as readily, certainly minor adjustments can be carried out without undue difficulty. The secret of altering the contour of a chromium-cobalt clasp is to achieve the desired modification with a series of minute bends, accomplished by the application of moderate, controlled force with the contouring pliers. The beaks of the pliers should have beveled edges so that the clasp is not forced against an angular surface. It bears repeating that the beaks of the pliers should not be serrated.

Adjusting the Framework

If an obstruction is caused by a part of the inner surface of a clasp wedging against a tooth surface, the metal in the area involved must be relieved. The general area suspected of harboring the obstacle should be dried off, and a pressure-indicating substance painted on the metal. Jeweler's rouge in chloroform or one of the commercial disclosing waxes may be used (Kerr Disclosing Wax, Kerr Dental Manufacturing Co., Detroit, Mich.). If the occlusal rests are being prevented from complete seating by what is obviously a very small discrepancy, it may require a considerable amount of pressure, applied to the occlusal rest, to disclose the offending spot. Pressure may be applied with a serrated instrument handle or with a pegwood stick. This will generally result in some of the disclosing agent being rubbed off the metal, thus revealing the precise point of overpressure. The disclosed mark should be relieved with a mounted stone, the disclosing agent and the residue from the grinding should be wiped off the metal with a cotton pledget, and the frame again should be tried on the teeth. If it is still slightly short of seating completely on the teeth, the procedure must be repeated until it glides smoothly to its seated position with the application of moderate pressure. Common areas of interference are the internal surface of the shoulders of the clasp, the clasp body, and the minor connector, in that order, although it is conceivable that an obstruction can occur at any area of the metal which contacts a tooth surface. When the framework does glide smoothly into place, all parts of the metal that contact tooth surfaces (clasp arms, rests, etc.) should be examined carefully to ensure that they are in tight contact with the tooth surface, thus indicating complete seating and an accurate fit. Each occlusal (incisal or cingulum) rest should fit snugly into its prepared recess. When inspecting the framework for proper fit, the junction of metal and tooth surface should be dried with a gentle stream of air to remove bubbles of saliva which might otherwise mask a discrepancy. If the rest fits down into the prepared recess but there is a slight discrepancy between the margins of the metal and the peripheries of the recess, it may indicate that the metal has been overtrimmed during the finishing operation in the laboratory. An explorer dragged across the margin of the tooth surface and the metal should reveal a smooth junction with no intervening crevice.

Adjusting for Over-Retention

It might be well to note that the framework should never snap into place with a discernible click. When this does occur, it indicates that there is too great a resistance to flexure of the alloy of one or more clasp arms. Usually, it is due to the fact that the retentive clasp terminals have been designed into too great an amount of retentive undercut. If an excessive application of force is required to flex the clasp arm, and if the clasp is not balanced so that the flexure is opposed by a resistant reciprocal arm, the tooth will receive a whiplash stress which will be injurious to the periodontal apparatus. Such a clasp should be adjusted by loosening it slightly, so that it engages slightly less of the retentive undercut. This can often be accomplished by polishing the inside surface of the clasp terminal with a rubber polishing point or wheel. In some instances, the clasp terminal may be shortened a slight amount, and in addition the clasp may be altered slightly with the adjustment pliers, so that it does not contact the surface of the tooth quite as intimately.

Wedging Effect

When the framework has been completely seated, the patient should be questioned to determine whether he feels any sensation of pressure on the natural teeth, either when the framework is being seated or after it is in place. A partial denture which restores a tooth-bounded edentulous space frequently elicits a complaint of tightness when the prosthesis is seated on the teeth. The patient may complain of a sensation which he typically describes as "wedging." The sensation is characteristically felt on the weaker abutment (the bicuspid). The pressure which produces the complaint may be simulated by placing the finger on the abutment tooth and applying pressure first in a mesial direction, for example, while at the same time inquiring of the patient, "Is it a pressure like this?" Carefully applied pressure against each surface of the tooth in question is usually successful in identifying the area of the framework that is the source of the pressure. If the pressure is one that seems to be wedging the two teeth apart, it is an indication that the offending obstruction is located on the inner surface of the body or shoulders of the clasp or, much less commonly, on the inner surface of the minor connector. Such an obstruction can usually be pinpointed by means of the disclosing agent and eliminated by grinding with appropriate stones.

Adjusting the Framework to the Opposing Occlusion

When the framework has been adjusted so that it glides smoothly into place under moderate pressure, without the patient experiencing any disagreeable wedging sensation or discomfort, it should be adjusted so that it is in harmony with the opposing occlusion. If it is opposed by a prosthesis, any needed adjustments may be made on the teeth of the prosthesis. If there are interferences with natural teeth, the adjustments may be made on both the framework and the teeth. Markings which indicate interferences may be made with either articulating paper or with occlusal indicator wax. Although the carbon of the articulating paper does not readily transfer to the highly polished chromium-cobalt alloy, it will do so if the surface of the metal is roughened slightly with a carborundum stone. If unusual difficulty is experienced in obtaining markings on

the metal with articulating paper, jeweler's rouge and chloroform may be used as a disclosing agent.

The Objective

The intercuspation of the remaining natural teeth should be closely observed in centric occlusion. The objective of the

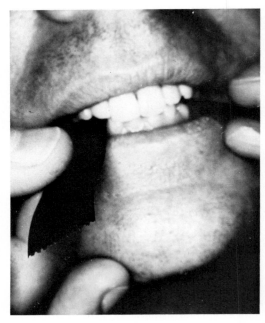

Fig. 11.2. Articulating paper may be employed to mark points of interference between the metal framework and the opposing teeth.

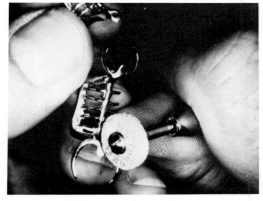

Fig. 11.3. Points of interference should be relieved with suitable stones followed by polishing.

equilibrating procedure is to adjust the occlusion so that the teeth occlude in all functional positions, with the partial denture in place, exactly as they do when it is out of the mouth.

The Equilibration Procedure

If articulating paper is employed, a strip should be placed between the teeth on both sides of the arch and the patient instructed to "close on the back teeth" (Fig. 11.2). When the teeth are tightly occluded in centric position, the patient is instructed to "grind" or "rub" the teeth slightly, from side to side, while at the same time maintaining them tightly together. The amount of mandibular movement should be small, and the interocclusal biting pressure moderately heavy. The markings thus obtained will be more representative of masticatory function than will markings obtained by having the patient execute wide movements of the mandible into lateral and protrusive positions. Areas of interference should be relieved with suitable stones (Fig. 11.3). When the occlusion has been adjusted so that all posterior teeth occlude simultaneously and uniformly, the patient should be instructed to move the mandible into lateral and protrusive relationships while the

intercuspation is closely observed for any sign of interference between the opposing teeth and the prosthesis. Any existing interferences should be eliminated. The metal should be polished at any point where it has been roughened by the grinding. Any part of an opposing prosthesis which has been roughened should likewise be smoothed and polished.

Fitting Two Frameworks

If both a maxillary and a mandibular framework are to be fitted to the mouth, the fitting of each one should be carried out individually. The task is much simpler if one framework is completely adjusted before work is begun on the second. When the second framework has been completely seated and adjusted, the occlusion should be such that the remaining teeth of both jaws intercuspate harmoniously in all functional movements and that no part of either framework interferes with normal closure or with any excursive movement within the patient's functional range.

Bibliography

Rudd, K. D., and Dunn, B. W.: Accurate removable partial dentures. J. Prosth. Dent. *18:* 559–570, 1967.

Chapter 12

THE FUNCTIONAL IMPRESSION
—THE ALTERED CAST

This chapter explains the rationale of functional basing of the removable partial denture. Two methods for accomplishing functional basing are discussed, and one technique, the altered cast method, is described in detail. Finally, the working characteristics of several impression materials, which may be employed to obtain the functional impression, are compared. Subject matter is arranged in the format which follows.

Introduction
Providing Support for the Prosthesis
The Principle of Functional Basing
The Altered Cast Method
The Functional Reline Method
Determining The Need for a Functional Impression
Impression Materials for the Functional
  Impression

Introduction

A widely accepted axiom of removable partial prosthodontics holds that it is fully as important that the denture be designed and constructed in such a way as best to preserve the oral structures as it is to restore function. The principle of functional basing is employed to create conditions which favor maximum longevity of the remaining structures.

Providing Support for the Prosthesis

Preservation of the remaining oral structures in such a state of health as to ensure their longevity is best achieved by exploiting tooth support to the maximum extent that it is available. In short, the prosthesis of ideal design is one that is entirely tooth-borne. Unfortunately, the number and distribution of the teeth remaining in the mouth of the typical candidate for a partial denture makes this not often possible of achievement. When complete tooth support is not available, stress should be distributed equally between the remaining natural teeth and all of the soft tissue support that is capable of bearing a portion of the masticatory load. A problem is encountered in employing this composite type of support, however, because the mucosa, as a result of its resilience and displaceability, provides an unstable foundation for the prosthesis. This is explained by the fact that the oral mucosa in stress-bearing areas of the mouth is capable of assuming two distinctly different contours. One is the form which it assumes when it is at rest—the resting or anatomic form; the other is its functional or supporting form, which it assumes when it is subjected to the pressure of an occlusal load.

This Jekyll-and-Hyde characteristic may be demonstrated by obtaining an alginate impression in a stock tray of a distal extension base type of partially edentulous mandibular arch and constructing, on the resulting cast, a metal framework with a lingual bar, two clasps, and acrylic resin bases. If this experimental prosthesis is placed in the mouth, and firm pressure is applied to the base with the finger, it will be found that the base usually can be depressed downward into the mucosa by a discernible amount. The movement occurs because the mucosa undergoes a change in form, when subjected to the pressure, from its resting to

comfort to the patient, or without exerting a dislodging force against the denture.

Note: The final impression may be registered with low fusing wax, with zinc oxide-eugenol paste, or with one of the rubber base impression materials. The technique for mouth temperature wax is described here.

2. The tissue surface of the resin tray is thoroughly dried, and a uniform layer of number 4 (extra soft) mouth temperature wax (Korecta Kerr Dental Manufacturing Co., Detroit, Mich.) is applied with a small brush. The framework should be seated in the mouth for approximately 5 minutes, being certain that all parts of the metal that contact tooth surfaces are precisely and accurately in position on the teeth.

3. The framework is removed from the mouth, and the impression is dried and inspected. Areas of the wax that are in good functional contact will appear glossy, while areas of insufficient contact will appear dull. Wrinkled areas indicate a lack of firm contact or insufficient time for the wax to flow. If the wax is penetrated by either the modeling composition or the impression tray, it indicates an area of over-pressure and should be relieved. The necessary corrections are made and the prosthesis is reinserted for a period of 10 to 12 minutes, to allow ample time for the wax to fill in voids, and to migrate to the periphery and be turned over the borders. The addition of wax to the borders creates the gentle distension needed to exclude air from the denture-tissue interface, thus providing a seal. The impression is complete when the entire tissue surface has a glossy appearance and the peripheries are rounded and smooth (Fig. 12.4).

Altering the Cast

The master cast is altered by substituting the denture-bearing areas, obtained with the corrective impression material, for the ones that were registered in the

* Note: University of Iowa Formula Wax (Kerr Dental Manufacturing Co., Detroit, Mich.) may also be used for this purpose.

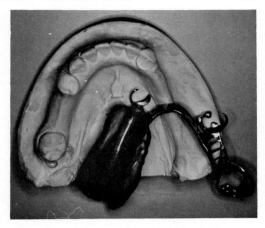

Fig. 12.4. Shown here is a functional impression obtained with low fusing wax after the borders of the tray were border molded with modeling composition. Note the full rounded borders. A functional impression is not needed on the opposite side of the mouth because the base is tooth-supported.

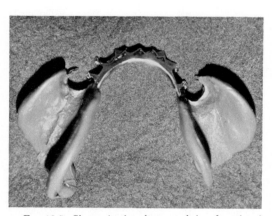

Fig. 12.5. Shown in the photograph is a functional impression which has been taken in rubber base impression material.

first (alginate) impression (Figs. 12.5–12.10).

The Functional Reline Method

When the reline method is followed, the denture is fabricated in the customary manner, with the sole exception that a layer of relief metal (Ash metal) approximately 1 mm. in thickness is burnished to the residual ridge area of the processing cast prior to final closure of the flask. The purpose of the metal is to provide a space on the tissue side of the denture for the reline material. The needed space could be provided by grinding the tissue side of the denture with stones and burs, but since the metal ensures a uniform depth, it is the preferred method. The denture is processed and fitted into the mouth in the customary manner, except that the relief metal is left in place (Fig. 12.11). When it has been worn for a trial period of a week or 10 days, and all needed adjustments have been accomplished, the relief metal is stripped from the acrylic resin and a reline procedure is carried out. The pe-

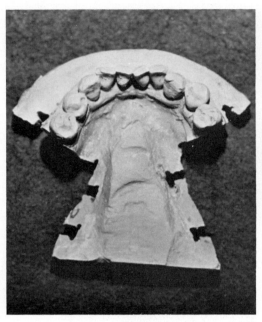

FIG. 12.6. The master cast is prepared for the alteration by making saw cuts to separate the denture-bearing areas from the rest of the cast.

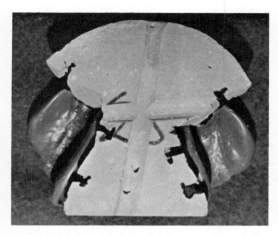

FIG. 12.8. The photograph shows a view of the assembly from the under side of the cast.

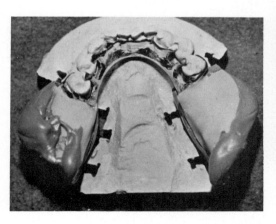

FIG. 12.7. The metal framework with the attached impression is positioned on the master cast. It is imperative that all occlusal (incisal-lingual) rests be properly seated in their prepared recesses.

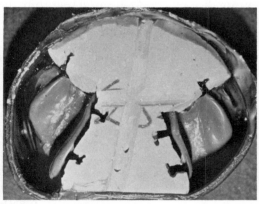

FIG. 12.9. The peripheral borders of the impression are protected with utility wax and the entire assembly is wrapped with boxing wax. Prior to pouring the stone the cast should be moistened by placing it in a shallow bath of slurry water for a few moments so that the new stone will more readily bond to it.

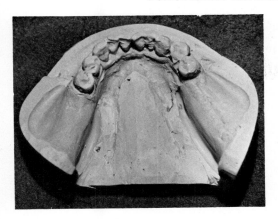

Fig. 12.10. Shown in the photograph is the altered cast. The newly added stone is customarily poured in a different colored stone than that of the original cast.

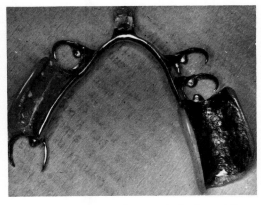

Fig. 12.11. A convenient method of providing a space of uniform thickness for the reline material, when the reline method of functional basing is to be carried out, is to burnish a layer of relief metal to the areas of the processing cast which will be occupied by the distal extension base. During processing the relief metal becomes a part of the denture base which the patient wears for a week or 10 days while the customary adjustments are made. At the end of that time, the relief metal is stripped out and a reline procedure is performed.

ripheries are refined by border-molding with modeling composition, after which the final impression is obtained with one of the corrective materials, fluid wax, one of the rubber base impression materials, or zinc oxide-eugenol paste. When the denture is inserted, with the impression

material inside it, due care should be exercised to ensure that the framework is in its proper position on the teeth. For this reason, the open mouth technique is preferred, since it permits observation of the framework on the teeth at all times. It is apparent that if the patient were permitted to exert pressure on the posterior teeth, the framework might rotate on the fulcrum (the abutments), thus distorting the relationship of the framework and bases to the teeth. When the impression has been obtained, a cast is poured and the reline is processed, either by flasking or by means of a reline jig.

A disadvantage of the reline method is that the occlusion, which has been so carefully developed, may be altered slightly by the reline impression and may require adjustment following the processing of the acrylic resin. Another drawback is the possibility of creating a visible junction line between the newly added acrylic resin and the original base material. However, these are relatively minor problems, not difficult to surmount, and the technique has much to recommend it.

Determining the Need for a Functional Impression

Since the displaceability of the mucosal covering of the residual ridge varies within a very wide range from mouth to mouth, it will be found that, as a practical matter, the degree of displacement is so slight in some mouths, with well formed ridges and a thick, healthy mucosal covering, that the functional impression is not essential. This is particularly apt to be true in the maxillary arch. The contour of some mucosal foundations may be virtually the same under an applied load as it is at rest. Accordingly, the decision as to whether or not to employ the functional impression technique in a given case may be based in part on the following test. Add acrylic resin bases to the framework by forming the resin base directly on the stone cast after a tinfoil substitute has been applied to it. Place the framework, with the attached resin bases, in the mouth and apply pressure with the fingers to each base. If the base can be depressed a discernible amount with finger pressure, a functional impression procedure should be carried out. If, however, there is no discernible movement of the base, consideration may be given to dispensing with the functional impression technique. When such a decision has been made, the resin bases can be used as record bases to obtain the required intraoral records. It must be pointed out, however, that dispensing with the functional impression procedure also eliminates the opportunity of establishing precisely accurate, functionally formed denture borders.

Impression Materials for the Functional Impression

Several impression materials are available for registering the functional impression, any one of which can be relied upon for recording accurately the mucosal tissues in their supporting form, provided they are properly manipulated. The materials vary widely in viscosity and, of course, the more viscous the material, the greater will be the tendency for compaction and displacement of the soft tissue. Materials of low viscosity are more accurate in recording fine tissue detail, since the mucosa is less prone to be distorted by pressure. It may be well to recall, in this connection, that tissue that has been displaced beyond a certain point has a tendency to rebound to its former contour. For this reason, overdisplacement of resilient tissue with the impression material should be avoided since, in service, the result may be an inflammatory reaction beneath the denture base. Overextension of the border tissues and excessive pressure on the primary stress bearing areas can be avoided by an understanding of the physical properties of the impression materials that are selected for use, and by manipulative techniques which are geared to these properties.

Fluid Wax

Fluid wax (Korecta Wax, Kerr Dental Manufacturing Co., Detroit, Mich.) is an excellent material with which to obtain the reline impression; its chief drawbacks

are the time required for its manipulation and the comparatively complex armamentarium needed for its use. In contrast, either zinc oxide-eugenol paste or the rubber base impression materials are instantly available for use, and the technique required for their manipulation is less time-consuming. It should be pointed out, however, that wax has certain virtues not possessed by any of the other impression materials. Perhaps its outstanding merit is the fact that it flows at body temperature. By virtue of this fact, it tends to flow away from points of pressure and to migrate into voids and areas of non-pressure. This is ideal for registering a type of tissue, such as the oral mucosa, which varies markedly in displacement in different regions of the mouth. A degree of mild compression and gentle displacement can be achieved with fluid wax that appears, from clinical evidence, to be exceptionally compatible with the mucosal tissue. The wax is applied layer-by-layer so that it is rarely, if ever, necessary to strip it out of the denture, although it can easily be removed if it should be desirable to do so for any reason. Fluid wax is the impression medium par excellence for obtaining an impression of either the markedly atrophic or the knife-edge residual ridge.

Zinc Oxide-Eugenol Paste

Zinc oxide-eugenol paste is an accurate impression material which is not unpleasant to the patient, and its employment requires a minimum of time. Although the impression must be obtained with a single insertion of the framework, most minor surface defects which occur can be patched by mixing a small amount of fresh material and inserting the impression a second time to accomplish their correction. Since the impression is obtained with a single insertion, the technique carries with it the hazard of failure to seat the framework on the teeth with precise accuracy, thus introducing a distortion that will result in an inaccurate altered cast.

A disadvantage of zinc oxide-eugenol

paste is that if the impression is not acceptable and must be remade, the removal of the material from the tray is an onerous, time-consuming chore. A caution that should be observed when zinc oxide-eugenol is employed for the reline impression is to ensure that all of the material is removed from the denture base before the new acrylic resin is added, since the eugenol can interfere with polymerization of the acrylic resin. Zinc oxide-eugenol is intermediate in viscosity between modeling composition, which has a very high viscosity, and alginate, which has a low viscosity.

The Rubber Base Materials

The rubber base impression materials, either mercaptan or silicone, are excellent materials for recording the reline-rebase impression. They are easy to manipulate and not unpleasant to the patient, and the procedure is not unduly time-consuming. If the impression must be retaken for one reason or another, the rubber can be readily stripped from the denture base. It should be noted, however, that the rubber is not easily patched if a void, bubble, or other surface defect is encountered. The viscosity of the rubber base materials is roughly comparable to that of zinc oxide-eugenol paste.

A special adhesive must be used to coat the tissue surface of the impression base to ensure that the rubber adheres to the acrylic resin as well as to the modeling composition.

Bibliography

Applegate, O. C.: The partial denture base. J. Prosth. Dent. 5: 636–648, 1955.

Hindels, G. W.: Load distribution in extension saddle partial dentures. J. Prosth. Dent. 2: 92–100, 1952.

Lytle, R. B.: Soft tissue displacement beneath removable partial and complete dentures. J. Prosth. Dent. 12: 34–43, 1962.

McCracken, W. L.: Partial Denture Construction, Ed. 3. The C. V. Mosby Company, St. Louis, 1969.

Chapter 13

INTERMAXILLARY RELATIONS

Introduction

The occlusion for the removable partial
denture may be basically similar to that
for a complete denture, or it may resemble more closely that for a fixed partial denture, depending on the number of
teeth being replaced, the design of the
prosthesis, and the nature of the opposing
occlusion. Accordingly, the methods used
to achieve an efficient occlusion may, in a
given set of circumstances, follow closely
those employed for the former, while in
other circumstances they may be more
nearly like those for the latter.

The Objective

The objective in developing an occlusal
scheme for the partial denture is the same
as for any oral prosthesis: to create an
arrangement of the opposing teeth which
is in harmony with mandibular movement, so as to provide the patient with a
masticating mechanism that is at the
same time efficient, comfortable, and esthetically pleasing. Equally important, in
the case of the removable partial denture,
is the need to distribute functional forces
between the remaining natural teeth and
the residual ridge in such a manner that
each shares a portion of the masticatory
load, commensurate with its ability to
withstand stress. A harmonious occlusion
will contribute materially to the control of
damaging, leverage-induced stresses,
while conversely, a faulty occlusion will
compound the destructive effects of these
stresses.

A partial denture with a hormonious
occlusion is one in which functional stress
is distributed among all of the occluding
teeth, and there are no deflective contacts
as the mandible moves through the
chewing cycle and into a position of tight
intercuspation.

Methods of Establishing the Occlusion

There are two principal methods of establishing the occlusion for a removable
partial denture: (1) the functionally generated path method, and (2) the articulator
or static method. Each method has advantages as well as disadvantages and limitations. Because of the enormous diversity
of partially edentulous jaws, and combinations of prostheses, the generated path

210

method is better suited to some conditions of partial edentulousness, whereas the articulator method may produce a better result for others.

The Functionally Generated Path Method

The generated path technique is based on the theory that the patient himself is the best articulator for developing the occlusion. Accordingly, the technique consists of having the patient create in wax his own individual pattern of jaw movement. The pattern which he creates in the wax is a negative record of the movement through space of each opposing tooth as the mandible executes its functional excursions. These generated pathways are then reproduced in stone so that each groove in the wax, representing the pathway of a cusp, becomes a ridge in the stone. The artificial teeth are then arranged on the partial denture framework to intercuspate with the pathways of their antagonists as represented by these stone ridges. Fundamental to the concept is the fact that the pathways are a dynamic, as distinguished from a static, representation of the opposing teeth.

The Articulator Method

The articulator method consists of attaching the maxillary and mandibular stone casts (one of which carries the framework of the prosthesis) to the upper and lower members of an articulator. The artificial teeth are then positioned on the framework so as to articulate with the stone teeth of the opposing cast.

The Functionally Generated Path Method

The functionally generated path technique consists in attaching a specially compounded hard-wax occlusion rim to an acrylic resin base which has been fastened to the retention latticework of the partial denture framework (Fig. 13.1). The assembly is placed in the mouth and the patient is instructed to simulate chewing movements for a period of from 20 to 30

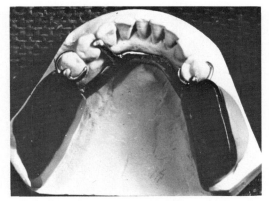

FIG. 13.1. The functionally generated path method is accomplished with a specially compounded hard-wax occlusion rim, luted to an acrylic resin base that has been attached to the retention latticework of the partial denture framework.

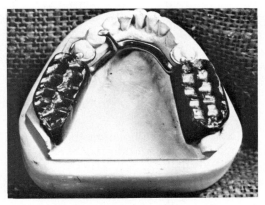

FIG. 13.2. The assembly is placed in the mouth and the patient is instructed to perform chewing movements for from 20 to 30 minutes. He is directed to bite and grind in all extremes of his functional range. The pattern which he wears into the wax will resemble a slightly widened version of the teeth which once occupied the edentulous spaces.

minutes. The pattern that is created in the wax will resemble a slightly widened version of the teeth which once occupied the edentulous spaces (Fig. 13.2). The occlusal surfaces will appear larger, because the pathway in the wax represents the teeth in their various extreme lateral, protrusive, and retrusive positions. The wax pattern is boxed (Fig. 13.3) and poured in

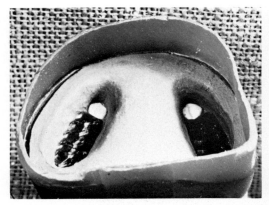

FIG. 13.3. The wax pattern is boxed with wax and poured in stone to create a countercast.

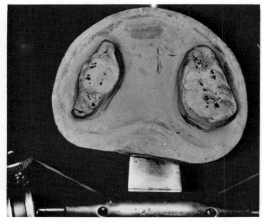

FIG. 13.4. The resulting stone countercast represents a positive reproduction of the cuspal pathways which were fashioned in the wax.

stone, to produce a positive representation of the opposing cuspal pathways (Fig. 13.4). The opposing cast, with the framework of the prosthesis, is mounted on the articulator, and the prosthetic teeth are fitted to articulate with the pathways (Fig. 13.5).

Advantages of the Generated Path Technique

Advocates of the functionally generated path technique maintain that there is reasonable doubt that any articulator exists that is capable of simulating, with complete fidelity, all of the complex movements that the mandible is capable of making. Moreover, should such an instrument exist, there remains the difficult question of whether intraocclusal records are sufficiently precise to make possible a reliably accurate adjustment of the instrument so that it will copy all of these movements. The generated path technique does not rely for its accuracy and effectiveness on the type or complexity of the articulator, or upon the skill of the clinician in obtaining, interpreting, and effecting the transfer of intraoral records. The method also eliminates the need for tracing devices or for a facebow transfer.

To summarize: (1) the method makes unnecessary the registration of intraocclusal records or a facebow transfer and dispenses with the need for a complicated

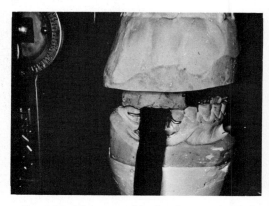

FIG. 13.5. The cast with the framework of the prosthesis is mounted on an articulator to oppose the stone pattern (the countercast), and the prosthetic teeth are arranged to articulate with the pathways.

articulator, and (2) jaw movements and tooth pathways are reproduced under more nearly functional conditions than is the case when static registrations (intraoral records) are transferred to an instrument.

Limitations of the Generated Path Method

The generated path method does not lend itself to use when the opposing occlusion is provided by a complete denture, or when all of the teeth (or replacements for them) are not present in the opposing occlusion. It should be noted, however, that when two removable partial dentures are being constructed, one may be completed by using the articulator method, after which the second may be made to oppose it by means of the functionally generated path method. Sometimes cited as a disadvantage of the generated path method is the fact that resistance may be encountered by the mandible, as the teeth shear through the wax, which might serve to deflect it from its natural path. Should this occur, it would create a discrepancy which would be impossible to detect, since there is no way that the accuracy of the generated path can be verified. Similarly, the patient's masticating force and direction may vary with foods of different types and textures. Thus, it may be postulated that the masticatory pattern of the teeth during actual function probably differs from that which they follow as they generate pathways in the wax. Finally, it should be pointed out that the generated path technique does not lend itself for use when the prosthesis is to replace anterior teeth.

The Articulator Method

Two objectives are fundamental to employment of the articulator method. The first objective is that the static relationship of the maxillary and mandibular casts to each other be accurately established. This relationship must be the same as that of the maxilla and the mandible in the three planes of space, i.e., horizontal, frontal (or coronal), and sagittal (Fig. 13.6). This is accomplished clinically by establishing the sagittal relationship (vertical dimension), followed by the horizontal relationship (centric relation). A final relationship is that of the two casts to the center of movement (the condyles) which is accomplished by means of a facebow transfer.

The second objective is that the dynamic relationship of the two casts be established. This refers to their relationship to each other as the mandible moves in space. In satisfying this objective, intraoral records of mandibular movement

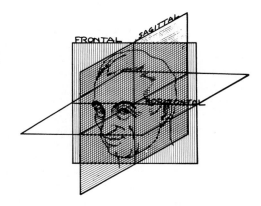

FIG. 13.6. One of the prime requirements, when the articulator method of developing the occlusion for the removable denture is followed, is that the casts of the mandible and maxilla be accurately related to each other on the instrument in the three planes of space designated as horizontal, frontal (or coronal), and sagittal.

must be made by means of which the articulator can be programmed to simulate the natural movements of the lower jaw.

Advantages of the Articulator Method

Summarized briefly, the advantages of the articulator method are as follows. (1) It is the method of choice when the edentulous areas to be restored are opposed by edentulous areas in the opposing jaw. (2) It is a better method when the prosthesis is opposed by a completely edentulous arch. (3) The occlusion can be developed rather simply for the typical partial denture, in a minimum of time. (4) It does not require the degree of cooperation by the patient that is required in generating the functional pathway. (5) It is the preferred method when anterior teeth are being replaced.

Limitations of the Articulator Method

The articulator method has few if any limitations, insofar as either the type of partial denture or the combination of prostheses for which the occlusion is to be developed is concerned. Assuming an articulator with a level of sophistication commensurate with the intraoral records that are to be used, the only limitations imposed would be related to the skill and care with which the intraoral records are obtained and to the accuracy and thoroughness with which they are used to program the instrument.

Vertical Dimension

Vertical dimension, as the term implies, is a relation of the two jaws in a vertical (sagittal) plane. Establishment of the correct vertical relation in construction of a removable partial denture is crucial, not only to the development of a harmonious occlusion, but to the comfort and well-being of the patient as well. If it is incorrectly established, the result may be not only a loss in masticating efficiency, but damage to the residual ridges and the remaining teeth, as well as to the temporomandibular joint. If the vertical dimension of occlusion is too great, the result

may be strained, tired muscles and irritated mucosa accompanied by rapid bone resorption. If it is too little, there may be a loss of efficiency, often coupled with an appearance of facial imbalance, and there may be temporomandibular joint symptoms. The vertical dimension is inseparably linked with the horizontal relation; both must be accurately determined if the patient is to regain his former masticating proficiency.

The Two Vertical Dimensions

The term "vertical dimension" is used to designate a vertical measurement of the face between two arbitrary points, one above and one below the mouth, usually selected as a point on the chin and a point on the nose or the upper lip near the midline. Two different vertical dimensions are commonly referred to (Fig. 13.7) as (1) the vertical dimension of occlusion,

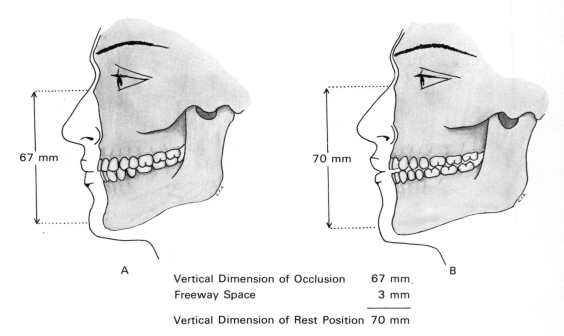

67 mm

70 mm

A

B

Vertical Dimension of Occlusion	67 mm
Freeway Space	3 mm
Vertical Dimension of Rest Position	70 mm

Fig. 13.7. The term "vertical dimension" is used to designate a vertical measurement of the face between two arbitrarily selected points (often a point on the nose and a point on the chin) at or near the midline. There are two vertical dimensions: A, the vertical dimension of occlusion which is the measurement between the two points on the face when the teeth (or the occlusion rims) are in centric occlusion and B, the measurement between the two points when the teeth are slightly apart and the mandible is in rest position. The vertical dimension of occlusion may be established clinically by subtracting 3 mm. (an average amount of freeway space) from the vertical dimension of rest position.

which is the vertical dimension of the face when the teeth or the occlusion rims are occluded, or (2) the vertical dimension of rest position, which is the vertical dimension of the face when the teeth are apart and the mandible is in rest position.

The resting position of the mandible is dependent upon a balance among several important muscle groups; hence it must be considered a postural position. The muscles involved are the postcervical group, the infrahyoid and suprahyoid groups, and the muscles of mastication (Fig. 13.8). It is the position customarily assumed by the mandible when it is not performing functional movement. Since the mandible must travel upward from rest position to bring the teeth into contact, it is apparent that the vertical dimension of rest position is always greater than the vertical dimension of occlusion.

The Freeway Space

The space which exists between the teeth when the mandible is in rest position is termed the "freeway space," the "interocclusal gap," or the "interocclusal clearance." The relation of the vertical dimension of rest, the vertical dimension of occlusion, and the freeway space may be summed up in the following equation: the vertical dimension of rest position is equal to the vertical dimension of occlusion plus the freeway space. An average amount of freeway space is generally considered to be from 2 to 4 mm.

Establishing the Vertical Dimension Clinically

Establishing the vertical dimension of occlusion for the average partially edentulous patient is simply a matter of relating the casts to each other in the vertical relationship at which the posterior teeth occlude. The patient who has lost all of the teeth in one arch, however, has for all practical purposes lost his vertical dimension of occlusion, and it must be rediscovered by methods which resemble very closely those employed with complete dentures.

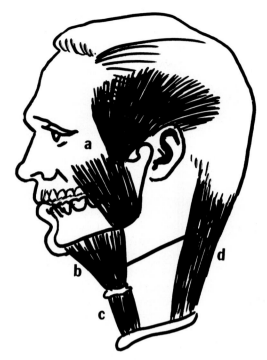

FIG. 13.8. The rest position of the mandible is dependent on a balance among several important muscle groups of the head and neck. These are the muscles of mastication (*a*), the suprahyoid group (*b*), the infrahyoid group (*c*) and the postcervical group (*d*).

The Basis for Methods of Establishing Vertical Dimension

Fortunately, the work of Niswonger and other investigators has formed the basis for clinical methods which make it possible to determine the vertical dimension of occlusion with an acceptable degree of clinical accuracy. Niswonger, one of the pioneer workers in devising methods for establishing the vertical dimension for edentulous patients, measured the freeway space between the natural teeth of 200 patients between the ages of 37 and 83 years of age. His study revealed that 83% of these individuals had a freeway space of $4/32$ inch, or approximately 3 mm. None had less than $1/32$ inch, and none more than $7/32$ inch of interocclusal clearance. Niswonger postulated that, since the relation of the vertical dimension of rest position and the vertical dimension of occlusion bear a constant relationship to one another in patients with natural teeth, he could devise a method of establishing vertical dimension for the edentulous individual by securing one measurement, and from it computing the other. The technique, which he conceived and perfected, was to determine the vertical dimension of mandibular rest position by making chin-nose measurements on the face. He could then subtract 3 mm. from it to arrive at the correct vertical dimension of occlusion. To prove his theory, he constructed 50 sets of complete upper and lower dentures in which he incorporated a freeway space of 3 mm., and all of the dentures were successful.

The Effect of Posture on Vertical Dimension. Because the vertical dimension of rest is essentially a postural position in which several large muscle groups of the head and neck are in a state of tonic equilibrium, it follows that the position of the head at the time that the rest position is determined is critical. Translated into clinical terms, this means that the amount of interocclusal clearance can be altered by the attitude of the head at the time that the measurement is made. If the head is thrown back, the mandible will tend to drop, thus creating an increased amount of freeway space. If it is pitched forward, the reverse is true. It should be apparent then that determining the vertical dimension of rest position should be accomplished with the patient's head erect (in the Frankfort plane), unsupported by the headrest. The head is in the Frankfort plane when a line which extends through the lowest point in the margin of the orbit (orbitale) and the highest point in the margin of the external auditory meatus (tragion) is parallel with the floor (Fig. 13.9).

Altering the Vertical Dimension of Occlusion

A problem frequently encountered, in developing the occlusion for a removable partial denture, is a loss of interridge

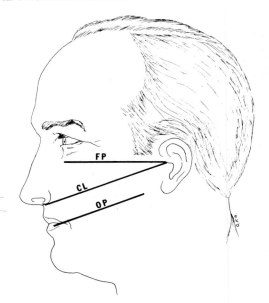

FIG. 13.9. The head is in the Frankfort plane (*FP, above*) when a line extending through the lowest point in the margin of the orbit and the highest part of the external auditory meatus is parallel to the floor. Camper's line, which is the line running from the inferior border of the ala of the nose to the superior border of the tragus of the ear, is designated *CL*. The occlusal plane, which is customarily made to parallel Camper's line, is designated as *OP*. The landmark used for locating the facebow to the condyle is 11 to 13 mm. anterior to the upper third of the tragus, on a line extending to the outer canthus of the eye.

space, so that there is inadequate space to accommodate the prosthesis or to establish an acceptable occlusal plane. There may be complete obliteration of the space between the teeth of one arch and the opposing residual ridge (Fig. 13.10), or between two opposing residual ridges. Contact between the tuberosity and the retromolar pad is a common example. The obvious conclusion would appear to be that the jaws have closed together as a result of a combination of the loss of natural teeth and attrition of the ones which remain. If this were true, the solution would be to retrieve the lost space by increasing the vertical dimension of occlusion with a prosthesis or a combination of prostheses. However, it cannot be taken

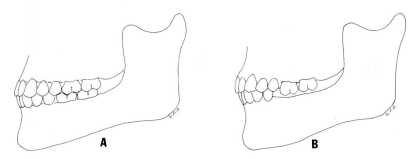

Fig. 13.10. A common clinical finding is the collapsed occlusion illustrated in these sketches. It results from the premature loss of posterior teeth without prosthetic replacement; the earlier the loss of the teeth, the more prone is the patient to this dental disablement. *A* depicts a normal occlusal relationship prior to extractions, *B*, after extractions. Factors which have been postulated in the etiology are (1) extrusion of the teeth which have no opponents, (2) overgrowth of the bone in the arch with the remaining teeth, (3) a change in the mandibular angle in which it becomes less acute, and (4) migration forward of the mandibular condyle. The probabilities are that, in most instances, the etiology is multicausal.

for granted that because there has obviously been attrition and tooth loss, and the jaws appear to be overclosed, that the vertical dimension of occlusion has been reduced. It must be remembered that teeth continue to erupt as attrition occurs and that they tend to extrude when they have lost their antagonists, thereby preventing what might otherwise be a diminished vertical dimension of occlusion and an increased amount of freeway space. If the dimension of the freeway space has not increased, then obviously a prosthesis which raised the occlusal level of the teeth or "opened the bite" would encroach on this space, thereby interfering with the rest position of the mandible. Reducing the patient's freeway space would mean that the closing muscles of mastication would be in a constant state of contraction as they attempted to return to their normal resting length. The result would be tired, sore muscles, and this would not be all of the problem. The unnatural pull of the muscles would impose stresses on the occluding teeth and on the temporomandibular joint which, given time, would very likely exceed their tolerance level. Quite apart from the discomfort, the result might be intrusion of the teeth, rapid resorption of the bone around the teeth, resorption of the bone of the residual ridge, and/or temporomandibular joint symptoms.

Diagnostic Signs of Overclosure

Although it is true that a loss of teeth and attrition of the remaining teeth is usually not accompanied by a corresponding increase in freeway space, there are exceptions in which the freeway space is obviously in excess of what is normal for the patient. Given these circumstances, the vertical dimension of occlusion can be increased with removable partial dentures, provided there has been a genuine overclosure, and the procedure is approached with understanding and accomplished with clinical skill.

While the most significant diagnostic sign of overclosure is an excessive amount of freeway space, it is usually accompanied by one or more additional clinical signs, such as (1) an acquired imbalance of facial dimension, which creates an appearance of premature aging (a shortened nose-chin distance), (2) a complaint of discomfort or pain in the region of the temporomandibular joint, (3) an occlusion in which the loss of posterior teeth has permitted the mandibular incisors to contact the palatal mucosa when the mandible is in closed position, and (4) a response from the patient that the "bite feels better" when the occlusal level is raised with temporary bite blocks, or even with cotton rolls.

Patient Selection

Increasing the vertical dimension of occlusion with a removable partial denture or dentures is, by its very nature, a quasi-experimental procedure. Hence, it is important that the patient for whom this service is to be provided be selected carefully. The ideal patient is one in good health and not over 30 years of age. Increasing the vertical dimension will probably not be successful if attempted for the elderly individual or for the one in poor health.

The Clinical Procedure for Altering the Vertical Dimension

Mandibular overclosure occurs very slowly, over an extended period of time and, as a result, the muscles and ligaments that are affected have gradually accommodated to a decrease in their former length. Unless the increase is to be no more than 1 or 2 mm., it would be ill-advised to return these muscles suddenly to the length that they once were. A better approach would be to accomplish the alteration in small increments, so that the patient can be closely observed for signs or symptoms which may offer clues as to the efficacy of the therapy. Accordingly, it is good clinical procedure to construct a removable treatment prosthesis in which the occlusal surfaces of the teeth are built up no more than 2 mm. (measured in the bicuspid region) with acrylic resin overlays which are an integral part of a metal framework. The patient can then be kept under observation for evidence of adverse symptoms, such as tired muscles, sore teeth, bone loss, temporomandibular joint tenderness, or any other untoward effects. When an occlusal level has been established at which the patient functions comfortably and efficiently, a more definitive type of prosthesis may be prescribed.

When the vertical dimension is to be altered, the facebow should be used to transfer the casts to the articulator. Changing the vertical dimension between casts that have been arbitrarily mounted on the articulator is to run the risk of error (see the facebow discussion in this chapter).

Horizontal Relationships

When the vertical relationship of the mandible to the maxilla has been established, the proper horizontal relationship can be determined. There are two horizontal relationships that are of importance in developing the occlusion: (1) centric relation and (2) centric occlusion.

Centric Relation

Centric relation is the most retruded, unstrained relation of the mandible to the maxilla from which lateral movement can be made at an established vertical dimension. It is constant throughout life except in the case of traumatic injury or inflammation in the temporomandibular joint. It is the customary reference point in developing the occlusion for an oral prosthesis. It is a bone-to-bone (condyle of the mandible to glenoid fossa of the maxilla) relation.

Centric Occlusion

Centric occlusion is a relationship of the jaws in which there is maximum intercuspation of the teeth. It is a tooth-to-tooth relationship.

The Relationship of Centric Relation to Centric Occlusion

In an ideal occlusion, centric relation and centric occlusion are one and the same. That is, when the jaws are in a position of centric relation the teeth are, at the same time, in a position of centric occlusion. Unfortunately, these two clinical entities often do not coincide in the natural dentition, particularly in the mouth of the candidate for a removable partial denture.

Methods of Retruding the Mandible

Establishing centric relation may sometimes be difficult, particularly when the patient has lost many natural teeth, in a random pattern, over a period of years. It may be especially difficult for the patient who is completely edentulous in one or both jaws, because often he has partially lost the proprioceptive sense which normally helps to guide the mandible into a proper closing position. There are many methods that may be employed clinically to retrude the mandible into its terminal (centric relation) position. The method of choice may be quite simple, or it may be rather complex, depending on the number of natural teeth remaining and their distribution, coupled with the acuity of the patient's proprioceptive sense.

The least complicated method is simply to have the patient relax the jaw muscles and then to bring the jaws together so that the mandible is in its most retruded, unstrained position. This method is most apt to be successful with the patient who has retained most of his natural teeth. Other methods of retruding the mandible into a position of centric relation are:

1. By instructing the patient to place the tongue as far back in the roof of the mouth as he can while he closes his jaws. (Retruding the tongue has the effect of retruding also the mandible). As an aid to the patient in orientating his tongue when a record base is being used, a small ball of wax may be affixed to the palatal surface of the record base near the posterior border, and the patient instructed to touch the "ball" with the tip of his tongue.

2. By having the patient tap the teeth (or occlusion rims) together very rapidly. (Tapping the teeth together usually has the effect of retruding the mandible into centric relation.)

3. By instructing the patient to relax the jaw musculature, "let the jaw hang loose," while the mandible is gently guided back into its most retruded, unstrained position.

4. By using a central bearing tracing device. In constructing a large mandibular Class I removable partial denture to occlude with a maxillary complete denture, a central bearing tracing device might be employed to advantage to ensure that the mandible is retruded. However, if a larger number of teeth remained in the lower arch there probably would not be sufficient space to accommodate the tracing device, and some alternative method would be a better choice.

Developing the Occlusion for the Mouth in Which Centric Relation and Centric Occlusion Do Not Coincide

In the construction of a removable partial denture in which centric occlusion and centric relation do not coincide, two different courses of action may be considered, (1) to accept the centric occlusion essentially as presented, perhaps equilibrating to eliminate minor interfering, deflective contacts, or (2) to modify the occluding surfaces of the teeth by a combination of equilibration and restorative procedures, in order to establish an occlusion in which centric relation and centric occlusion do coincide. The decision as to whether or not to embark on this latter, more involved course must be based on these three important considerations. (1) The comfort of the patient with the occlusion which he now possesses. If he is functioning comfortably with his present occlusion, this would clearly argue for leaving it undisturbed. (2) The health of the periodontium. Certainly, traumatogenic contacts which jeopardize the well-being of the remaining teeth should be eliminated, by whatever means are required. (3) The extent of the alterations to the tooth surfaces that would be necessary to effect the desired change. If the treatment involved would be extensive, it would militate for acceptance of the occlusion "as-is," and this would be especially true if the patient is happy and comfortable, and the mouth is in a state of health. It bears emphasis that the most opportune time to make this decision is at the time that the treatment plan is formulated.

Whichever course is pursued, minimum goals should be to reduce the length of extruded teeth which have been out of occlusion and received no wear, to level and smooth rough, worn incisal edges, and to eliminate hypercontacts that cause a forward or horizontal slide of the mandible.

Establishing the Horizontal Relationship at Which the Occlusion Will Be Developed

Relating the opposing casts on the articulator, for the purpose of developing the occlusion, may be as simple as hand-articulating the casts, or as involved as employing a central bearing point tracing and intraoral checkbite, depending on the number of remaining teeth and the nature of the opposing occlusion.

Relating the Casts by Hand Articulation

When at least one natural tooth is present in each of the four quadrants of each jaw, and these teeth occlude with opponents, the task of relating the casts in centric occlusion is comparatively simple. Generally in such an instance, the casts can be simply hand-articulated (Fig. 13.11) into what coincides unmistakably with centric occlusion. This will be done following close observation, in the mouth, of the natural teeth in occlusion. Casts thus related can be mounted on the articulator arbitrarily or by means of the face-

bow, as deemed most appropriate (see the facebow discussion in this chapter).

Registering Centric Relation with Record Bases

When positive occlusal stops (occluding tooth surfaces) are not present in each quadrant of the mouth (Fig. 13.12), so that the casts cannot be unmistakably related by hand articulation, it becomes necessary to make occlusion rims to substitute for the missing teeth and, of course, record bases must be made to support the occlusion rims (Fig. 13.13).

Shellac-Gutta-Percha-Acrylic Resin Record Bases. Record bases may be constructed of either shellac or gutta-percha baseplate material, or of acrylic resin. Temporary clasps to stabilize the record bases may be made of wrought wire if desired, or prefabricated clasps, which are economical and lend themselves readily for the purpose, may be preferred (Fig. 13.14).

Record Bases Attached to the Framework. If the metal framework has already been constructed at the time that jaw relation records are being obtained,

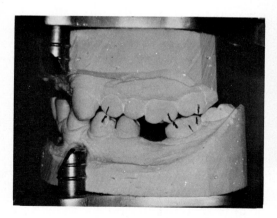

FIG. 13.11. When at least one natural tooth occludes with an opponent in each quadrant of both arches, the casts may be accurately related to each other in a relationship of centric occlusion by simple hand articulation.

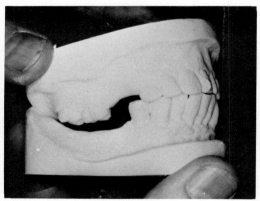

FIG. 13.12. When positive occlusal stops (natural occluding teeth) are not present in each quadrant of the mouth, so that the casts cannot be unmistakably related by hand articulation, it becomes necessary to substitute occlusion rims for the missing teeth, and record bases must be made to support the occlusion rims. The casts shown here could not possibly be accurately related to each other by hand articulation.

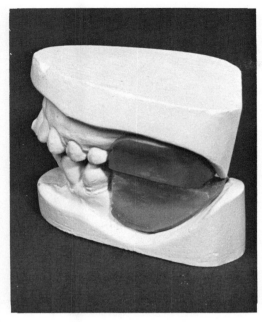

FIG. 13.13. Record bases may be constructed of either shellac or gutta-percha baseplate material, or of acrylic resin. The record bases shown here are made of shellac resin and the occlusion rims of baseplate wax.

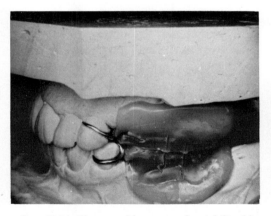

FIG. 13.14. The record bases may be stabilized by means of clasps made of wrought wire or with prefabricated clasps.

tional baseplate, the record base attached to the metal framework more nearly simulates conditions as they will be when the prosthesis is finished. A further advantage is that the occlusal rests tend to prevent overdisplacement of the mucosa under the bases, which is a common occurrence when conventional record bases are employed. Clearly it is the method of choice when it can be used, although it obviously cannot be employed to relate the planning casts to each other. Accordingly, planning casts are customarily related to each other by means of shellac or gutta-percha baseplates, whereas an acrylic resin base attached to the metal framework is the method of choice for relating the master cast to its opponent.

The Stabilized Record Base. When a functional impression has been obtained and the altered cast has been prepared, time can be saved by converting the acrylic resin tray, in which the impression was obtained, into the record base. The method consists in refitting the base to the cast with zinc oxide-eugenol impression paste.

All impression material must first be removed from the tray and the resin must be clean and dry. Tinfoil is adapted to the

the record bases and occlusion rims can be attached to the retention latticework of the framework (Fig. 13.15). This is the preferred method for obtaining intraoral records. In addition to fitting well and being better stabilized than a conven-

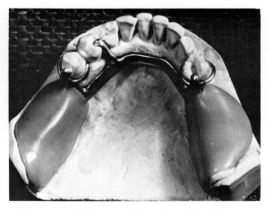

FIG. 13.15. If the metal framework has been constructed by the time that the jaw relations are to be obtained, the record bases and the occlusion rims can be attached to the retention latticework of the framework, to provide an excellent method of establishing the jaw relationships.

areas of the cast which will be occupied by the denture base. Zinc oxide-eugenol impression paste is mixed and placed in the tray, and the framework and tray are seated on the cast over the tinfoil. When the impression material has hardened, the framework is removed from the cast. The tinfoil which adheres to the zinc oxide-eugenol paste is left in place to provide a smooth surface to contact the mucosa.

Establishing Centric Relation for the Partial Denture Which Opposes an Edentulous Maxilla

When a mandibular removable partial denture is being constructed to oppose a complete maxillary denture, the problem of relating the two casts accurately on the articulator will require a different approach from that employed to oppose either natural teeth or another partial denture. The procedure requires that record bases with attached occlusion rims be fabricated for both arches. The mandibular record base is, of course, attached to the metal framework.

Vertical Dimension

The vertical dimension is first established following Niswonger's precepts.

Vertical Dimension of Rest Position. The vertical dimension of rest position is first established without either record base in the mouth. Two dots are placed on the patient's face, one on the chin and one on the upper lip, in approximately the midline or close to it. A skin pencil, or small adhesive markers may be used. Sites for the marks should be selected that are on areas of skin which are relatively immobile and that can be easily contacted with whatever measuring device is to be used. This may be a celluloid millimeter ruler (Fig. 13.16), an outside caliper, or a Boley gauge. The patient is instructed to count from 1 to 10, and to hold the jaw at the position it has assumed at the count of 10 while the distance between the dots is measured. The patient is now instructed to pronounce several words containing sibilants ("S" sounds) such as "Mississippi," "San Fran-

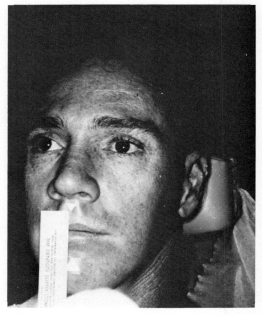

Fig. 13.16. The vertical dimension may be determined clinically by placing two marks on the patient's face, either on the skin or with adhesive tape as shown here. Measurements are made between the two points with a suitable measuring device such as a modified Boley gage, a millimeter rule (as shown here), or an outside caliper. If the patient is edentulous in one jaw, or completely edentulous, the vertical dimension of rest position can be determined and the vertical dimension of occlusion then computed by subtracting 3 mm. from this measurement.

cisco," or "success," and again to hold the jaw steady at the position reached following the last word pronounced. A measurement is again made between the dots. The patient may now be instructed to swallow and relax the mouth muscles while a third measurement is made. If the three measurements correspond, the distance may be accepted as the vertical dimension of rest position. If the three measurements are close together, but not identical, an average may be computed and accepted as the vertical dimension of rest position.

Vertical Dimension of Occlusion. The maxillary record base is placed in the mouth and the labial surface of the wax occlusion rim is contoured so that the upper lip drapes naturally over the labial flange. The anterior length of the flange should be adjusted so that its edge assumes the position to be occupied by the incisal edges of the anterior teeth. The mandibular record base is placed in the mouth and the occlusion rims of both bases are adjusted until the patient contacts the opposing teeth or occlusion rim at a measurement 3 mm. less than the vertical dimension of rest position. This is the relationship at which the occlusion will be developed.

Centric Relationship

If the edentulous spaces permit, an intraoral tracing device may be employed to establish the horizontal (centric) relationship (Figs. 13.17–13.19). If there is not sufficient space in the partially edentulous ridge to accommodate the tracing device, the relationship may be obtained by retruding the mandible into its retruded position and recording the relationship with interocclusal check-bites.

The Effect of Pressure on Interocclusal Records

It is important, when interocclusal records are being obtained by means of a

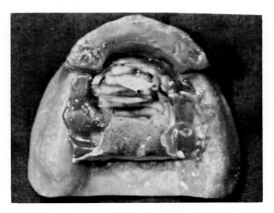

Fig. 13.18. A metal recording plate can be attached to the maxillary record base upon which to scribe the arrow point tracing. A section of occlusion rim may be attached in the cuspid-to-cuspid area upon which can be recorded the midline and any other reference marks that are desired.

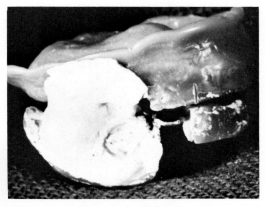

Fig. 13.19. Plaster checkbites have been used here to register the centric relationship so that it can be transferred to the articulator.

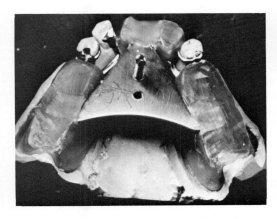

Fig. 13.17. In registering centric relationship for the partial denture which opposes a complete maxillary denture, a central bearing point-arrow point tracing device may sometimes be employed to advantage, if the edentulous spaces and the remaining teeth are so located that the tracing device can be accommodated.

record base (Fig. 13.20), that excessive pressure on the displaceable tissues of the denture-bearing area be avoided. If interocclusal records for a distal extension base type of partial denture are obtained under pressure, the soft underlying mucosa will be flattened out or compressed as the record base is forcibly displaced downward (Fig. 13.21). When an occlusal record which has been obtained under pressure is subsequently placed on the stone cast, the

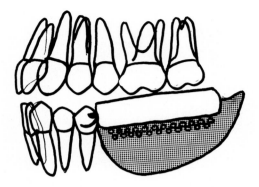

FIG. 13.20. It is very important, when intraoral records are obtained for a partial denture with a distal extension base, that pressure on the record base be avoided. The sketch depicts the wax occlusion rim ready for use in obtaining an intraoral record of centric occlusion.

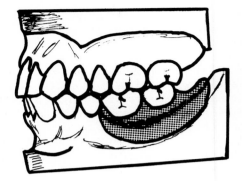

FIG. 13.22. When these record bases are placed on their respective casts, the record bases cannot, of course, displace the surface of the stone cast in the manner in which the mucosa was displaced and so the relationship that is transferred to the articulator will not be accurate.

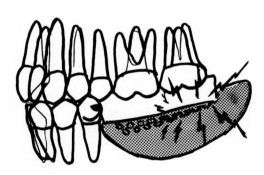

FIG. 13.21. Excessive pressure will depress the record base by displacing the underlying resilient mucosa.

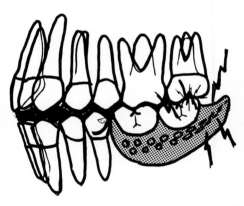

FIG. 13.23. When the teeth are arranged between the incorrectly oriented casts and taken to the mouth for trial, the posterior teeth will be in hyperocclusion. This may or may not be clinically apparent, depending on the magnitude of the discrepancy.

record base cannot, of course, depress the unyielding surface of the stone and, as a result, the relationship of the two casts to each other will be inaccurate (Fig. 13.22). If the casts are mounted on the articulator in this incorrect relationship (Fig. 13.23), the posterior teeth will always be in hyperocclusion by the amount that the soft tissue has been displaced. The disparity may or may not be apparent when the denture is tried in the mouth, or even when the finished denture is inserted,

because the soft tissue may be displaced under the denture base in the same way that it was under the record base. However, the occlusion will be faulty, nonetheless, and is very apt to be the root cause of intractable soreness when the denture is subjected to the rigors of mastication.

This undesirable sequence of events can be avoided by employing a medium other than baseplate wax for the interocclusal record. Baseplate wax cannot be relied on for this purpose because it is so difficult to soften it uniformly throughout its mass. As a consequence, it offers more resistance to closure in one area of the mouth than in another. Such unequal resistance has the effect not only of displacing the record base into the mucosa but possibly of causing the mandible to be shunted from its normal path of closure as the proprioceptors seek to guide it through a pathway that avoids interference.

Another reason for avoiding pressure when the interocclusal record is made is the fact that the mucosa varies in its displaceability from one area of the mouth to another, depending on its thickness, its resiliency, and its tone. As a result, excessive pressure may allow the record base to be depressed more in one area than another so that it is canted to one side or the other, or anteroposteriorly. Clearly there are compelling reasons for employing a material for the final registration that exerts an absolute minimum of resistance to closing pressure (Fig. 13.24).

Establishing the Occlusal Plane

Establishing the occlusal plane for the removable partial denture seldom poses any problem, since the presence of only a few natural teeth provides an adequate guide to its proper orientation. The plane should ideally be located, insofar as possible, in the same position that it occupied prior to the loss of teeth, since all masticatory and phonetic function is programmed by the neuromuscular mechanism to take place with the incisal and occlusal surfaces of the teeth at this level. When one jaw is edentulous and some of the anterior teeth are still present in the opposite arch, their incisal edges will provide a reference for the anterior level of the occlusal plane. The remainder of the plane is established for the mandibular teeth by extending a line posteriorly to the upper third of the retromolar pad.

Mounting the Casts on the Articulator

The casts may be transferred to the articulator for mounting either by the arbitrary method or by means of the facebow.

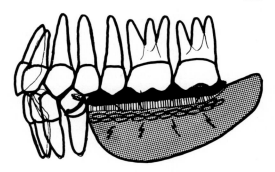

Fig. 13.24. To avoid an inaccuracy due to pressure, a soft substance such as bite registration wax, plaster, stone, or bite registration paste (zinc oxide-eugenol paste) should be used as an intervening medium. Thus, records can be obtained with a bare minimum of pressure, so as not to depress the base into the displaceable underlying tissue.

In the former method, the casts, properly related to each other in the horizontal and vertical planes, are secured together and mounted in the center of the articulator, with the midline of the casts aligned with the incisal pin and the occlusal plane parallel with the bench top.

The Facebow

In discussing the relationship of the maxilla and mandible earlier in the chapter, it was stated that the two casts must be related to one another in the three planes of space, i.e., frontal, horizontal, and sagittal. One other relationship must be considered, that of the teeth to the center of movement which is located in the temporomandibular joint, or more specifically in the mandibular condyle. The facebow is an instrument which makes it possible to relate the jaws to the mandibular condyles, and to transfer this relationship to an articulator. The purpose is to transfer a radius (condyle to a given point on the cast) from mouth to articulator. When the mandible opens and closes, it moves on an arc of closure which, when viewed in the sagittal plane, has its center in the condyle. Thus it follows that the distance from the center of rotation of the arc to the teeth in either arch will have relevance in the development of the occlusion for an oral prosthesis.

There are two types of facebows used in prosthodontics; the simple or arbitrary facebow and the hinge axis or kinematic bow. The simple facebow is designed to be placed on the face over the condyles, which have been arbitrarily located and indicated by marks on the skin of the face. It is attached to a maxillary record base or to a wax or modeling composition "clutch" of the teeth. The hinge axis bow, on the other hand, is designed so that the precise point which overlies the hinge axis of the mandibular condyle can be located on the skin of the face. Use of the hinge axis facebow is not considered essential to development of an efficient, harmonious occlusion for the removable partial denture.

The Value of the Facebow Transfer

Because of the nature of the facebow and of what it purports to contribute towards a harmonious occlusion, it may be fairly contended that its potential value to the occlusion of the average partial denture will be in direct ratio to the number of teeth being replaced by the prosthesis. This is true because the fewer the remaining teeth, the more mandibular movement will be influenced by the condyles and the less by the natural teeth, and thus the greater the potential contribution of the facebow. Conversely, the greater the number of remaining teeth, the more the direction and extent of mandibular movement will be influenced by these remaining teeth, thereby diminishing the potential value of the facebow transfer. Virtually all authorities are in agreement that the simple facebow is sufficiently accurate for removable partial denture construction.

Accomplishing the Facebow Transfer Clinically

The facebow transfer may be made rather simply and quickly if an orderly sequence of steps is followed. The first requirement is that certain reference points be placed on the skin of the face.
Locating Reference Points. The reference points which represent the approximate center of the condyles should first be located on the sides of the face and marked with a skin pencil. This may be done in one of three ways, of which one is the hinge axis method which will not be discussed since it is not customarily employed in developing the occlusion for the removable partial denture. The other two methods follow.

1. Measure 11 to 13 mm. anterior to the upper third of the tragus of the ear, on a line extending from the upper margin of the external auditory meatus to the outer canthus of the eye. A condyle marker (Richey Condyle Marker, Hanau Engineering Co., Buffalo, N.Y.) is a handy device (Fig. 13.25) for making this measurement.

2. Palpate the area by having the patient open and close the jaw several times while the area just anterior to the tragus is palpated with the index finger. As the condyle moves forward and downward on the slope of the glenoid fossa, it creates a depression which may be readily felt with the finger. The center of the depression is marked with the pencil as representing

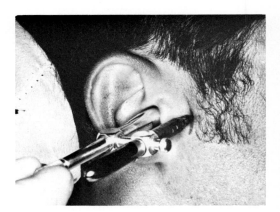

FIG. 13.25. A condyle marker is a handy device for locating the center of the condyle on the skin of the face. The device scribes an arc 13 mm. anterior to the upper third of the tragus. The condyle is then located on the skin of the face at the point on the scribed line which is on a line drawn between the upper third of the tragus and the outer canthus of the eye.

the approximate center of the condyle. The distance from the surface of the skin to the bone of the condyle, which is about 12 mm. on the average is ignored as having no bearing on the success of the technique.

Either of these two arbitrary techniques of employing the facebow is considered sufficiently accurate for orienting the casts in the development of the occlusion for the removable partial denture.

The Axis-Orbital Plane. A refinement to the facebow is the axis-orbital pointer which makes it possible to orient the casts on the articulator to a third reference point on the skull such as the oribtale, which is the lowest point in the margin of the bony orbit (Fig. 13.26). Thus, the relationship of the occlusal plane to the Frankfort plane (orbitale to tragion) is transferred to the articulator. This has the effect of relating the occlusal plane to the articulator approximately as it is viewed in the mouth. The advantage is that it is somewhat easier to relate the occlusal plane of the teeth on the articulator to the way that they will appear in the mouth.

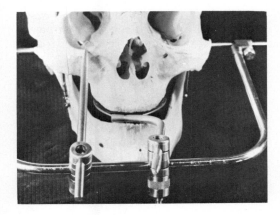

FIG. 13.26. If the casts are to be related to the axis-orbital plane, a third reference point on the skull is needed. The orbitale is commonly used for this purpose. It is located by palpating the lower border of the orbit and establishing the reference point at the lowest point of the orbital margin, on a line with the center of the pupil of the eye as the patient stares straight ahead.

Programming the Articulator to Simulate Mandibular Movement

When the casts have been correctly related to one another on the articulator in a position of centric occlusion as well as in relation to the center of movement (the condyle), they represent the two jaws as they are related to one another (and to the mandibular condyle) in the mouth. When movement is introduced, however, the accuracy of this tooth-to-tooth relationship may cease to exist, unless the movements which the articulator is capable of making are identical to the movements which the mandible makes in function. Simulating this movement in the articulator is complicated by the fact that the temporomandibular joint is the most complex bony articulation in the body. Consequently, this joint is capable of executing an intricate range of movements which involve all three spacial planes.

Protrusive Movement

When the mandible is brought forward with the anterior teeth edge-to-edge, the mandibular condyles glide downward and forward along the surfaces of the glenoid fossae. The angulation of the downward, forward path traversed by the two condyles can be registered with a fair degree of accuracy and transferred to an articulator by means of a protrusive checkbite.

The Protrusive Record. The intraoral protrusive record is obtained by placing soft wax or bite registration paste between the posterior teeth, or occlusion rims (Fig. 13.27), and having the patient close with the anterior teeth edge-to-edge as in biting a thread. If this interocclusal record is carefully made, it will register the angulation that the condylar path makes with the horizontal plane, and this angulation can be transferred to an articulator which has an adjustable condylar guidance. Movement of the articulator will then more closely simulate the natural condylar movement of that particular patient. The condyles should be brought forward at least 4 to 6 mm., which is con-

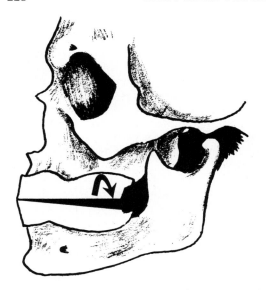

Fig. 13.27. The downward-forward movement of the mandible into a protrusive position has the effect of bringing the condyles downward and forward on the articulating surface of the glenoid fossa. If wax is interposed between the teeth (or occlusion rims), the angulation that the condylar path makes with the horizontal plane can be measured and transferred to an articulator.

sidered minimal in order to create a recordable amount of angle from the horizontal plane.

Lateral Movement

When the mandible moves laterally, the condyle on the side towards which the movement is directed, i.e., the working side, rotates around a vertical axis while the opposite condyle, often referred to as the orbiting condyle, moves downward, forward, and medially. The working-side condyle not only rotates around a vertical axis, however, but simultaneously with this rotational movement there is a bodily side-shift of the mandible, which has been named the Bennett movement after the man who first called attention to the phenomena. This lateral shift of the condyle on the working side may be in a horizontal direction, upward, downward, backward, or a combination of directions, depending on the anatomy of the joint. In a hori-

zontal plane the Bennett shift may take the form of either an immediate side-shift, or a more gradual and progressive one. The Bennett movement, then, is a component of the lateral excursion of the mandible. This lateral movement of the jaw may be recorded and transferred to an articulator, provided the articulator has been designed to accept such a record. Although the most accurate method of registering the Bennett component (the lateral side-shift) is generally conceded to be by means of a pantographic tracing, it can be accomplished with a fair degree of accuracy by means of intraoral checkbites.

Lateral Checkbites. Lateral checkbites may be made in a manner similar to those described for the protrusive checkbite, although it should be borne in mind that all articulators cannot be adjusted to simulate this movement and unless the articulator has this capability such records would be useless.

Placing the Matter in Perspective

The variety of methods and instrumentation which may be employed in developing the occlusion for the partial denture ranges all the way from the static relationship of hand-articulated casts mounted on a simple hinge instrument, through the functionally generated path, to what is generally regarded as the most sophisticated method, the pantographic tracing employed with a three-dimensional articulator. This naturally raises the question: What are the criteria which govern the choice of method? Because of the myriad variables, most important of which are the type of prosthesis and the nature of the opposing occlusion, the answer is too complex to be reduced to a simple formula. However, some logical conclusions can be drawn by using the occlusion of the complete denture as a frame of reference.

The patient who is completely edentulous presents with only one of the five major factors which govern occlusion, namely the horizontal condylar guidance. The other four factors, i.e., orientation of the occlusal plane, the prominence of the compensating curve, the inclination of the cusps, and the angle of the incisal guidance, can be established in a manner which best achieves an ideal balance among them, in harmony with the condylar guidance (Fig. 13.28). Quite the opposite is true in the case of the partial denture which opposes natural teeth (Fig. 13.29). In this instance, all of these factors have already been established by nature and cannot be modified, no matter how advantageous it might be to do so. This draws attention to the important role played by the natural teeth in influencing jaw movement. The muscles of mastication and the temporomandibular joint govern mandibular movement until the teeth come into contact, at which time the teeth take over as the dominant influencing factor. Therefore, in developing the occlusion for the prosthesis in which natural intercuspating teeth are an integral

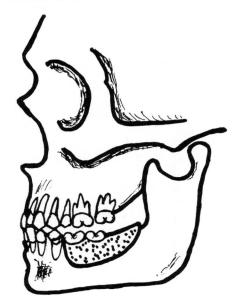

FIG. 13.29. When the partial denture in the lower arch is opposed by a complete arch of natural teeth, all five of the factors which influence occlusion have already been established and cannot be modified, no matter how advantageous it would be to do so.

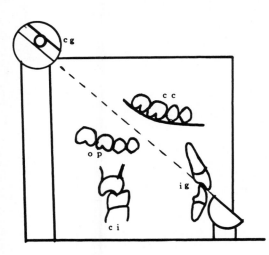

FIG. 13.28. In developing the occlusion for complete dentures, the dentist has under his control four of the five major factors which control occlusion. They are illustrated above as *cc*, the compensating curve; *op*, the occlusal plane; *ci*, cusp inclination; and *ig*, incisal guidance. The fifth factor, *cg*, condylar guidance cannot be altered or controlled. In contrast to this, in construction of the removable partial denture the dentist seldom has this degree of control over the influencing factors because they usually are already established by the remaining natural teeth.

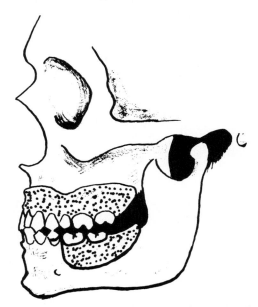

FIG. 13.30. In developing the occlusion for the mandibular partial denture that opposes a complete maxillary denture, a harmonious occlusion is a more readily attainable goal if it is developed on an articulator that closely simulates the jaw movements of the patient.

part, the powerful influence which they exert must not be overlooked.

From the foregoing it may be concluded that the fewer the number of natural teeth which remain, the greater will be the degree of control that can be exercised on the development of the scheme of occlusion. In the case of a mandibular partial denture that opposes an edentulous maxilla (Fig. 13.30), development of a harmonious occlusion is a more readily attainable goal if the occlusion is developed on an articulator which closely simulates the movements of the patient's mandible. In this case, the orientation of the occlusal plane, the degree of curvature of the compensating curve, and the types of posterior tooth cusps would be, to some degree, controllable for the purpose of achieving the most harmonious intercuspation.

The occlusion for opposing Kennedy Class I partial dentures would benefit similarly, although the degree of control would, perforce, be more limited because the incisal guidance, in addition to the horizontal guidance, would already be established and so, not be amenable to modification. In contrast, the Kennedy Class III or Class IV denture would permit virtually no modification of any of these factors and, as a consequence, the use of jaw relation records with a complex articulator would be of questionable value.

Bibliography

Beck, H. O.: Choosing the articulator. J. Amer. Dent. Ass. 64: 468–475, 1962.

Beck, H. O.: Selection of an articulator and jaw registration. J. Prosth. Dent. 10: 878–886, 1960.

Christensen, C.: The problem of the bite. Dent. Cosmos 47: 1184–1195, 1905.

Coleman, A. J.: Occlusal requirements for the removable partial denture. J. Prosth. Dent. 17: 155–162, 1917.

Craddock, F. W.: The accuracy and practical value of records of condyle path inclination. J. Amer. Dent. Ass. 38: 697–710, 1949.

Craddock, F. W.: Recording procedures in partial denture construction. Int. Dent. J. 8: 367–369, 1958.

Craddock, F. W., and Symmons, H. F.: Evaluation of the facebow. J. Prosth. Dent. 2: 633–642, 1952.

Fish, W. E.: A new principle in partial denture design. Brit. Dent. J. 92: 135–144, 1952.

Hughes, G. A., and Regli, C. P.: What is centric relation? J. Prosth. Dent. 11: 16–22, 1961.

Kraus, B. S., Jordan, R. E., and Abrams, L.: Dental Anatomy and Occlusion. The Williams & Wilkins Company, Baltimore, Md., 1969.

Lytle, R. B.: Vertical relation of occlusion by the patient's neuromuscular perception. J. Prosth. Dent., 14: 12–21, 1964.

Niswonger, M. E.: The rest position of the mandible. J. Amer. Dent. Ass. 21: 1572–1582, 1934.

Schuyler, C. H.: Fundamental principles in the correction of occlusal disharmony, natural and artificial. J. Amer. Dent. Ass. 22: 1193–1202, 1935.

Tench, R. W.: Dangers in dental reconstruction involving increase of the dimension of the lower third of the face. J. Amer. Dent. Ass. 25: 566–570, 1938.

Thompson, J. R.: The rest position of the mandible and its significance to dental science. J. Amer. Dent. Ass. 33: 151–180, 1946.

Thompson, J. R., and Brodie, A. G.: Factors in the position of the mandible. J. Amer. Dent. Ass. 29: 925–941, 1942.

Westbrook, J. C.: A pattern of centric occlusion. J. Amer. Dent. Ass. 39: 407–413, 1949.

Chapter 14

SELECTION AND ARRANGEMENT OF TEETH—THE DENTURE BASE

*This chapter is concerned with the selection
and arrangement of the teeth, both anterior
and posterior, for the different types of
removable partial dentures. Design and
construction of the denture base are also
discussed. Subject matter is organized in the
following manner.*

Introduction

The teeth are important components of
the removable partial denture, from a
standpoint of both esthetics and function.
The posterior teeth restore the ability to
masticate, maintain interarch distance,
and contribute towards the restoration of
lost facial contour. The anterior teeth assist in restoring masticatory function,
play a major role in satisfying the cosmetic requirements, and are of pivotal
importance to the phonetic function.

The enormous array of possible combinations of missing teeth and edentulous
spaces, combined with the striking differences in partial denture designs, creates a
requirement for a prosthetic tooth having
a combination of qualities impossible for
any one tooth to satisfy. In order to meet
these demands, the ideal prosthetic tooth,
in addition to being pleasing in appearance, would have to satisfy a formidable
list of requirements. It would need to be
adaptable to any edentulous space, easily
attached to the prosthesis, unbreakable,
resistant to wear, and capable of articulating with teeth of any occlusal pattern
or material without adverse effects to either. Such an ideal tooth, of course, does
not exist. However, a variety of different
types of teeth is available, and collectively
they satisfy the demands of the removable
partial denture quite well, whatever its
requirements. Each type of prosthetic
tooth has advantages as well as limitations. One who understands the strong
and weak points of each type of tooth is in
a position to select the most suitable one
for the prosthesis being constructed.
Clearly, this responsibility is not one to be
delegated to the laboratory technician.

The Types of Prosthetic Teeth

Replacement teeth for the removable
partial denture are, for the most part,
supplied by tooth manufacturers, although
some types of teeth can be, and often are,
fabricated in the dental laboratory. The
manufacturers market teeth of various
types, which are made of either porcelain

or acrylic resin, as well as combinations of the two. The laboratory-crafted type of tooth is made either by casting the tooth in metal as an integral part of the framework, or by casting a retentive element on the framework to which a resin or porcelain tooth can be attached. The post tooth is an example of the latter construction. It consists of a small, upright metal post, onto which a resin tooth can be processed or a porcelain tooth can be attached with cement.

Selection of the most suitable replacement tooth for a prosthesis will have far-reaching effects on the success or lack of success with which the prosthesis is worn. Upon this choice may hinge (1) the efficiency of mastication, (2) the esthetic excellence, (3) the comfort with which the prosthesis is worn, and (4) the longevity of the teeth and restorations that articulate with the prosthetic teeth.

Characteristics of Acrylic Resin Teeth

Although the tooth made of methylmethacrylate has certain physical properties that make it uniquely suitable for use with the partial denture, it also has some disadvantages, as well as some limitations. The following paragraphs will enumerate some of the more important physical properties of the plastic tooth.

Strength. Acrylic resin teeth are not dangerously weakened when ground thin in circumstances where interridge space is severely limited or when extensive grinding is required to fit the tooth around an adjacent clasp. Plastic teeth lend themselves well to the recontouring which is sometimes necessary to reduce the size of the food table.

Percolation. Percolation is the leakage of liquids into a space between the tooth and the denture base. The danger of percolation is virtually eliminated with plastic teeth, because the tooth material and denture base material bond together chemically.

Stain Resistance. Although not a frequent problem, plastic teeth may absorb stain under some circumstances.

Abrasion Resistance. The plastic tooth has a comparatively low resistance to wear, the tendency being more marked in some mouths than in others. The variance in rate of tooth wear among different individuals is due to differences in diet, chewing patterns and, perhaps even more important, the presence or absence of bruxing and clenching habits. Often overlooked is the fact that wear of the plastic tooth occurs on the labial aspect of anterior teeth, as well as on the occlusal surfaces of posterior teeth. Thus, not only is vertical dimension lost as a result of wear of the posterior tooth, but the esthetic quality of the anterior teeth may also slowly deteriorate for the same reason. There is evidence to suggest, however, that wear of posterior plastic teeth may not be quite the detriment to the removable partial denture that it is in complete dentures, since plastic teeth typically wear up to the point where the natural teeth come into occlusal contact, at which time the rate of wear of the plastic may virtually cease. It is important to note also that the poor abrasion resistance of plastic may be an advantage when the denture tooth is opposed to a gold crown or a natural tooth, since the plastic bears the brunt of the wear, thereby minimizing wear of either the gold or the enamel.

Ease of Fabrication. The denture with plastic teeth is more difficult to rebase than is the one with porcelain teeth. The explanation for this is that porcelain teeth are comparatively easy to remove from the denture base by the application of heat, whereas the plastic tooth must be cut away from the denture resin with a bur. In addition, the denture with plastic teeth is more difficult to wax up in the laboratory, since the teeth are more vulnerable to damage by the flame which is customarily used to smooth the wax. Similarly, more care is required in polishing the denture with plastic teeth, because the plastic tooth may be abraded by the action of the revolving wheels and the polishing medium, and hence must be carefully protected when these procedures are being performed.

Characteristics of Porcelain Teeth

Porcelain teeth are unexcelled in appearance and are very high in abrasion resistance. However, there are other physical properties in which porcelain suffers by comparison with the plastic tooth.

Wear Resistance. Resistance to wear of porcelain is excellent. This means that the labial surface of the porcelain anterior tooth will retain its life-like appearance for many years of service, and vertical dimension will not be lost as a result of occlusal wear of posterior teeth. On the other side of the coin, the porcelain is capable of causing wear of both enamel and gold when it is opposed to either material.

Stain Resistance. Porcelain is impervious to stain, which must be counted an important advantage in some mouths.

Ease of Fabrication. The denture with porcelain teeth is easier to wax up, as well as to polish, in the laboratory than is the one with plastic teeth. On the other hand, it is somewhat more difficult to process, since the porcelain is subject to breakage during flasking operations. Already noted is the fact that the denture with porcelain teeth is easier to rebase.

Strength. Porcelain is notably weak in thin sections and, if the diatorics are partly effaced, the tooth may not be mechanically anchored in the denture base. Such a tooth may loosen and drop out after a brief period of service.

Friability. Porcelain teeth are more subject to breakage as a result of careless handling by the patient, because the porcelain is much more friable than is plastic.

Noise, Clicking. Porcelain is more apt to produce clicking noises in the mouth of the patient who does not possess good neuromuscular control. This is most often encountered with the senescent individual, and is normally not as apt to be a problem with the removable partial denture as it is with complete dentures.

Percolation. Percolation around the necks of porcelain teeth may occur, unless avoided by careful technique. Percolation occurs as follows. When acrylic resin polymerizes, the methyl-methacrylate expands upon reaching a certain temperature in the curing cycle. Then, at another point in the cycle, it contracts. The net effect of this dimensional change, although actually miniscule in amount, may be to create a hairline crack between the acrylic resin of the denture base and the porcelain, since there is no chemical bond between the two materials. This tiny crevice may become discolored by food and liquids after the denture has been in service for a brief interval. The stain will be unsightly if it occurs in the anterior part of the mouth, and will likely be repugnant to the patient whether or not it is visible to others. Percolation is avoidable by careful laboratory technique, but the threat of its occurrence must be counted a shortcoming not shared by plastic teeth.

Trauma. It is the opinion of some authorities that the porcelain tooth generates greater trauma against the residual ridge than does the plastic tooth, because of its hardness. A contrary view is that since porcelain is more efficient in penetrating the bolus, it is, therefore, less traumatic to the residual ridge. Since the teeth are occluded many times each day with no food in the mouth, the postulation that porcelain is more traumatic to the ridge would seem to have the firmer basis in logic. This is a moot point which does not lend itself well to the usual investigative techniques of conventional research.

Selection of Teeth for the Anterior Edentulous Space

Although the prosthesis of choice for restoring the anterior edentulous space is normally the fixed partial denture, there are many circumstances where the removable prosthesis may be superior for one reason or another. Generally it can be said that, from a standpoint of esthetics, anterior teeth replaced with the removable type of partial denture may be more pleasing in appearance than those replaced with the fixed partial denture, provided the clasps need not be displayed. The types of teeth available for the replacement of missing anterior teeth are (1) the denture tooth, either porcelain or acrylic resin, (2) the interchangeable facing, either porcelain or acrylic resin, and

(3) the post, or pressed-on, tooth which is customarily fabricated of acrylic resin.

The Denture Tooth

Denture teeth, properly arranged, are the most esthetic type of anterior substitute by any yardstick (Fig. 14.1). Almost any combination of desired shade, size, or contour is readily available, as are characterized teeth, also. Moreover, individual characterizing touches may be added by simulating wear, flattening contacts, and the like. A marked advantage of the denture tooth, over any other type of anterior replacement, is the fact that when there has been excessive loss of alveolar bone in the anterior region of the mouth, the teeth may be positioned in a flange of acrylic resin of whatever thickness is needed to restore symmetry and a pleasing natural contour to the lip (Fig. 14.2). On the other hand, an extremely pleasing composition may be achieved by abutting the tooth directly to the residual ridge, when the plumping effect of the flange is not needed.

The denture tooth is ordinarily not the replacement of choice for the single missing tooth, because of its vulnerability to the shearing type of stress to which it will be exposed in the incising segment of the occlusion.

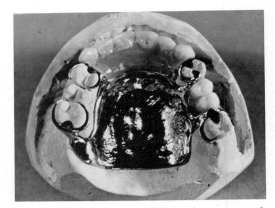

Fig. 14.2. If the necks of the replacement teeth need to be brought out labially so as to be pleasingly aligned with the adjoining natural teeth, it is best accomplished by employing a flange of acrylic resin.

The Interchangeable Facing

The interchangeable facing is the strongest type of anterior tooth replacement, and hence should be employed for most single tooth replacements, since a denture tooth so employed must be attached to the prosthesis by a relatively narrow strip of acrylic resin that is vulnerable to fracture.

Another indication for this type of construction is when the interridge space is severely limited, because of an excessively deep vertical overlap of the maxillary teeth, or in instances where the alveolar ridge is overly bulbous, to the extent that space to accommodate the retention latticework of the metal framework is restricted (Figs. 14.3 and 14.4). Either plastic or porcelain facings may be used. The plastic is, of course, stronger, hence less prone to fracture, although some wear of the labial surface is a reasonable expectation. On the other hand, porcelain has an extremely low resistance to the shearing type of stress to which it may be exposed, and so is vulnerable to fracture unless the incisal edge is well protected by the metal backing. Protection is provided by extending the metal backing slightly beyond the porcelain incisally, so that contact with the teeth in the op-

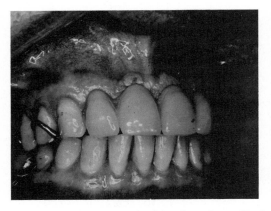

Fig. 14.1. Denture teeth abutted to the residual ridge are the most esthetic substitute for missing natural anterior teeth.

posing arch, during excursive movements of the mandible, is made by the metal instead of the porcelain. The interchangeable facing may be refitted when the contour of the residual ridge is altered by resorption, which may be counted an important advantage for this type of tooth replacement.

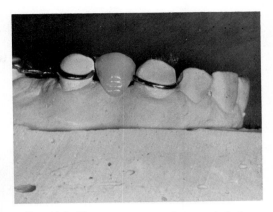

FIG. 14.5. The post or pressed-on tooth is intermediate in strength between the interchangeable facing and the denture tooth, being somewhat weaker than the former but stronger than the latter. It can be quite acceptable esthetically, if carefully fitted to the mucosa and properly matched in shade with the adjoining teeth.

The Post or Pressed-On Tooth

The post tooth is intermediate in strength between the denture tooth and the interchangeable facing, being much stronger than the former but not quite as strong as the latter (Fig. 14.5). The post tooth requires at least an average amount of interocclusal space, however, and so cannot be used to best advantage in an extremely close occlusion. The post tooth is generally not as pleasing esthetically as the denture tooth, but may, under some circumstances, be superior to the interchangeable facing in this regard. See Table 14.1 for a summary of anterior tooth selection.

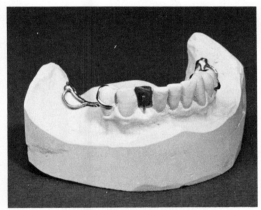

FIG. 14.3. The interchangeable facing may be used to replace anterior teeth on the removable partial denture when maximum strength is required. The photograph shows the metal backing which is manufactured to fit the channel in the facing. Note that the cast has been scraped where it will be contacted by the ridge lap of the facing, so that it will be in intimate contact with the oral mucosa.

Shade Selection

If natural anterior teeth are present, the shade of the prosthetic teeth is decided by matching the appropriate shade-guide tooth with the natural teeth, preferably the ones directly adjacent to the edentulous space. The shade-guide tooth should be moistened with saliva and the matching should be done in natural light rather than under the operating light. (Northern light is to be preferred if it is available.) It is not unusual to find that

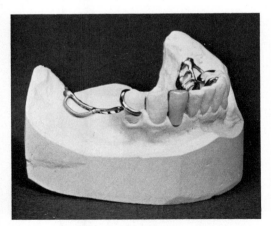

FIG. 14.4. This photograph shows the facing (which may be either porcelain or plastic) in place on the backing. Note the close adaptation of the ridge lap to the stone cast.

TABLE 14.1.

Selection of anterior tooth replacements

Tooth Type	Indications	Strong Points	Weak Points
Acrylic denture tooth	Most anterior spaces Excellent when labial contour must be built out with a flange	Good esthetically Strong in thin sections Durable in close bite	The labial surface wears excessively in some mouths so that esthetic excellence may deteriorate
Porcelain denture tooth	For most anterior spaces provided adequate space exists Excellent with a flange to restore labial contour	Excellent esthetics	Not as strong as plastic or an interchangeable facing
Interchangeable facing	For the close bite occlusion For the single tooth replacement	Strongest of the replacement teeth Facing is easily replaced if broken	Not as good esthetically as denture teeth
The pressed-on or post tooth	Generally same as interchangeable facing	Strong in restricted space	Fair esthetically

the patient's remaining teeth vary in shade from one another. When this is the case, a shade should be chosen which enables it to blend best with the teeth which adjoin the space it is to occupy.

The procedure of shade selection is unlike almost any other decision that is made in prosthodontic practice, in that one's snap opinion is very likely to be more accurate than one based on a more deliberative judgment. The reason for this is that the optic nerve characteristically becomes quickly fatigued, and when it does, its ability to discriminate between closely similar shades is greatly diminished. Thus, it is best to select a shade rather quickly by relying on one's initial judgment. If the shade proves to be unusually difficult to decide, a tentative selection should be made, after which the eyes should be rested for a short period before an attempt is made to corroborate the judgment with another matching procedure.

Selecting the Mold

Anterior teeth should be selected which are in harmony with the patient's fea-

tures, and which blend with any remaining natural teeth that are present (Fig. 14.6). It should be kept in mind that a tooth may be anomalous in appearance as an individual entity, yet altogether pleasing in its harmony with the overall composition. The opposing teeth, as well as those adjacent to the edentulous space,

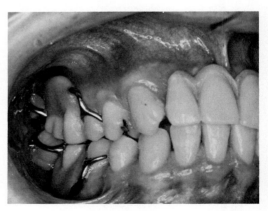

FIG. 14.6. Anterior teeth should be selected which fit the edentulous space and which blend harmoniously with the adjoining teeth in form (mold) and color (shade).

may be used as guides for the proper size and contour. Generally, the anterior edentulous space will be found to be slightly smaller than the combined widths of the natural teeth that are being replaced. As a result, replacement teeth will need to be chosen which are slightly smaller than were the natural teeth. In some instances, needed space can be created by disking the natural teeth which adjoin the edentulous space. In addition, it will often be necessary to reduce the mesiodistal width of each of the replacement teeth, in order to fit them into the available space and to achieve the most balanced and pleasing composition (Fig. 14.7).

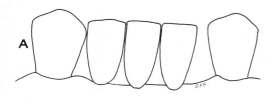

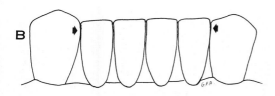

FIG. 14.7. Generally, the edentulous space will be found to be slightly smaller than the space occupied by the natural teeth because of drifting of the adjoining teeth. Additional space can oftentimes be created by disking the natural teeth which adjoin the space, and by reducing slightly the size of the replacement teeth. *A*, the natural teeth have migrated into the edentulous space with the result that teeth of the same size as the lost natural teeth are too large for the space. *B*, the mesial surfaces of the cuspids have been disked and each replacement tooth has been narrowed slightly, so as to fit into the space.

The Patient's Viewpoint in Tooth Selection

If a previous prosthesis which supplied anterior teeth, has been worn by the patient, it is important to ascertain his opinion of the esthetic effect which these teeth created. His remarks will establish a useful point of reference from which to proceed in the selection of the anterior teeth. Beauty is in the eye of the beholder, and the very essence of good esthetic achievement is the creation of a dental composition in which the interplay of detail is both pleasing to the viewer and consistent with the patient's self-image. The key to accomplishment of this objective is an insight into the patient's hopes and expectations in regard to the appearance of his mouth. Acquiring this knowledge demands a high level of communicative skill, combined with astute psychological insight.

Many times, when queried as to his opinion of anterior tooth replacements, the patient will simply state that he would prefer that the dentist use his professional judgment, and that he (the patient) will abide by that judgment. Given this challenge, one cannot do less than bring to bear one's utmost creative skill and artistic perception.

Establishing the Midline

Nature does not always locate the natural central incisors precisely on either side of the midline of the mouth, and more often than not, the midline of the maxillary teeth does not coincide with the midline of the mandibular teeth. However, in arranging artificial teeth in the maxillary arch when the maxillary central incisors have been lost, it is generally best to establish the central incisors on either side of the midline. It should be noted that there is only one reliable method of establishing a midline accurately, and that is by observation of the mouth, particularly the upper lip. If an attempt is made to employ various other anatomical landmarks as reference points, such as the maxillary frenum, the center of the cast, or the midline of the mandibular teeth, the result is very apt to be inaccurate. Although the philtrum is the most helpful anatomic guide, the only reliably accurate reference point is the mouth itself. When the midline has been established on the wax occlusion rim, it should then be transferred onto the art portion of the master cast as a permanent record. Should the anterior teeth need to be removed from the record base and rearranged at a later date, this mark will serve as a handy reference point.

Arrangement of the Anterior Teeth

When conditions permit some latitude in the arrangement of the teeth, as in replacement of all of the maxillary anterior teeth, for example, the same precepts may be followed that are applicable in tooth arrangement for the completely edentulous patient. Many times it will be possible for the clinician to contribute some individuality to the tooth arrangement which is especially fitting for the patient being served. For example, a natural lateral incisor with a diagonally worn incisal edge might be matched on the contralateral side of the arch with a replacement tooth which exhibits a similar diagonal wear pattern. On the other hand, when restoring the typical two or three tooth anterior space, the opportunities for creating a pleasing effect are much more limited.

When the mesiodistal dimension of the edentulous space is less than the width of the missing natural teeth, and it cannot be enlarged sufficiently to accommodate the usual number of teeth, it may be necessary to eliminate one tooth altogether, in order to compensate for the reduced dimension. Eliminating one of the anterior teeth, however, carries with it the risk of interfering with proper restoration of the midline. A decision must sometimes be made between using fewer but larger teeth (than those being replaced), or the same number of smaller teeth (than the size of those being replaced). Generally, it may be said that fewer, smaller teeth are the lesser of two evils, although certainly there are exceptions. While this can be a

vexing problem in the maxilla, it is normally of far less consequence in the mandible.

The very opposite of a restricted space may be encountered in the mouth in which diastemas were, or are, present between the natural teeth. In this circumstance, a slightly larger substitute tooth may be selected, or perhaps restoration of the diastemata between the substitute teeth will result in a more harmonious composition. It is important that the patient be consulted on questions of this kind, since spaces between the replacement teeth may appeal to some individuals while being distasteful to others.

When denture teeth are to be abuted to the ridge, the proper way to ensure that the tooth is well-adapted to the mucosa in the mouth is to scrape the surface of the processing cast at the site to be occupied by the ridge lap to a depth of at least 1 mm. (Fig. 14.8), so that when the prosthesis is inserted, the tooth will be snugly fitted to the alveolar mucosa (Fig. 14.9). The ridge lap may be further adjusted, at the time of insertion of the finished denture, so as to avoid undue pressure, which might cause discomfort, or even stimulate bone resorption. When arranging the teeth, it is generally more convenient to fit the tooth to the cast without the

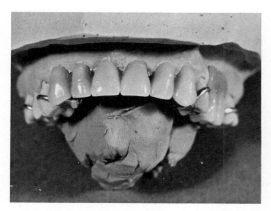

FIG. 14.8. When denture teeth are employed as replacement teeth, they should be individually fitted to the stone of the residual ridge. When carefully adapted to the mucosa, the denture tooth is the most natural appearing of replacement teeth.

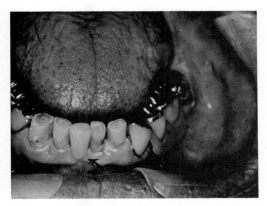

Fig. 14.9. The proper way to fit the replacement tooth to the mucosa of the edentulous ridge is to scrape the cast slightly in the area to be occupied by the ridge lap of the tooth. The replacement tooth is then carefully fitted to the cast. A tooth so prepared will make intimate contact with the mucosa and will appear in the mouth as a natural tooth (*arrow*).

framework in place. Following adaptation of the teeth to the cast, the framework can be replaced and the teeth can then be modified to accommodate to the retention latticework. Carefully fitted to the mucosa in this manner, a denture tooth of the proper shade will appear virtually indistinguishable from the adjacent natural teeth.

Try-in of Anterior Teeth

Many times it will be prudent to try the tooth arrangement in the mouth, so that the esthetic effect can be assessed and approved by the patient before the denture is processed. This is especially applicable when (1) the position, size, or arrangement of the missing natural teeth is not being faithfully reproduced because of space limitations, (2) natural diastemas are not being reproduced in the tooth arrangement, (3) there is a mutual agreement with the patient that a change in size, shape, or arrangement of the teeth (from what he is presently wearing) is desirable, or (4) there is reason to doubt the accuracy of the midline. Moreover, the patient may have worthwhile suggestions for improving the arrangement, and certainly it would be preferable to hear any

such suggestions before the prosthesis is processed rather than afterwards. It should be noted, in this regard, that when the patient does not seem to be in complete accord with a tooth, or color, or arrangement, at the time of try-in, it is imprudent to employ subtle suasion to gain his approval. An acquiescence so obtained is almost certain to be transitory. When he has worn the prosthesis for a short time, he may very well become convinced that he has made a mistake, which will lead to the altogether logical conclusion that he was "talked into it."

Try-in for the Exacting Type of Patient. It may on occasion be desirable, when serving the very exacting type of patient, to permit him to take the trial denture home for a leisurely examination of the anterior tooth arrangement in familiar, private surroundings. Equally important, it affords an opportunity for another person, a spouse, for example, whose approbation may be important to the patient, to express his opinion. The private try-in is especially recommended when a complete denture is being made to oppose a removable partial denture, and the patient has exhibited some indecision in placing his stamp of approval on the tooth arrangement, yet has no concrete suggestions for modification or improvement. Until the patient grants his unequivocal approval, the denture should not be processed.

Selection of Posterior Teeth

Posterior replacement teeth should be selected which fit into the available edentulous space and which also are harmonious in composition, size, and occlusal anatomy with the teeth which they are to oppose, whether natural or artificial. It may be well to point out that the replacement teeth need not precisely duplicate the missing natural teeth in type and number; indeed, it will not often be possible to do so. For example, the most suitable replacement tooth for a space formerly occupied by a first molar and second bicuspid might be two bicuspids, and similarly, two second molars might best fit a space vacated by a natural second bicuspid, first molar, and second molar. Prosthetic teeth, as supplied by the manufacturer, may be regarded as blanks to be fitted into edentulous spaces of varying length, height, and breadth, and to intercuspate with opposing teeth of myriad cusp-fossae patterns.

A fundamental consideration in the selection of posterior teeth for the partial denture is the size of the food table. Leverage exerted on the abutment tooth, as well as stress applied to the residual ridge by the distal extension base type of partial denture, is profoundly affected by the size of the collective occlusal surfaces of the denture teeth. The larger the food table, the greater will be the load on the ridge, and the more the stress on the abutment teeth. A smaller food table can be achieved by employing smaller teeth, by eliminating a bicuspid or a molar or, in some circumstances, by substituting a bicuspid for a molar. Smaller teeth can penetrate the bolus with less force than is required for larger teeth, hence stress exerted on the denture base will be less. The teeth should be narrow and sharp, rather than wide and flat, so that they can cut and shred the food, rather than crush it (Fig. 14.10).

The type of posterior tooth most often used for the removable partial denture is the denture tooth, either porcelain or plastic. They are provided by the manufacturer in anatomic, semianatomic and nonanatomic occlusal patterns. The all-metal tooth is also used with some frequency, while the pressed-on, or post tooth, and the interchangeable facing are less often indicated.

Acrylic Resin Denture Teeth

The plastic denture tooth is the most commonly employed posterior tooth in removable partial denture construction because it is uniquely suited for the purpose. It is not dangerously weakened by the grinding that may be necessary to fit the tooth into the restricted interridge spaces so often encountered in the partially edentulous mouth, and the plastic does not abrade either gold or enamel.

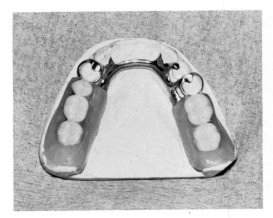

FIG. 14.10. To reduce the stress on the residual ridges to a minimum, posterior replacement teeth should be selected which are smaller mesiodistally and narrower buccolingually than the natural teeth. The teeth on the right of the photograph are too large in all dimensions, the teeth on the left side are a much more suitable size.

The anatomic occlusal pattern is generally preferred to either the semianatomic or the nonanatomic tooth because it can be more readily adapted to a cusp-fossa or cusp-embrasure relationship with the occlusal surfaces of opposing natural teeth. The reason for this is that the cusps of the anatomic tooth can be readily modified to intercuspate with opposing grooves and fossae, whereas cusps must be created in the nonanatomic tooth by grinding grooves and spillways in the occlusal surface.

The Porcelain Denture Tooth

The porcelain tooth should not be opposed to either natural teeth or to gold alloy because of its tendency to abrade these substances. Although the use of porcelain for the removable partial denture is somewhat restricted for this reason, it may be employed with gratifying results when opposed to porcelain or to plastic denture teeth.

The Metal Tooth

The all-metal tooth is an excellent replacement for the restricted posterior space which is not readily visible in the mouth. It is particularly well suited for the first molar space in the mandibular arch (Fig. 14.11) that has been partially closed by the mesial drift of the second molar. Its use is generally restricted to the edentulous space that measures from 3 to 8 mm. in mesiodistal width. If the framework is made of one of the chromium-cobalt alloys, the metal tooth should not be permitted to occlude heavily with a gold restoration, because of the wear of the gold which will ensue.

The Post Tooth

The post tooth is commendably strong and reasonably esthetic. It may be employed for the narrow posterior space, although it requires at least an average amount of interocclusal space. Its most common application is to replace a single maxillary bicuspid.

The Interchangeable Facing

The interchangeable facing is sometimes employed in the maxillary first bicuspid space when interocclusal space is

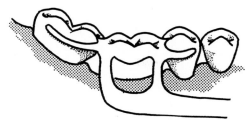

FIG. 14.12. The one- or two-tooth space in the posterior part of the mandible may be difficult to restore satisfactorily, when atrophy of the residual ridge has been extensive, without creating food traps between the prosthesis and the adjoining teeth. Such a space may be restored by employing a metal occlusal surface which is an integral part of the metal framework, thus eliminating potential areas of food entrapment and permitting saliva to flow under and around the pontic, so that the area is to some degree self-cleansing.

at a premium. Facings may be selected of either porcelain or acrylic resin.

The Self-Cleansing Pontic

The small one-tooth space, in the posterior part of the mouth, is sometimes difficult to restore without creating food traps between the denture and the adjoining teeth when atrophy of the residual ridge has been extensive. This is especially true when the adjoining teeth have tipped or rotated so that the edentulous space is smaller at the occlusal level than it is at the level of the residual ridge. If the space is restored with the conventional denture tooth and an acrylic resin base, food traps are unavoidably created between the proximal surfaces of the teeth and the denture. A better solution may be to restore the space with a self-cleansing occlusal surface which is an integral part of the metal framework (Fig. 14.12). Such a restoration may be easily maintained in a state of cleanliness by the patient, and restoration of function is as complete as it would be with any other type of pontic or replacement tooth. This method of replacement may also be employed when the mandibular molar has an extreme mesial tilt and disking cannot be expected to eliminate the undercut between the proximal surface of the tooth and the framework.

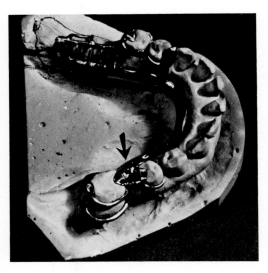

FIG. 14.11. The all-metal tooth is particularly well suited to the small (less than 8 mm.) space in the mandibular arch. It should not be in heavy occlusion with an opposing gold restoration, if the prosthesis is to be made of one of the chromium-cobalt alloys, since the gold may be abraded by the chromium-cobalt.

Plastic Opposed to Porcelain

There is abundant clinical evidence that plastic teeth wear rather rapidly in some mouths. Although this poses a much greater threat to complete dentures than to the typical removable partial denture, it may create a problem in the case of two long-span Kennedy Class I partial dentures. One solution to the problem of low abrasion resistance of the acrylic resin tooth is to employ the plastic tooth in one arch and porcelain in the other. Research studies indicate that when porcelain maxillary posterior teeth are opposed to plastic mandibular posterior teeth, or vice versa, wear of the plastic is reduced by a significant amount. The physical principle here demonstrated is that the coefficient of friction of like materials is often greater than that of unlike materials. The example is often cited of the diamond phonograph needle acting on the comparatively much softer record, which produces no demonstrable wear of the softer material over prolonged periods of frictional contact. By employing such a technique, one may take advantage of some of the desirable physical properties of each material while circumventing in large part the disadvantages. It is important to note that the research study alluded to was conducted with glazed porcelain teeth, and that porcelain which has been roughened by grinding is extremely abrasive. Thus it follows that any benefit to be gained by employing the two materials together would be lost if the surface of the porcelain were roughened. Therefore, when this technique is followed (i.e., plastic opposed to porcelain), any needed grinding should be accomplished on the plastic teeth and the areas roughened by the grinding should afterwards be polished.

Gold Occlusal Surfaces

A method can be employed which retains most of the advantages of the plastic tooth while eliminating entirely its poor wear resistance. The technique consists in replacing the occlusal surfaces of the plastic denture teeth with gold alloy. The plastic teeth are arranged in whatever oc-clusal scheme is desired, and the denture is fabricated and delivered in the usual manner. The patient is permitted to wear the prosthesis for several weeks, during which period final occlusal adjustments are accomplished. When all needed adjustments have been completed, the occlusal surfaces of the plastic teeth are reproduced in gold by means of stone dies and counter dies, the teeth are prepared with modified three-quarter crown preparations, and the gold occlusal surfaces are cast and cemented into place (Fig. 14.13). The combination of gold and plastic makes possible a highly efficient, as well as long wearing, occlusion, although it must be conceded that the gold does add some additional weight to the prosthesis.

Amalgam Occlusal Surfaces

Silver amalgam can be employed to reduce wear of the plastic tooth, and thus prolong its period of usefulness. The acrylic teeth are arranged and articulated in the usual manner, and the denture is processed. One-surface amalgam cavity preparations are then made in the occlusal surfaces of the teeth and filled with amalgam. The patient wears the prosthesis for at least 24 hours before the amalgam is polished. Although resistance to wear of the amalgam is substantially less than that of gold alloy, it is nevertheless much greater than that of acrylic

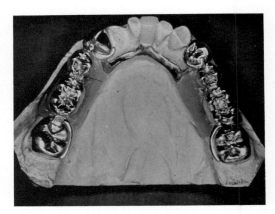

Fig. 14.13. Gold occlusal surfaces fitted to acrylic resin denture teeth make an excellent posterior tooth for the removable partial denture.

resin and, of course, the technique is much simpler and less costly than is the use of gold alloy.

Selecting a Posterior Tooth Form for the Patient Who Already Wears a Prosthesis

In deciding whether to employ a porcelain or an acrylic tooth with either an anatomic or a nonanatomic occlusal pattern for a patient who is presently wearing a prosthesis, one should be mindful of the fact that change is not always welcome to individuals in the denture-wearing age groups. Accordingly, when a prosthesis is being made over and a change in posterior tooth type or form is contemplated—from plastic to porcelain, for example, or from anatomic to nonanatomic—it is always in order to inform the patient of the proposed change and the reason for making it. If the patient is made to understand beforehand the differences that he can expect as a result of the change, he will be better prepared to adapt to it. (See selection of posterior tooth replacements, Table 14.2.)

Restoring Occlusal Surfaces with the Partial Denture

When the occlusal surfaces of one or two teeth in the arch being restored are in infraocclusion, and it is not feasible to restore the occlusion with conventional onlays or crowns, it may be possible, in selected instances, to realign the occlusal surfaces with an extension of the metal framework. The occlusal surface of the tooth that is to support the occlusal overlay should ideally be covered with an onlay or crown, although this is, of course, not always suitable. The refractory cast is articulated with a cast of the opposing arch, and the occlusal overlays are waxed into functional intercuspation as an inte-

TABLE 14.2.

Selection of posterior tooth replacements

Tooth Type	Indications	Strong Points	Weak Points
Resin denture tooth	Opposed to gold Opposed to natural teeth Opposed to resin or porcelain teeth	Easiest to fit to the residual ridge and around a clasp	Poor abrasive resistance
Porcelain denture tooth	Opposed to porcelain, or to resin teeth	Excellent esthetics Excellent wear Highly efficient	Subject to breakage Weak in thin sections More difficult to process because of the danger of breakage
Acrylic with gold occlusals	Where plastic is indicated but will wear too rapidly	Excellent wear, efficiency, and resistance to breakage	Additional time and expense required to fabricate Increased weight
Cast metal	In the small restricted posterior space that will not detract esthetically	Clean and will wear indefinitely Not subject to breakage Easily maintained	Very hard surface May add slightly to the weight
Pressed-on acrylic	Any posterior space	Can be fitted into narrow or short edentulous spaces Has ample strength	Not as good esthetically as the denture tooth

gral part of the framework (Fig. 14.14). This procedure should be employed only in a caries-resistant mouth where oral hygiene is of a very high order. A prosthesis which has been designed to overlie the occlusal surface, or surfaces, of natural teeth should be left out of the mouth for at least 8 of the 24 hours. If deep pits and fissures are present on any of the occlusal surfaces to be covered with the metal overlay, they should be widened, smoothed, and then treated with stannous fluoride. The light weight of the chromium-cobalt alloy makes it particularly suitable for this method of restoring the occlusion, although the hardness of the alloy must be counted a disadvantage.

While this method of realigning an occlusal plane is not as ideal as accomplishing it with conventional restorations, it does, nonetheless, fulfill a need in selected cases. The patient for whom this service is provided should be seen periodically, so that, should any decalcification occur beneath the overlay, it will be discovered early.

Rules for Arranging Posterior Teeth

In general, the same rules apply to the arrangement of the posterior teeth for the partial denture as those which apply to

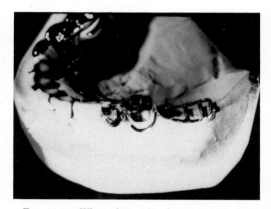

FIG. 14.14. When the occlusal surfaces of one or two teeth in the arch being restored with the partial denture are in infraocclusion as a result of tipping or intrusion, it may be feasible to restore the occlusion with an occlusal overlay that is an extension of the metal framework. The second bicuspid has been so restored. The first bicuspid space in the photograph will be restored with a post tooth.

the complete denture. Since the occlusal surfaces of most natural teeth have been altered by wear, it should be anticipated that the prosthetic teeth will have to be altered with suitable stones and burs so that the two will probably intercuspate.

Positioning the Tooth Adjacent to the Clasp

The posterior tooth that is to occupy a position immediately adjacent to the clasp must be adapted to three different structures: (1) the clasp, (2) the residual ridge, and (3) the opposing occlusion. The task can be simplified somewhat by fitting the tooth first to the opposing teeth and to the ridge, with the framework off the cast. When this has been accomplished, the framework is returned to the cast and the tooth is fitted to the metal framework.

Positioning Maxillary Bicuspids for Maximum Esthetic Effect

When the maxillary edentulous space begins distal to the cuspid, the arrangement of the bicuspids is so crucial to a pleasing appearance that it is deserving of special comment.

If the bicuspids are positioned in a buccal flange, the patient may exhibit a variety of colors and textures when this area is glimpsed during conversation. On display are the natural teeth, the metal clasp, the denture flange, the artificial tooth, and the mucosa. If crowns or other restorations are present in the area still another color and texture must be added to the melange. As expected, the overall cosmetic effect may fall far short of the patient's expectations. A more pleasing composition can often be achieved by eliminating a portion of the buccal flange and abutting the denture tooth directly to the mucosal covering of the alveolar ridge. If only the bicuspids are being replaced, the buccal flange may be eliminated altogether for maximum esthetic effect. If the edentulous span extends distally into the molar area, the flange may be omitted in the bicuspid region and added in the molar area, where it will be much less in evidence.

When a buccal flange must be employed, it is important to the appearance that the cervical line of the denture teeth be at a vertical level which is in harmony with those of the adjacent natural teeth. A frequent mistake, from a cosmetic standpoint, is to select a replacement bicuspid which is so much shorter than the adjoining natural teeth that the cervical lines do not blend harmoniously.

Intercuspating Posterior Teeth

As a general rule, the classic pattern of intercuspation of the maxillary and mandibular teeth should be strived for, i.e., mesiobuccal cusp of the maxillary molar in the buccal groove of the mandibular molar (Fig. 14.15). However, this classic relationship is not essential to good function and, of course, cannot be achieved in many instances (Fig. 14.16).

Generally, the lower posterior teeth should be positioned with the central grooves over the crest of the mandibular ridge (Fig. 14.17), unless the maxilla and mandible are in a Class III relationship, in which case the buccal cusps often should be placed over the ridge instead of the central groove. Placing lower teeth with the cusps buccal to the crest of the mandibular ridge is a root cause of disbalancing stresses on the residual ridges, as well as torsional forces on the abutment teeth, and should be avoided.

The occlusal surfaces of posterior teeth should have grooves, ridges, and spillways which enable them to function against their antagonists with harmony and efficiency, whatever the occlusal scheme. Flat, abraded occlusal surfaces of natural teeth should not be opposed by flattened artificial teeth, because of the loss of efficiency and the magnified stress which two

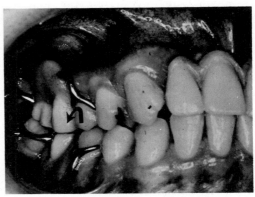

FIG. 14.16. Oftentimes it is not possible to achieve an ideal intercuspation of the prosthetic teeth with either the natural teeth or with opposing denture teeth. However, a harmonious occlusion can be developed irrespective of the fact that opposing tooth relationships are not ideal.

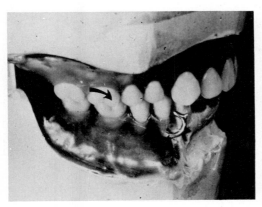

FIG. 14.15. In arranging posterior teeth, the classic pattern of intercuspation is an ideal to be strived for. Although it cannot always be achieved, it was accomplished in the occlusion shown here. Note that the mesiobuccal cusp of the maxillary first molar (arrow) occludes with the buccal groove of the mandibular first molar.

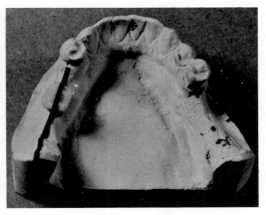

FIG. 14.17. Lower posterior teeth should be positioned with the central groove over the crest of the mandibular ridge, in most instances, although in some Class III occlusions it may be necessary to place the buccal cusps instead of the central groove over the crest of the ridge.

such surfaces generate. Instead, cutting edges and escape-ways for the food should be provided in the artificial teeth. Tooth surfaces which have been recontoured or altered by grinding should always be smoothed and polished prior to mouth service. This applies, with special emphasis, to porcelain, which is extremely abrasive when the glaze has been lost as a result of grinding.

If the distance between the bows of the articulator is increased approximately ½ mm. prior to arranging the posterior teeth, it will contribute toward achieving a tight intercuspation of the teeth in the finished prosthesis. Fine adjustments can then be accomplished by intraoral equilibration. It should be borne in mind that when artificial teeth are articulated against the stone teeth of an opposing cast, the stone is easily abraded, which may introduce discrepancies into the occlusion.

The Partial Denture Base

Although the primary role of the denture base is to provide support for the replacement teeth, a properly designed base can, in addition, contribute materially not only to the comfort with which the prosthesis is worn but to its stability and retention as well. By means of accurate extension of the peripheries, functionally formed borders, and intimate adaptation to the underlying mucosa, the base can assist substantially in neutralizing the twisting, tilting types of stresses to which the prosthesis is subjected; stresses that would otherwise be transmitted unabated to both the residual ridges and the abutment teeth. The important role of the denture base as a stabilizing influence is sometimes overlooked and frequently underestimated.

The partial denture base may be constructed of (1) metal (Fig. 14.18), (2) acrylic resin, or (3) a combination of metal and acrylic (Fig. 14.19).

The Acrylic Resin Base

The denture base made of acrylic resin possesses the eminently desirable attribute of being easily refitted at a rela-

tively moderate cost to the patient, which is not true of either the metal base or the metal-plastic combination. Since the overwhelming majority of removable par-

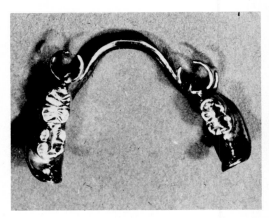

Fig. 14.18. The denture shown here is made entirely of metal (chromium-cobalt). Although worn with satisfaction by the patient for several years, it could not be relined or rebased when it no longer fit so it was necessary to remake it. It was remade with conventional acrylic resin bases. Following a brief period of wear of the new prosthesis the patient voluntarily stated that he preferred the acrylic resin bases because they were so much lighter in weight.

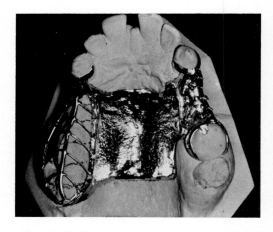

Fig. 14.19. The base shown on the reader's left will be made of acrylic resin attached to the retention latticework. The base on the right will be made up of a combination of metal and acrylic resin. Note the finish lines on both sides and the retention studs in the metal of the right side. The metal base is employed on this side of the mouth because the ridge is well healed and it will be entirely tooth-supported so that the need for a future refitting operation is not likely.

tial prostheses—particularly those with a distal extension base—are almost certain candidates for future rebasing or relining, the acrylic resin should be the material of choice in all but a few exceptional instances.

The Metal Base

The metal base does have certain advantages, although they seldom transcend the fact that it cannot be refitted. Perhaps most important, metal has the property of transmitting the sensation of heat and cold to the underlying tissues. There is reason to believe that this more closely simulates natural conditions than acrylic resin and, if this be true, the metal may be more compatible with the mucosa than is the acrylic resin. There does appear to be clinical evidence that tissue change beneath a metal denture base may be somewhat less rapid than is the case with the resin base, perhaps because of the stimulation produced by temperature change. There is evidence, too, that the sense of taste may be improved because the sensation of heat and cold is keener. These postulations are admittedly empirical, there being no reliable research to support them.

An important disadvantage of the metal base for the mandibular denture is the fact that proper extension onto the buccal shelf cannot be as readily accomplished with a thin metal border as is possible with the rounded, relatively thick border of acrylic resin. Similarly, the contour of the lips or cheeks cannot, as a rule, be restored as well with a metal base as with acrylic resin. Finally, not to be overlooked is the higher cost of the metal base because of the increased amount of time required for its fabrication.

The Metal-Acrylic Resin Base

The combination metal and acrylic resin base consists of a cast metal base (Fig. 14.20) which fits the residual ridge, and onto which is attached an acrylic resin superstructure that retains the teeth. It has essentially the same advantages and disadvantages as the all-metal base, although it may be slightly lighter in

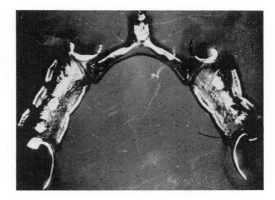

Fig. 14.20. The combination metal-acrylic resin type of denture base shown consists of a metal section which fits the ridge onto which will be attached an acrylic resin portion which will hold the teeth. Note the nailhead type of retention to hold the resin.

weight. Since it shares with the metal base the fact that it cannot be readily resurfaced, it is not often indicated for use.

Acrylic Resin versus the Metal Base

To summarize the pros and cons of metal versus the acrylic resin base: acrylic resin is generally the material of choice for the removable partial denture base, although the metal base may be indicated (1) when the patient has a strong preference for metal for personal reasons, (2) in order to reduce the risk of breakage when an abnormally heavy bite is coupled with limited intermaxillary space, (3) when tongue room is at a premium and the additional space made possible by the relatively thin metal flange will afford the patient more comfort, (4) in the extremely rare instance of sensitivity of the patient to acrylic resin, and (5) for the compulsive brusher. The metal will resist abrasion of the toothbrush when the patient cannot be dissuaded from this destructive practice.

Design of the Denture Base

A time-honored principle of partial denture base design is that the base should cover as wide an area as the limiting structures will permit and that the patient can comfortably tolerate (Fig. 14.21). The biomechanical principle here

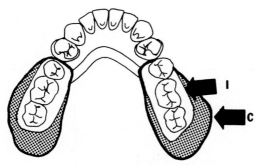

FIG. 14.21. The partial denture base should cover as much area as the patient can comfortably tolerate. The mandibular base should cover the retromolar pad and extend onto the buccal shelf. The bases indicated by white, *i* in the sketch, are not adequately extended. The coverage indicated by the dotted area *c* shows the area that should be covered.

operant is that occlusal forces will be distributed over a wider area, so that stress per unit of area will be minimal.

The importance of proper extension of the denture base was highlighted by an investigative study conducted by Lytle in which he sought to study the magnitude of soft tissue displacement beneath dentures. In one part of the study he measured the displacement of the soft tissues beneath a partial denture with a distal extension base which did not cover the retromolar pad and found that the tissue was displaced more than 3 mm. under an occlusal load. As might be expected, the greatest amount of displacement occurred in the area farthest from the rest support.

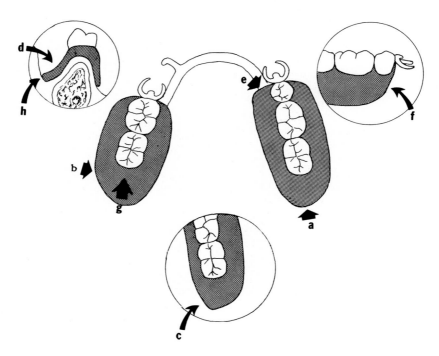

FIG. 14.22. The mandibular base should cover the retromolar pad (*a*) and extend buccally onto the buccal shelf (*b*). From the distal terminus, the distolingual border should drop straight down into the mylohyoid area; the distolingual flange should be tapered laterally and the distal edge beveled (*c*). The lingual flange should be thin enough to allow maximum tongue room; it may be made slightly concave but should not be carried beneath the teeth. The buccal flanges should be made slightly concave to provide a "grip" for the buccinator muscles (*d*). The metal finish lines, both internal and external, should be neatly trimmed to form a sharp straight junction so as to create no thin feathers of acrylic resin to overlap the metal (*e*). The anterior border of the buccal flange should taper distally and should be beveled (*f*). The acrylic resin should be trimmed to form a neat junction with the teeth and this includes the distal surface of the last tooth (*g*). All peripheries should be round, smooth and well polished. The buccal peripheral border should be at least 2 mm. in thickness (*h*).

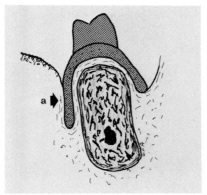
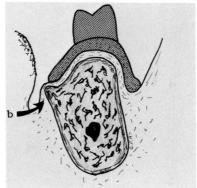

FIG. 14.23. The configuration of the lingual flange of the mandibular base in the area of the mylohyoid ridge will depend on the anatomy in this region of the mouth. If the ridge is neither excessively prominent nor undercut, the flange may be extended below it as shown at *a* in the sketch (*left*). If it is prominent and undercut, the flange may have to be terminated at or near its crest as shown at *b* in the sketch (*right*).

Extension of the Mandibular Base

The total area of the maxilla that is capable of providing support for the denture is greater than that of the mandible, in a ratio of approximately 1.6:1 (Personal communication from T. Fischer and W. D. Sweeney, Department of Biomaterials, University of Alabama School of Dentistry) because of the differences in structure of the two. This points up the importance of exploiting all possible means of support for the mandibular base. In applying the principle of maximum coverage, the mandibular distal extension base should be extended to cover the retromolar pads, and extended laterally to include the buccal shelf (Fig. 14.22). Both of these areas are more resistant to alteration in contour as a result of bone resorption than are the residual ridges, and a base which receives a portion of its support from these structures will be more stable, over a longer period of time, than one which does not. The distolingual border should extend vertically downward from the top of the retromolar pad into the alveolingual sulcus. There is nothing to be gained by extending the lingual flange distally into the retromolar space beyond the retromolar pad. The amount of vertical extension of the flange inferiorly will depend, to an important degree, on the anatomy of the mylohyoid ridge. If this structure is sharp and markedly undercut, the lingual flange may have to be

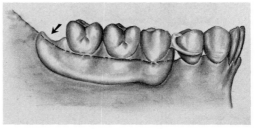

FIG. 14.24. Proper extension of the mandibular base, to cover the retromolar pad confers an additional benefit when the ascending ramus forms an acute angle with the body of the mandible. The distal extremity of the base will turn upward as it covers the pad, thus contributing to stabilization of the prosthesis against distal displacement.

terminated at its crest (Fig. 14.23). On the other hand, if the ridge is not sharp and does not create an undercut beneath it, the flange may be extended a moderate amount into the alveolingual sulcus. The distal border of the lingual flange should curve slightly laterally, and the distal edge should be beveled so as to be as innocuous as possible to the tongue. The peripheral borders of the buccal and labial flanges should be extended into the vestibules, so as gently to distend the tissue of the resilient mucobuccal fold. Properly extended in this manner, the base will contribute optimally to retention.

It is worth noting that proper extension of the mandibular base, to cover the retromolar pad, confers an additional ben-

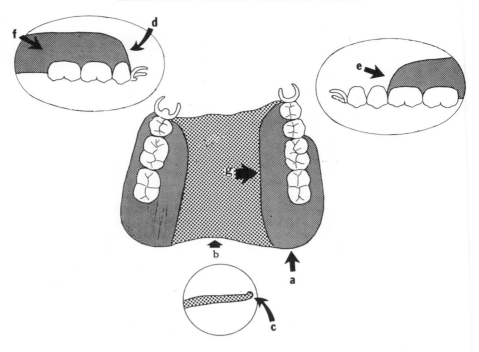

Fig. 14.25. The maxillary full coverage base should be extended to cover the tuberosity and the hamular notch (*a*). The posterior palatal border should terminate on tissue that is resilient but not movable. This will be on or close to a line which passes through the hamular notch on each side and the fovea palatinae (*b*). The tissue surface should be lightly beaded if it is metal and post-dammed if it is acrylic resin. The posterior border as viewed from the polished surface of the prosthesis should taper slightly and be beveled (*c*). The anterior border of the buccal flange should taper slightly posteriorly and be beveled whether the bicuspids are positioned in a flange (*d*) or abutted as shown at (*e*). The buccal flange should be slightly concave to provide a "grip" for the buccinator muscle (*f*). The metal finish lines should be neatly formed so that there is no overlap of the resin onto the metal (*g*). The buccal flanges should be at least 2 mm. in thickness, rounded, smooth, and well polished.

efit when the ascending ramus forms an acute angle with the body of the mandible. The distal extremity of the base will turn upward as it covers the pad, thus stabilizing the base against distal displacement (Fig. 14.24).

Extention of the Maxillary Base

The greater the number of teeth that are being replaced by the removable partial denture, the nearer to a complete denture should be the configuration of the maxillary denture base. The full coverage base should be extended to cover the tuberosity and the hamular notches (Fig. 14.25). The palatal border should terminate on tissue that is resilient but not movable. The posterior border, as viewed from the polished surface, should be slightly beveled so as to merge smoothly with the resilient soft tissue. When the denture has buccal flanges that begin in the bicuspid region, the anterior border of the buccal flange should be tapered posteriorly, and the edge should be beveled. The buccal flange should be slightly concave to provide a "grip" for the buccinator muscle. The peripheral borders of the denture flanges which extend into the vestibules should be at least 2 mm. thick, rounded, smooth, and polished. When the denture is retained and supported primarily by natural teeth, it is not essential that the peripheral borders be extended

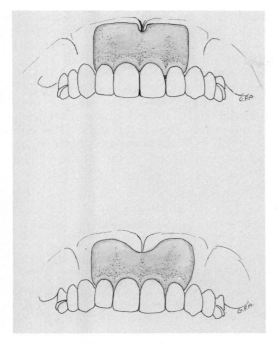

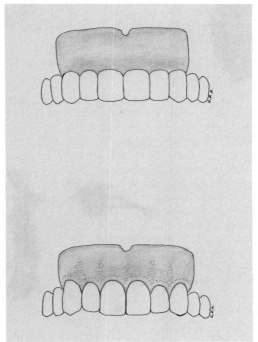

FIG. 14.26. When a labial flange is employed, it must provide clearance for the labial frenum. The amount of clearance should not exceed the exact amount required by the frenum for functional freedom (*upper sketch*). An excessive amount of clearance (*lower sketch*) will create an air leak and may allow the ingress of food.

FIG. 14.27. When anterior teeth are supplied by means of a labial flange, they should be made to appear as natural as possible. One way to contribute to a pleasing dental composition is to avoid the use of stereotyped, half-moon shaped scallops of the cervical borders of the teeth (*upper sketch*). If the festooning is varied in height and contour so that each tooth appears as an individual entity the overall appearance will be much more lifelike (*lower sketch*).

into the vestibular fornix in the manner required with complete dentures. However, there will be less likelihood of food accumulation beneath the base that is well extended into the vestibules than with one with borders which terminate short of the mucobuccal fold.

The Labial Flange

If an anterior flange is to be employed, it should be formed so as to permit freedom of movement of the labial frenum, but this should not be accomplished by gouging out an oversized opening in the acrylic resin. The aperture for the frenum should allow complete freedom for this structure, but there should be no excess clearance which

would allow the ingress of air, as well as providing a gathering point for food and debris (Fig. 14.26).

The anterior teeth should be made to appear as natural as possible. To be avoided is the creation of a series of stereotyped half-moon shaped scallops, which is the benchmark of a "production line" prosthesis. When several anterior teeth are being replaced, the cervical junction of tooth and resin should be made to simulate nature by varying the height of the gingiva-tooth junction as well as its configuration from tooth to tooth. It is important, too, that the height of the cervical line be commensurate with that of the adjoining natural teeth (Fig. 14.27). If the denture base is visible during conversation, characterization of the acrylic resin may add to the naturalness of the oral composition.

The Problem of the Resin Base in Flasking Operations

In articulating the teeth with their opponents, the acrylic resin record base that was used to register the intermaxillary relationship may be used as a temporary denture base. However, when the resin base is so employed, it will create a problem in the laboratory, since elimination of the resin from the denture mold after it has been flasked is a difficult, onerous task. The problem may be avoided by removing the acrylic resin from the framework prior to arranging the teeth, and substituting in its place a wax-tinfoil base in which the teeth can be arranged and tried in the mouth. When this procedure is followed, tinfoil should be adapted to the areas of the cast to be occupied by the denture base. The framework is then placed on the cast (over the tinfoil) and sticky wax applied to the metal latticework and to the tinfoil to help bind the materials together and impart strength. Baseplate wax is then added to create the remainder of the base. If reasonable care is exercised, the wax base will be durable enough to withstand the stress of normal handling during the try-in.

Bibliography

Lytle, R. B.: Soft tissue displacement beneath removable partial and complete dentures. J. Prosth. Dent. 12: 34–43, 1962.

Myerson, R. L.: The use of porcelain and plastic teeth in opposing complete dentures. J. Prosth. Dent. 7: 625–638, 1957.

Wallace, D.: The use of gold occlusal surfaces in complete and partial dentures, J. Prosth. Dent. 14: 326–333, 1964.

Chapter 15

Insertion, Counseling, Complaints, and Adjustments

This chapter deals with the insertion (delivery) of the prosthesis, counseling of the patient, the complaints which are most commonly heard, and the adjustments which are an integral part of the partial denture service. Inflammations induced by the prosthesis which often elicit no complaint from the patient are described. The discussion is organized under the subject headings which follow.

Introduction
The Insertion Procedure
Counseling
Post-Insertion Follow-up
Common Complaints of the Partial Denture
*   Wearer*
Factors in Assessing the Need for Adjustments
Hints for Accomplishing Adjustments
Inflammations Caused by the Prosthesis
*   Which Often Elicit No Complaint*

Introduction

While the insertion appointment usually represents to the patient the culmination of his hopes and expectations, there still remain several objectives to be achieved which are very much a part of the overall treatment, and it is important that sufficient time be set aside for their accomplishment. These objectives are (1) to make the prosthesis as comfortable as it is possible to make it, (2) to teach the patient how to insert and remove it and otherwise care for it, (3) to instruct him in the proper methods of maintaining the oral cavity and the remaining teeth in an immaculate state of cleanliness, and (4) to reinforce the education which has been ongoing, up to this juncture, in regard to the minor annoyances and vexations that

he may experience as he becomes accustomed to the prosthesis.

The Insertion Procedure

The Appointment

The appointment for the insertion should be made early in the day, if at all possible, so as to leave ample time for the patient to call back for guidance, should some question arise following a brief period of wear, or even for his return to the office in the unlikely event that unusual discomfort is experienced. A further consideration is the fact that most people tend to be more cheerful and optimistic in the early part of the day and to become progressively less so as the day wears on. The day of the week should also be considered. Delivery of the denture should not be scheduled on the last day of the work week, because the patient should be seen 24 hours following insertion. Although the prosthesis ofttimes will require no adjustment at that time, it is comforting to most patients to be reassured following a day of wear that they are doing well and that everything is in order intraorally. Another factor which merits consideration in arranging the appointment for insertion is to avoid, if possible, a time when the patient will need to transact business or fulfill a social engagement immediately following the insertion. The patient who wears an oral prosthesis for the first time needs an interval of privacy in which to accustom himself to the strangeness of the bulky foreign body before exposing himself to the additional stress of appearing before the public. Certainly, most individuals will not wish to eat in public until they have first had an opportunity to practice in privacy.

Inserting the Partial Denture

Normally, the metal framework will have been tried in the mouth, at a previous appointment, and any needed adjustments accomplished on this part of the prosthesis. Hence, the adjustments which will be required at the insertion appointment will be limited to the denture base and to the occlusion. Prior to the appointment, the completed partial denture should be carefully examined under good light and magnification. The intaglio (tissue surface) should be scrutinized critically for blebs, bubbles, blisters, or artifacts in either the metal or the plastic. It should be felt with the fingers to detect sharp edges which might be sources of irritation when placed against the mucosa under pressure. Sharp, knife-like edges of acrylic resin will not be well tolerated by the delicate oral tissues, and this type of border should be avoided.

The First Seating of the Prosthesis. When the denture is first seated in the mouth, it should be "felt" rather than thrust to place. Undercut areas in the mouth, which presage interference to insertion, will have been noted at the time of examination. Those which have not been eliminated by surgery should be recalled to mind at the time of insertion, so that suitable precautions can be taken not to force the prosthesis over a prominence, which might cause abrasion of the tissue and pain to the patient. When an obstacle to easy insertion, is discovered, the approximate area of the prosthesis which corresponds to the interference should be painted with a pressure-indicating medium (such as P.I.P.—Pressure Indicating Paste, Mizzy, Inc., Clifton Forge, Va.), and the area of the resin which is responsible for the frictional contact should be relieved sufficiently to permit comfortable seating. A maxillary prosthesis, with acrylic resin in the palate and over the tuberosities, will frequently scrape the lateral surfaces of the tuberosities even

though they may not be bulbous. One reason for this is that the acrylic resin typically contracts across the palate during polymerization, thus bringing the flanges inward. Another region that sometimes interferes with comfortable seating of the maxillary denture is the labial plate of bone, when a labial flange makes up a portion of the denture. Mandibular areas that frequently impede insertion and removal are the mylohyoid ridge area and the area buccal to the mandibular bicuspids (Fig. 15.1).

Providing Interocclusal Clearance for the Denture. The heels, or posterior extremity, of a mandibular partial denture should be carefully observed for interference with the maxillary posterior teeth, the tuberosity, or the maxillary denture, as the case might be. When the posterior extremity of a mandibular base makes

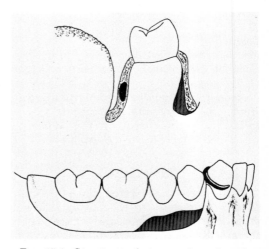

Fig. 15.1. Structures that sometimes interfere with seating of the lower partial denture are the mylohyoid ridge and the area buccal to the mandibular bicuspids. The latter area is shown in this sketch. The *upper sketch* shows a cross section of the mandible through the bicuspid area. Note that the residual ridge is thicker in cross section at the crest than it is lower in the vestibule. Thus, if the flange is made to fit the mucosa snugly in the vestibule, it will be too tight to slip over the wider area near the crest of the ridge. If acrylic resin is removed from the inside of the denture, it will leave a void as shown by the shaded portion. The *bottom sketch* shows the denture base from a lateral view. The shadowed area overlies the undercut.

contact with a maxillary base which covers the tuberosity when the jaws are in closed position, some clearance between the two must be established. The routine for accomplishing this follows. The acrylic resin of the maxillary base at the area of interference should first be thinned as much as possible without weakening it structurally. If the interference is still present, the mandibular base should be shortened the amount required to provide clearance in centric position as well as in all functionally excursive movements.

Flange Extension and Frenulum Clearance. The flanges of the denture should be observed for evidence of overextension and adjusted accordingly. Each of the frenula should be inspected to ensure that it has adequate clearance. It must be emphasized that frenulum clearance that exceeds the minimum required to clear the structure will allow air to gain entry beneath the denture, thus decreasing retention. When the denture can be comfortably inserted and removed, the occlusion should be carefully examined.

Inserting the Denture with an Interchangeable Facing

When interchangeable facings are a part of the denture, they should not be cemented into place until the prosthesis has been completely seated and adjusted. The facing is then slid onto the backing and adjusted so that it fits the mucosa. Contact with the mucosal tissue should be firm, but excess pressure should be avoided because of the danger that it will stimulate bone resorption. Excessive pressure is indicated by blanching of the mucosal tissue and by signs of discomfort from the patient. The facing should be free to slide on and off the backing, without any binding contact with the adjoining teeth. If it does make forceful contact with one of the adjacent teeth, the offending area of contact on the facing should be relieved, so as to preclude the likelihood of breakage of the porcelain after it has been cemented to the backing, or of transmitting a horizontal thrust against the natural teeth.

Equilibration of the Occlusion

Either articulating paper or occlusal indicator wax (Fig. 15.2) may be used to disclose premature contacts. Small discrepancies may be difficult to detect, because of movement of the base and the fact that some parts of the tooth surfaces cannot be viewed intraorally. They can be disclosed with an acceptable degree of accuracy if the task is approached with an understanding of the objectives and reasonable care is exercised.

Short strips of articulating paper or equilibration wax should be placed between the occlusal surfaces of the posterior teeth, and the patient should be instructed to close firmly and rub the teeth together while still keeping them in contact. The objective in refining centric occlusion is to create even contact among all of the maxillary and mandibular posterior teeth, both natural and artificial, on both sides of the mouth. On a distal extension base type of partial denture the occlusion should ideally be adjusted so that the second bicuspid-first molar areas bear the

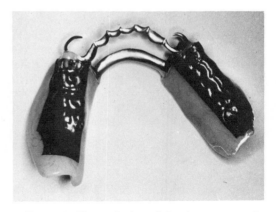

FIG. 15.2. The occlusion of the denture must be adjusted to eliminate interferences and deflective contacts, so that the upper and lower teeth, both natural and artificial, intercuspate harmoniously. In this sketch, equalizing wax has been applied to the denture teeth. The denture is inserted, and the patient is instructed to bite and rub the teeth together. The wax will be pierced at areas of heavy contact. These areas of the teeth are marked with a special marking pencil, the wax is removed, and the offending surfaces are relieved with suitable stones.

brunt of the occlusal load. It will not, of course, be possible to attain the type of balanced occlusion with most partial dentures that is strived for with complete dentures. However, the replacement teeth should not be permitted to interfere with the patient's ability to make excursive movements of the mandible freely, within his functional range.

It should be noted that when a complete maxillary denture opposes a mandibular partial denture, in which the mandibular anterior teeth are still present, the natural teeth should not be permitted to contact the maxillary teeth because of the damage which they are capable of inflicting on the anterior portion of the maxilla.

Final Polishing

A roughened surface of metal or acrylic resin, besides being annoying to the patient, tends to attract and retain stain, and to act as a nidus for bacteria. Therefore, the final step in the insertion is to smooth and polish any surface, whether metal, porcelain, or acrylic resin, which has been roughened by the adjustment procedure. Porcelain teeth which have been effaced by grinding become extremely rough and abrasive and should receive special attention to restore, as nearly as possible, the original surface smoothness. This can be done with pumice-impregnated hard rubber wheels, followed by buffing, with a rag wheel and fine pumice, at high speed on the polishing lathe.

Counseling

The dentist's total familiarity with all aspects of the wear and maintenance of an oral prosthesis may cause him to overlook the fact that to most patients the wearing of an oral prosthesis is a completely new experience. Accordingly, it may be taken for granted that he needs to be told (1) the proper way to insert and remove the prosthesis from the mouth, (2) how to maintain the natural teeth and the prosthesis in a state of meticulous cleanliness, (3) the pros and cons of night wear, and (4)

the importance of periodic maintenance of the prosthesis. Instruction on inserting and removing the prosthesis must be done by means of demonstration before a mirror. Further recommendations may be either verbal or written or, preferably, a combination of the two.

Written Instructions

Verbal instructions are sometimes incomplete, oftentimes misunderstood, and, all too often forgotten by the time the patient is ready to put some of the advice into practice. Written instructions have a further advantage in that psychologically the printed word carries more authority than does the spoken word. It scarcely needs to be said that instruction should be in nontechnical, easily understood terms and that it be concise and to the point. The following format covers the subject rather thoroughly and has been used by the author in pamphlet form for a number of years.

GETTING THE MOST FROM YOUR REMOVABLE PARTIAL DENTURE

Because of the many different types and designs of removable partial dentures (removable bridges), it isn't possible to make very many general statements which will apply in every respect to the partial you have just received. The following remarks, however, are applicable, in varying degrees, to all removable dental appliances.

Why Wear a Partial?

Aside from the obvious benefits of returning the mouth to a condition of healthful function by replacing the missing teeth, there are other compelling reasons for wearing a partial denture. When one or more teeth are removed from the upper or lower jaw, the teeth next to the extracted ones tend to drift, tip, and rotate, while the teeth in the opposite jaw move up or down into the space thus created. This results in a bite in which the teeth come together in an unnatural manner, much like two cog wheels which do not intermesh properly. When the teeth are brought together (as in chewing and swallowing), unbalanced, harmful stresses are developed in teeth and bone, and this results in loosening of the teeth, as well as loss of bone around the teeth. You probably would be unaware of the condition until it is quite advanced, but the destruction will become progressively worse unless some treatment is instituted. A properly designed and fitted partial denture can halt this breakdown and help to maintain the mouth in a state of health.

The Difficult "Break-In" Period.

A partial denture or removable bridge can succeed only if you contribute your maximum effort and cooperation during the difficult break-in period. The time required to learn to use an appliance with deftness and assurance will depend to a large degree on your personal attitude, although such factors as age, temperament, the shape and size of the abutment teeth and the gums, and the length of time you have been without teeth are important factors. A positive attitude and a sincere desire to master the problem are essential ingredients for success.

Learning to Speak Clearly.

You may experience some difficulty in speaking clearly right at first, particularly if you have an upper partial which covers all or part of the roof of the mouth. The tongue may find itself somewhat restricted, and needs time to adapt itself to the changed environment. This condition is temporary, and will improve rapidly, almost without conscious effort on your part. You can, if you like, speed up the process by reading aloud and repeating several times the sounds which give you most difficulty.

Learning to Eat

Learning to eat will take considerably longer, depending on the number of teeth replaced. Of course, if you have two partials (an upper and lower), your patience may be taxed to the utmost. Two weeks is perhaps about average for most individuals to learn to eat with ease and complete comfort. Try to select soft foods right at first, take small bites and eat slowly. Sticky foods will almost surely unseat the appliance, and should be avoided until you are more experienced. Anticipate some awkwardness at first, but do not be discouraged. Some 35,000,000 Americans are wearing complete artificial dentures (with no natural teeth to help hold them in), and you can certainly master your partial denture if you have the will to do so. Success with a partial will help you immeasurably to master the wearing of a complete denture if it ever becomes necessary. Incidentally, wearing a partial will help preserve the health of your remaining teeth, and thus postpone (perhaps forever) the time when you might be faced with the choice of either wearing a complete denture or going without teeth altogether.

How About Sore Spots?

Sore spots frequently occur as the partial settles into place, since nature did not design the teeth or gums to withstand the stresses of chewing with an artificial appliance. Sometimes this soreness will disappear as the tissues accustom themselves to their new role. If soreness persists for more than 24 hours, however, return to your dentist so that a trained person can determine what adjustment is needed.

Care of the Partial

A partial denture is a precision appliance, and should be treated as such. It will withstand heavy biting stress when it is in place in your mouth. However, it is very likely to bend or break if it is dropped. A bent or broken partial can seldom be returned to its original state of usefulness, so treat it as you would a fine watch. Be very careful in placing and removing it from the mouth. Never bite it into place. Occasionally, a clasp may become loose or slightly out of adjustment. Don't attempt to adjust it yourself. Return to your dentist so that he can decide what needs to be done to correct it.

Maintenance

The belief that a partial denture is permanent is a myth, since mouth tissues, like all body tissues, are undergoing constant change. Your partial should be examined periodically to determine whether or not undue settling has occurred. If the partial has changed position to any extent because of shrinkage of the underlying tissue, it can be quite serious, and will almost certainly place undue strain on the abutment (the clasped) teeth. Some types of appliances will need relining from time to time to compensate for tissue shrinkage. If the change is extensive, the partial may have to be reconstructed. Your dentist will advise you as to the treatment that is needed.

Should I Wear My Partial at Night?

It is much better to leave your partial out of the mouth at night while you sleep, in order to give the mouth tissues a chance to rest and recuperate. When it is left out of the mouth, it should be immersed in water, since most partials are constructed, at least partly, of a plastic material which will warp if permitted to dry out.

Mouth Hygiene

Now that you have a partial, it becomes doubly important that you maintain your mouth in a state of meticulous cleanliness. The teeth under the clasps are especially susceptible to decay, since they no longer receive the same cleansing action of the cheeks, tongue, and saliva. Never allow food to accumulate around the abutment teeth or on the partial denture for any length of time. The partial should be brushed under cold water after every meal and also at bedtime, along with your regular tooth brushing routine. Rinsing is not enough. You may use your regular toothbrush and any mild toilet soap or, if you prefer, use the toothpaste or powder which you normally use for your natural teeth. You may prefer to soak the partial in a special cleaning solution to maintain its cleanliness. If you do immerse it in a solution, do not use one which contains chlorine (such as Clorox), as the chlorine can damage the metal. To be safe, do not immerse it for more than 15 minutes. If you brush the partial, fill the sink with water so that if it slips out of your hands the water will break the fall and minimize the chance of breakage. A partial denture brush, especially designed to clean the inside of the clasps, is a good investment and may make the cleaning job easier than when a regular tooth brush is used. If you smoke, your denture may become stained with the heavy, dark tobacco tar which settles out of the smoke. You can remove this stain by periodically immersing the appliance overnight in white vinegar. Once a week is usually often enough to maintain cleanliness, although it may have to be done oftener. You will be the best judge of this.

Summary

So have patience, and do not be discouraged by temporary discomfort at first. Millions have mastered the wearing of a dental prosthesis, and you can certainly do it too if you have the will.

How to Insert

The patient should be rehearsed before a mirror in the proper method of inserting and removing the prosthesis from the mouth (Fig. 15.3). He should be cautioned never to "bite" the prosthesis into place, but instead to guide it firmly into a seated position along its path of insertion, with the balls of the fingers applied to the clasps. Pressure should be applied gradually as it slips into place along its planned path. In removing the prosthesis, he should be instructed to apply force to the clasps with the thumbnails for the lower denture and with the second or index fingers for the upper denture. The pressure should be concentrated near the shoulders of the clasps rather than at the terminals, and the same amount of force should be applied on both sides of the prosthesis simultaneously. Force applied near the shoulders, rather than at the terminals, will minimize the possibility of distorting the clasp arm. This precaution applies, with increased emphasis in the case of the combination clasp, since the wrought wire retentive arm is much more vulnerable to distortion than is the arm of the cast clasp. If one or more clasps are retained with a lingual retentive arm, a method must be devised for the patient to apply the necessary dislodging pressure to the lingual surface of the tooth. This may be difficult when the clasp is located on a mandibular second molar. Indeed, removing the partial denture with such a clasp may test the digital dexterity of the patient, as well as the ingenuity of the dentist, and draws attention to the fact that lingual retention should not be used whimsically, but only when there is no better alternative. The patient should be permitted to practice before a mirror, until he can demonstrate an acceptable level of proficiency in inserting and removing the prosthesis, before he is dismissed.

Oral Hygiene

The patient who is partially edentulous has, with few exceptions, arrived at this unfortunate state as a result of carelessness or disregard for or ignorance of the basic fundamentals of oral hygiene. Unless he can be motivated to change long-standing personal habits and can be encouraged to attain and to maintain a high level of oral cleanliness the prognosis for the prosthesis must be very guarded. An important responsibility of the dentist is to attempt to kindle a sincere desire on the part of the patient to practice good oral hygiene (Fig. 15.4).

The problem of oral cleanliness is compounded for the patient with a partial denture because, when the typical partial prosthesis is in position on the remaining natural teeth, it creates crevices and crannies which are traps for the accumulation of oral debris and sanctuaries for the bacteria which form the dental plaque. As

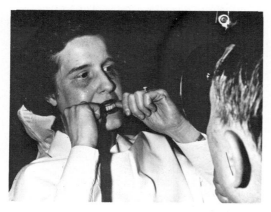

FIG. 15.3. The patient should be rehearsed before a mirror in the proper method of inserting and removing the prosthesis from the mouth. In the photograph shown here, the dentist is holding the mirror so that both can observe and discuss the patient's performance.

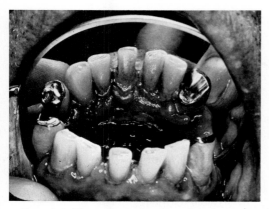

FIG. 15.4. The patient whose mouth is shown here was fitted with a mandibular prosthesis approximately 9 months prior to the time this photograph was made. The instruction which the patient received in oral hygiene at the time of insertion, if any, is not known. The treatment was a failure, as evidenced by the inflammation and pathology, despite well prepared abutments, and good design and structuring of the partial denture.

such they abet the prolonged contact of food substances with the surfaces of the teeth as well as with sheltered areas of the mucosa. Debris tends naturally to lodge in the protected nooks and crannies created by the prosthesis, and accumulation is encouraged because the denture interferes with the natural self-cleansing action of the lips, cheeks, and tongue. If food substances are permitted to accumulate undisturbed, some or all of the usual sequelae may be confidently predicted, i.e., decalcification of enamel under the clasps, inflammation of the marginal gingiva, recurrent decay around fillings, and erosion and caries of root surfaces. Clearly, motivation and education of the patient in averting these calamatous consequences warrant unremitting efforts.

Although the patient with a removable prosthesis has a unique oral hygiene problem, it need not be an insurmountable one. If he approaches the problem with understanding, and performs faithfully and unfailingly a properly prescribed regimen, the average patient can do a creditable job without undergoing any hardship. When the appliance is out of the mouth,

most tooth surfaces will be at least as accessible to the toothbrush and other cleansing aids as they were before he began wear of the prosthesis. As for the prosthesis itself, it should not tax his ingenuity to cleanse it while it is out of the mouth. The key to success is an understanding of the problem, regularity, and thoroughness. Dental floss is an indispensable aid in cleaning the proximal surfaces of all abutment teeth that are contacted by a minor connector. The most effective method is to "saw" the floss back and forth (buccolingually) against the abutment tooth surface until there is a discernible "squeak." Brushing of the teeth and the prosthesis should ideally be done after every meal and snack.

There is a wide divergence of opinion concerning the various mechanical aids to oral hygiene. Three of these, which commonly stimulate much interest and elicit questions, are the electric toothbrush, the water spray, and the ultrasonic cleaner. The following paragraphs are not intended to give a full account of these innovations, but rather to assess their value to the partial denture wearer.

The Electric Toothbrush. Generally, it can be said that the electric toothbrush will do nothing that a motivated patient with average manual dexterity and coordination could not do as well with a conventional toothbrush. However, it must be conceded that a great many patients are not motivated to achieve excellence in oral hygiene, and as for manual dexterity and coordination, these unfortunately are attributes not shared equally by all, particularly by the elderly and the handicapped. For these reasons, the mechanical toothbrush does have a place in the oral hygiene armamentarium, and it should be prescribed when there is reason to believe that the patient will, or can, do a better job of maintenance with its help.

The Water Spray. The water spray has a basic weakness in that it will not remove the bacterial plaque from the tooth, and it is obvious that any tooth-cleaning technique which does not remove the plaque certainly leaves much to be desired. Although it does an excellent job of removing loose debris and seems to exert a beneficial effect on the gingival tissues, there is a very real risk that it will give a patient an unwarranted feeling of security, and so it should not be prescribed without adequate safeguards. The patient must ·not be under the illusion that the water spray can substitute for a good toothbrushing routine. If it is prescribed, it must be made unmistakably clear that it is an adjunct which does not, and indeed cannot, supplant the toothbrush and dental tape or floss.

The Ultrasonic Cleaner. A comparative newcomer to the field of denture cleaners is the sonic cleaner which is marketed by several manufacturers under their individual brand names. The operating principle is this: sonic waves which are high frequency sound waves (above the range of normal hearing) produced by an electromagnetic transducer, form millions of microscopic bubbles in a liquid. The bubbles burst inwardly to create a scrubbing action on any object immersed in the solution. The scrubbing action of the tiny bubbles lifts food particles from the smallest and deepest crevices of the prosthesis. Most of these cleaners do a creditable job, as attested to by independent testing organizations, although certainly they are not essential to maintaining a prosthesis in an entirely acceptable state of cleanliness. Still, this device may be a boon to the ultrafastidious individual to whom the mere thought of cleaning an oral prosthesis is repugnant or to the handicapped patient who is not physically able to accomplish the task satisfactorily by conventional means.

Soaking versus Brushing the Prosthesis. Whether to brush or to soak the prosthesis is often debated among dental authorities, which would seem to indicate that the answer is not a simple one. Because of the fact that the commercial cleansers are advertised so extensively through the mass communication media, the answer is especially pertinent.

There is little question that brushing of acrylic resin with a toothbrush and a cleansing agent over a prolonged period of time will abrade the resin, and it is equally apparent that any change in surface contour of the tissue surface of the resin will have a deleterious effect on its adaptation to the mucosa. Abrasion is particularly apt to occur to the denture of the compulsive brusher who wields the denture brush with an exaggerated gusto several times a day. Indeed, there is abundant evidence to indicate that the gradual loosening of some dentures after a relatively short period of wear is due, in part, to a loss of resin from the tissue surface caused by the abrasive action of the toothbrush. When the risk of abrasion is coupled with the fact that the brushing operation is much more apt to expose the prosthesis to the possibility of dropping or mishandling, it would appear that the soaking solution has much to recommend it. However, some of the commercial cleansers presently on the market contain substances which tarnish the chromium-cobalt alloy. Although many of them are perfectly harmless to the alloy, as well as effective cleansers, this cannot be said of all of them. A further complicating factor is that some of the manufacturers have a penchant for changing the formulation of their product from time to time.

Therefore, if a soak type cleanser is recommended, the patient should be cautioned not to leave the prosthesis in the solution for more than 15 minutes per 24-hour period. If brushing is recommended, a mild toilet soap should be used and the patient should be warned not to scrub the tissue surface of an acrylic resin base and never to use an abrasive type of cleanser on it. A partial denture brush which is shaped to fit the inside of the clasps is a worthwhile investment. Also strongly recommended are bristles with rounded ends, because their abrasive action is less severe. The patient should be instructed to fill the sink partially with water, to break the fall should the prosthesis slip from his grasp.

Night Wear of the Prosthesis

Purely from a standpoint of physiology

and preservation of mouth tissues, there is no question whatever that the prosthesis should be left out of the mouth at night while sleeping, so as to give the recuperative powers of the body an opportunity to rehabilitate the oral tissues. Equally important, it provides the tongue, cheeks, and lips with an opportunity to exert their cleansing action on areas of the teeth which are not self-cleansing because of the presence of the prosthesis. However, there are circumstances which alter this general rule. One example is the bruxist who will probably inflict more damage on the oral structures with the prosthesis out of the mouth than he would with it in place, where it can carry a portion of the occlusal load. Another example is the patient who wears a maxillary complete denture and a mandibular partial denture, and who insists on wearing the complete denture during sleep either for cosmetic reasons or for comfort. If he cannot be persuaded to change this practice, it is better that he wear both dentures, so as to preclude the damaging effects on the anterior portion of the maxilla which would otherwise result from contact with opposing natural mandibular teeth.

Periodic Maintenance

The need for periodic maintenance should be explained to the patient early in the doctor-patient relationship. He should be made aware of the irreversible damage which can accrue from wearing a prosthesis which no longer accurately fits, and it bears emphasis that he will seldom be aware of the loss of fit until it is quite advanced, because of the slow, gradual nature of bone resorption. The fee for the refitting service, if there is to be a fee, should be mutually understood, lest the patient assume that the original fee included refitting procedures. It should also be pointed out to the patient that at the time of the refitting, the prosthesis must remain with the dentist while the laboratory work is performed. (This does not apply if a chairside reline is employed.) This could be profoundly important information for the patient whose prosthesis

replaces one or more anterior teeth, and who must deal directly with the public in earning his livelihood.

From a standpoint of maintaining the patient's oral health, an efficiently administered recall system is far superior to advising the patient merely to "return in six months" or (what has even less to recommend it) to advise him to "get in touch when it gets loose." Human nature being what it is, most individuals are much more likely to keep an appointment that has been made for them by the dentist than they are to telephone the office on their own initiative at some future date to arrange for one. Most individuals who wear a removable partial prosthesis should receive a dental prophylaxis at approximately 6-month intervals. This time interval is a good rule of thumb to use for the average patient.

A definite appointment should be set aside for the first post-insertion visit and, except in unusual circumstances, it should be made for the day following delivery of the denture. Clearly, there are major flaws in the practice of instructing the patient to return if he feels a need to be seen, instead of scheduling a definite appointment. A patient, thus instructed, may assume that he is going to be seen at any time he decides he needs attention. If it happens that he cannot be seen at the time that he selects, because of a crowded appointment schedule, he is very apt to be disgruntled.

Post-Insertion Follow-up

The Twenty-Four Hour Post-Insertion Appointment

The patient should be questioned to determine whether there are specific complaints and, if so, these should be evaluated and resolved to his satisfaction. If there are no complaints, the mouth should be examined carefully with the prosthesis in place as well as out of the mouth. Any erythematous area should be noted and its cause established. The areas immediately surrounding the abutment teeth, in particular, should be inspected for evidence of pressure. The occlusion should be carefully examined since some minor change in interocclusal relationships is to be expected following a brief period of wear.

Subsequent Adjustments

Although a single post-insertion check may suffice for the typical tooth-borne denture, most extension-base dentures will require two or more post-insertion appointments, the second scheduled 48, or perhaps 72, hours following the first. In general, the fewer the remaining natural teeth and the larger the prosthesis, the more likely the need for post-delivery adjustments. If the patient does not seem to be in an optimistically confident frame of mind at the end of 24 hours, he should be seen again in 48 to 72 hours, even though he may have had no specific complaint and have demonstrated no clinical signs of inflammation. Certainly, no patient, who has any unhealed lesion caused by the prosthesis should be dismissed without another appointment. The patient should be impressed with the fact that the dentist is available to minister to his needs in connection with the wear of the prosthesis. He should never be given reason to draw the inference that the dentist is discouraged by his ineptitude or impatient with his complaints. This is important because some individuals are acutely sensitive lest they be classified as "chronic complainers" or "sissies" incapable of bearing even moderate discomfort. Not to be lost sight of, as a factor in the patient's adaptive capacity, is the healing effect of time.

Common Complaints of the Partial Denture Wearer

In addition to dissatisfaction with the appearance of the partial denture, complaints may be classified under the headings of either discomfort or inefficiency. A third category, labeled "miscellaneous," will also be discussed.

Discomfort

Tooth Soreness. Discomfort, ranging in intensity from slight tenderness to outright pain, is occasionally encountered from teeth which have recently assumed the burden of supporting a removable partial denture. This is a serious development which demands early attention. The most common cause of tooth pain, from a removable partial denture, is hyperocclusion caused by an occlusal rest which interferes with normal closure into centric occlusion. The interference may be so slight that the patient is not even aware of it at the time of insertion, but the repeated trauma to the tooth over a period of several hours has the cumulative effect of making the tooth tender and sore to bite on. The remedy is to provide the required interocclusal clearance. It may be necessary to reduce the bulk of the rest, to grind off part of an opposing cusp, or perhaps to accomplish a combination of the two procedures. Following the occlusal adjustment it may be well to leave the prosthesis out of the mouth for 24 hours or longer if need be, depending on the severity of the symptoms. Another cause of tooth "lameness," only slightly less common, is an overly tight clasp or one that has become distorted. The "too tight" clasp should be loosened slightly, and the bent clasp should be straightened if it can be done successfully. Any manipulation of the clasp should be accomplished with smooth-beak pliers (Fig. 15.5). Serrated beaks will scratch or mar the clasp alloy, and beaks with sharp edges on the working surface are very apt to nick the clasp if a bend of any magnitude is performed. A nick caused by the contouring pliers will typically escape notice at the time the adjustment is made, but the clasp arm may rupture at a grain boundary later. Ironically enough, the breakage typically occurs while the patient is eating soft food. It is preferable that the operation with the pliers not be performed in the presence of the patient, if it is possible to avoid it. He may interpret it as the correction of a mistake or, even worse, may conclude that adjusting a clasp is a simple operation which he can perform very well for himself the next time the prosthesis feels too tight or too loose.

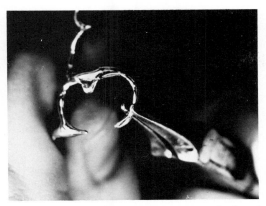

FIG. 15.5. The working surfaces of the beaks of the contouring pliers used to adjust the clasp should have no sharp angles, since bending the wire against an angular surface is very apt to damage it. Neither, should the beaks have a serrated surface, for the same reason.

Abrasion and Laceration of Soft Tissues. Two basic types of traumatic ulcers are produced by the wear of an oral prosthesis. One is the laceration of the mucosa caused by pressure from the border of a denture. The second is the bruising of tissue caused by the slight rubbing movement of the denture against it during function. While the root cause of the former is simply an overextended border or one that is rough or sharp (or a combination of these), the factors involved in the latter are much more numerous, as well as considerably more complex. Most prominent of these are (1) a rough uneven contour of the bone of the residual ridge as an aftermath of tooth removal, (2) the presence of blebs of resin or other roughness of the tissue surface of the denture base, (3) a lack of precise adaptation of the base to the mucosa, with the result that areas of mucosa beneath zones of overpressure are traumatized, (4) the presence of a thin, atrophic mucosal covering in the stress-bearing areas which has too little connective tissue stroma to protect it from trauma, (5) the presence of sharp protuberances or ridges of bone (mylohyoid ridge) often covered with a too-thin mucosal covering, and (6) a lack of occlusal harmony. Whether or not the occlusion is a primary or merely an exci-

tative cause of a traumatic ulcer may be debated. However, there is no disputing the fact that occlusal disharmony is a factor in a very high proportion of instances of soreness beneath dentures (Fig. 15.6).

The "Loose Denture." The most common cause for this complaint is simply a loose fitting prosthesis which is not well adapted to the mouth. Less commonly, loose clasps permit too great a degree of movement, and the patient does not have the neuromuscular skill to compensate for the lack of retention. Loose clasps may sometimes be made more retentive by adjusting the retentive tip more closely into the undercut. However, a denture with a distal extension base which is no longer well-adapted to the mucosa of the ridge may have rotated the retentive clasp arm out of the undercut so that it no longer contributes retention, and such a clasp cannot be satisfactorily adjusted. The remedy for this is refitting.

When examining a partial denture which the patient considers to be "loose," there is no standard scale upon which the degree of retention can be measured. A rule of thumb is to place the ball of the finger under the retentive arm of the clasp

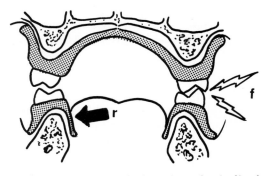

FIG. 15.6. Force applied against the inclined plane of a denture tooth on one side of the arch produces a horizontal resultant force which shunts the denture laterally. As a result, a force is transmitted against the lingual surface of the ridge on the contralateral side. In the sketch above, *f* is the force (an interceptive contact), and *r* is the resultant stress applied against the lingual surface of the residual ridge on the opposite side of the mouth. Interceptive contacts are a root cause in a high percentage of complaints of soreness beneath the denture.

in question and to apply a force in an occlusal direction. If the clasp passes this "test," i.e., resists this modest amount of unseating force, it may be considered reasonably retentive, and the patient may be faced with a choice of overstressing the abutment teeth with overly tight clasps or of improving his neuromuscular skill to a point that he can manage the prosthesis with the clasps only moderately tight. The reality is that some persons never acquire the skill to eat caramel candy with their prosthesis without having it lift off the teeth, whereas other individuals may do so with ease by virtue of their splendidly coordinated neuromuscular control. It may be of interest to note that a few people are endowed with such a highly developed neuromuscular skill that they can handle the prosthesis with deftness shortly after insertion. Another group may gradually develop and improve their skill up to a satisfactory level over a period of time, while a third group may never attain a satisfactory degree of skill insofar as manipulating the prosthesis with the border muscles is concerned.

The patient who complains of looseness, but whose prosthesis appears to be quite stable and retentive, can be an enigma. He should be asked to describe the action or movement that triggers the dislodgment, and then be asked to demonstrate it. It is not unusual to discover that he is practicing some oral habit which exerts tremendous leverage on the denture, without being aware of it. The solution to a problem which is caused by a noxious oral habit is to bring the habit to the individual's attention, and to encourage him to break it forthwith, not only so that he can retain the denture successfully, but also to avert the harmful effects which he may be unconsciously wreaking on the supporting structures.

Still another possible cause of a complaint of looseness is a deflective occlusal contact that produces a torsional stress which dislodges the denture.

Inefficiency

Under the heading of inefficiency may be grouped several related complaints having to do with the patient's inability to masticate satisfactorily despite the fact that the prosthesis is reasonably tight and comfortable.

Inability to Chew. The patient who complains of an inability to eat following insertion of the prosthesis may be one who has had no posterior teeth for a number of years. As a consequence, his neuromuscular mechanism is programmed to incise and nibble food on the anterior teeth, but not to grind it in the posterior part of the mouth. A period of time may be required in such a circumstance for the patient gradually to relearn to execute the chewing pattern required to comminute food with the posterior teeth.

"Dull Teeth." It is not unusual for the patient who has worn a prosthesis for an extended period of time to complain of the teeth being "dull." He may state that he isn't able to eat as well as he could with a previous denture, or perhaps with the present denture when it was newer. Abraded plastic teeth are the most common cause of this complaint. Excessive wear of the occlusal surfaces may often be accompanied by a closure of the vertical dimension, which contributes further to the loss of efficiency. Reconstruction of the prosthesis may be the solution to this complaint, (see Chapter 16, Refitting Procedures).

Occlusal Disharmonies. Occlusal discrepancies which interfere with function may be apparent after only a brief period of wear, and it is noteworthy that while the patient may be aware that something is amiss, he will seldom complain of an uneven occlusion as such. Generally, premature contacts occur because of uneven settling of the denture bases. Less commonly, they may be due to a change in contour of the denture base itself. This may occur when the acrylic resin imbibes moisture for a period of time following insertion, which has the effect of expanding the resin slightly, thus altering the relative positions of the teeth.

Excessive Bulk. The patient should be conditioned to expect a temporary feeling of bulk when the prosthesis is first inserted. However, if there is a complaint of excessive fullness, after he has worn the appliance for a reasonable period, it may be necessary to reduce farther the thickness of a portion of the prosthesis in the areas in question, provided this does not weaken it structurally. As a general rule, this type of modification should be done very gradually, in small increments, allowing the patient time between adjustments to adapt to the change before further alteration is carried out. It should be borne in mind that the orbicularis oris muscle actually becomes smaller following the removal of natural anterior teeth, and that it requires from 3 to 5 weeks for this muscle to regain its former size, so that it can redrape itself naturally over anterior replacement teeth. In the interests of reducing bulk to a minimum, lingual flanges should be made as thin as feasible, to provide maximum space for the tongue. However, the borders must never be thinned to a knife-like edge. The post dam border of a maxillary partial denture, if it is acrylic resin, should be beveled so as to blend into the soft palate as unobtrusively as possible.

Miscellaneous Complaints

Gagging. This complaint is not often heard from the wearer of the removable partial denture because the maxillary denture which with rare exceptions is the cause of the complaint, can be made thin and, if need be, designed short of any contact with the soft palate, thus avoiding the usual trigger zone for the gag reflex. However, some removable partial dentures, for purposes of retention, must be extended onto the post dam area in the same manner as for a complete denture. When this is the case, the posterior border should be established in a palatal zone where the tissue is slightly displaceable but not movable, and it must fit snugly against the palatal tissue. When gagging is encountered in a denture of this type, it may be due to simple overextension onto the soft palate by an overly thick border or by the fact that the denture does not fit snugly against the tissue, so that a make-and-break contact is created which triggers the gag reflex. Such a discrepancy

may be due to an inaccuracy in the impression, or a failure to add a slight beading to the metal border or a post dam to the acrylic resin, as the case may be. This draws attention to the importance of accurately establishing this border in the design of the prosthesis. In determining the location of the posterior border, the patient should be instructed to say "ah" as the palatal tissue is observed closely for movement. The posterior border should be established just short of this movable tissue.

Failure to incorporate a post dam in the acrylic resin may be corrected by adding one to the denture with self-polymerizing resin. If the border is metal, however, there is no feasible alternative but to remake the framework.

Phonetic Problems. Phonetic problems caused by a removable partial denture are not commonly encountered, largely because of the phenomenal adaptive ability of the speech mechanism to function in almost any environment, however altered. Nevertheless, just as neuromuscular skills vary widely among a cross section of individuals, so too does the ability to articulate clear speech sounds. Well known is the fact that one individual can manage with apparent ease a loose denture which another individual simply could not tolerate. In a similar vein, the ability to produce clear speech sounds varies among individuals, and this is particularly true when the speech mechanism is handicapped by the presence of a foreign body overlying its field of operation. When a problem of phonetics does arise, it may be attributed to (1) a change in the contour of the speech area (the anterior part of the palate, (2) the maxillary anterior teeth not being positioned far enough labially, or (3) a combination of these two factors.

The problem of an altered contour of the speech area is virtually eliminated when a cast metal is employed which reproduces the natural contour of the palate. On the other hand, a problem may be created when acrylic resin must be used to cover the rugae area, since it must be substantially thicker, for strength.

Summary. If the anterior teeth are placed in the same position occupied by their natural precursors and the rugae area is covered with a thin layer of metal which reproduces the natural contour of the palate, the possibility of any serious phonetic problem is remote. On the other hand, if the teeth have been placed anteriorly or posteriorly to the position occupied by the natural teeth, there may be difficulty with the labiodental sounds "f," "v," and "ph," as well as with the dental sounds "ch," "j," "s," and "z." The patient should be given a reasonable period of time to overcome a problem of articulation prior to any modification of the denture. If mastery is not ultimately achieved, there will be need to reposition the anterior teeth or alter the contour of the palate, as the case may be. In determining whether a speech impediment is caused by the position of the teeth or by the contour of the palate, wax may be flowed onto the palate of the denture to create a temporarily altered surface. If overcontouring the incisive papilla or the anterior portion of the median raphe eliminates the speech difficulty, then the change of contour may be made permanent by substituting a permanent material for the wax.

Adhesion of Chewing Gum. Patients sometimes complain that chewing gum adheres to the appliance. Questioning will usually elicit the information that it is more prone to stick to the acrylic resin than to the metal. The patient can be told that some brands of gum are more adhesive than others, and advised to experiment a bit with several different brands until one is found which is minimally adhesive, hence less troublesome. Gum will adhere more readily to a rough or stained surface than to a smooth one, and so any surface roughness should be eliminated by smoothing and polishing. Another remedy which may be of help is to soak the prosthesis overnight in a half-and-half solution of water and household vinegar. This will make the surface of the resin extremely slick so that the two substances seem to have less affinity for each other.

Excessive Salivation. A copious flow of saliva is a common complaint when an oral prosthesis is first inserted, but it persists for only a few days at most and, more commonly, outflow is controlled in a matter of hours. It is a normal physiological reaction to a foreign body by the autonomic nervous system, and the patient can be assured that it is normal, as well as transitory, and no cause for concern. The probability of excessive salivation, immediately following insertion, underscores the importance of arranging the insertion appointment at a time which allows the patient a period of comparative privacy to get acquainted with and adjust to the prosthesis.

Burning Sensation in the Mouth. The patient with a prosthesis sometimes complains of a burning sensation which may emanate from either maxilla or mandible. The triggering mechanism(s) may have a physical basis, or may be attributable largely to systemic factors, perhaps coupled with a psychosomatic component. Generally, the cause of the sensation may be traced to pressure on the nerves which emerge from either the mental or the incisive foramina. Normally, the mental foramen is located on the buccal aspect of the mandible, near the apices of the bicuspids but, following advanced resorption of the alveolar bone, it may "migrate" to a position on the crest of the residual ridge, where it is protected only by a thin layer of mucosa. Because of this meager protection, the nerve is exposed to pressure from the denture, which produces a burning sensation. Less commonly, the sensation may be relayed to the patient's consciousness as pain, and it may, under some circumstances, be referred to the chin, the lip, and even the cheek. The diagnosis should be established by exerting pressure on the prosthesis over the foramen, in an effort to duplicate the sensation described by the patient.

The incisive foramen may be subjected to pressure in a similar manner. Although the nerve is normally well protected by virtue of its position under the thick padding of the overlying incisive papilla, it may, as a result of resorption of labial alveolar bone, become situated on the crest of the residual maxillary ridge, a location in which it is vulnerable to pressure from a prosthesis. When the cause of the sensation has been established as pressure from the prosthesis, the appropriate area of the denture must be relieved.

When no physical basis can be established to account for a burning sensation, the possibility of its being a local manifestation of a systemic condition must be given consideration. Endocrine imbalance (the menopause), and dietary deficiencies, as well as systemic disease (anemia, diabetes), are possible etiological factors. Not to be lost sight of is the psychosomatic factor. Some writers have pointed out the fact that this complaint comes, typically, from postmenopausal females, and contend that in this particular group it has essentially a psychosomatic basis, with overtones of cancerophobia. Accordingly, an important part of the therapy is the reassurance of the patient that the partial denture has not damaged the mouth, and that the discomfort does not portend the existence of a neoplasm. The recommendation should be made to remove the prosthesis for periods of rest during the day and, by all means, to leave it out of the mouth during sleep.

Food Accumulation Under the Denture. The complaint is sometimes heard that food accumulates under the denture. The most common cause of this annoyance is an underextended flange, assuming that the denture otherwise fits well. If it is determined that this is the case, the flange may be extended by building it out to the desired length with auto-polymerizing acrylic resin. Another cause of food accumulation, which is not as amenable to correction, is the denture flange which covers an undercut. Oftentimes an undercut requires the removal of base material from the tissue surface of the flange, so that the denture can be inserted and removed comfortably. The removal of the resin creates a void between the base and the mucosa into which food subsequently finds its way to the vexation of the patient. This is a difficult problem when it must be confronted following insertion, since the only completely satisfactory solution is prevention. The difficulties which are caused by undercuts in the denture bearing areas are well known and should be anticipated at the time of the examination and preliminary planning, so that proper steps can be taken to avert them.

Cheek or Tongue Biting. Cheek biting is caused by the buccal mucosa being trapped between the maxillary and mandibular posterior teeth. It is usually due to the fact that the teeth have been placed in the denture(s) without sufficient horizontal overlap. Also contributing is the fact that when the natural teeth are extracted, the buccinator muscle tends to sag into the space created by the lost teeth. When the edentulous space is subsequently filled with prosthetic teeth, it may require a period of wear of the prosthesis before the muscle regains its former tonus and no longer tends to droop inward from its original position. The palliative treatment for cheek biting is to pinpoint the precise tooth surfaces that are involved, and to round off the axial-occlusal line angles of the involved teeth, after which the altered surfaces should be highly polished.

When tongue biting is encountered, it usually indicates that the mandibular teeth have been positioned too far lingually. The problem can be alleviated by modifying the teeth to provide the needed clearance.

Unpleasant Taste. An occasional patient may complain of an unpleasant taste following insertion of the prosthesis. Generally, the patient with this problem is an adolescent with multiple amalgam restorations and a prosthesis fabricated of one of the chromium-cobalt alloys. The evidence suggests that the differences in electromotive potential of the two alloys plays an important role in the phenomenon, perhaps abetted by the patient's particular salivary chemistry. The treatment is to remake the prostheses with an acrylic resin base and gold wrought wire clasps.

Factors in Assessing the Need for Adjustments

The importance of prudent management of the patient whose oral tissue has been abused by denture trauma should not be underestimated. Indeed, the success of a prosthesis can very well hinge on the way that post-delivery adjustments are accomplished, since it is common for a prosthesis to fit so poorly, following several adjustments, that it requires refitting. Clearly, a high order of clinical judgment is required to accomplish the precise amount of relief required to achieve comfort, without creating a change in the prosthesis which jeopardizes its fit or its ability to function.

The objective to be sought in accomplishing adjustments of the removable partial denture is twofold: (1) to correct discrepancies in the prosthesis, and (2) to relieve discomfort or pain. When assessing need for adjustments, several pertinent considerations should be factored into the decision: (1) the phenomenon of differing pain thresholds, (2) the part played by the time frame, (3) the semantic factor, and (4) the existence of a systemic influence.

The Pain Threshold. One should keep in mind the vast differences in pain tolerance of different individuals. Given an identical stimulus, three individuals may respond in three entirely different ways. One may react violently, as though from intolerable pain, another as though it were an uncomfortable, entirely unpleasant sensation, while a third may react as though it were a minor annoyance of little consequence. The individual with a high pain threshold is customarily pictured as the brawny construction worker, but this is by no means a reliable criterion. It is not at all unusual for such an individual to have a lower threshold than a delicate, elderly female who appears to epitomize frailty.

The Time Frame. The amount of time that the irritant has required to produce its effect on the mucosa is significant. The mucosa may appear erythematous 6 hours following insertion but exhibit painful contusions 12 hours later.

The astute clinician will not overlook this important factor in assessing the amount of adjustment that is needed in the prosthesis.

Semantics. In assessing the patient's complaints and the extent of the therapy needed to return abused tissue to a state of health, the semantic factor should not escape notice. Terms such as "pain," "soreness," and "discomfort" do not have the same connotation to all people. One person may use the word "pain" to describe a sensation which, from all objective criteria, is identical to the signs observable in another who uses the term "soreness" to describe what he feels, or perhaps even the milder term "discomfort." All clinicians are familiar with the patient who complains of intolerable pain, but who demonstrates few, or at most mild, clinical signs of irritation, as well as with the one whose oral mucosa bears painful appearing abrasions and contusions, which he may describe on being questioned as "uncomfortable."

Systemic Influence. The root cause of discomfort under a prosthesis may have such a strong systemic component that any adjustment of the prosthesis itself is actually counterproductive. The fragility of the oral mucosa of the postmenopausal female and its low resistance to traumatic insult is a classic example. If such an individual is taking a drug such as Premarin, the irritability of the mucosa may even be increased, and it may be further aggravated by a diet of marginal quality. The anemic patient is another example, and the diabetic still another.

Hints for Accomplishing Adjustments

1. An appointment should be scheduled so that the patient can be seen 24 hours following delivery of the denture. Sufficient time should be set aside for an unhurried examination of the mouth and the prosthesis and to accomplish whatever treatment and adjustment is needed.
2. A standardized procedure should be followed which positively establishes

the nature of the complaint(s). This is best accomplished by obtaining an abbreviated history which includes such questions as: Exactly where does it hurt? When? What triggers it?

3. Tissue that has been lacerated usually indicates an overextension or an overly sharp border. Erythema and abrasion of mucosal tissue is most often indicative of a discrepancy in the tissue surface of the base, or a disharmonious occlusion.

4. Occlusion is the root cause of much denture-induced soreness. Hence, most adjustments should consist of minor modifications of the denture, combined with equilibration of the occlusion.

5. Acrylic resin that has been carried in a purse or stored in a dresser drawer will very likely to distorted from dehydration. Such a denture should be immersed in water for a 24-hour period before any evaluation is attempted, except in the case of a gross discrepancy which is readily apparent or which prevents the denture from being seated in the mouth.

6. When trauma produces inflammation, it is accompanied by swelling. If complete relief is provided for an irritated, edematous area, it will become an unwelcome void beneath the denture when the swelling subsides. Always undertrim rather than overtrim.

7. Nature is standing by to assist in the treatment, if given the opportunity. Removing the irritant, reassuring the patient, and then permitting Nature to exert its healing effect will solve a large percentage of complaints of soreness.

Inflammations Caused by the Prosthesis Which Often Elicit No Complaint

Denture Sore Mouth

Denture sore mouth, or "DSM," is not a frequent finding under a removable par-

tial denture, being much more common with complete dentures, but it may occasionally be encountered (Figs. 15.7 and 15.8). When it does occur beneath a partial denture, it is found most commonly beneath a maxillary prosthesis which has a palatal section made entirely of acrylic resin. Typically, the mucosa beneath the denture is red and smooth, and it may or may not be painful. The redness is confined to the precise outline of the prosthesis, and a diagnosis of allergy is some-

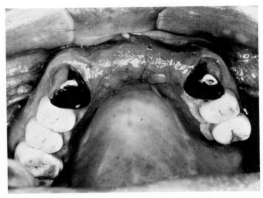

FIG. 15.7. The area of inflammation (darkened) shown in the photograph delineates precisely the outline of the removable partial denture that the patient was wearing as shown in the next sketch, Figure 15.8.

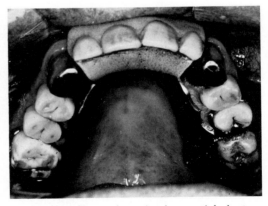

FIG. 15.8. Shown here is the partial denture which covered the red, erythematous area shown in Figure 15.7. Although the patient's oral hygiene was moderately good, he had worn the prosthesis for 24 hours a day, without a rest period for the tissues, over a period of approximately 4 years.

times erroneously made on this basis. The
patient may complain of a burning sensation, but more often he is not aware of the
mild inflammation. The condition is almost invariably associated with a faulty
fitting prosthesis, coupled with poor oral
hygiene, and there seems to be a correlation with 24-hour wear or the absence of a
rest period for the foundation mucosa.
Finally, there is good reason to believe
that, in some instances at least, nutrition
may play a role.

Treatment is to improve the oral hygiene habits and to insist that the prosthesis be left out of the mouth at night. A
well balanced diet, containing adequate
amounts of proteins, minerals, and vitamins should be part of the treatment, if
there is reason to believe that the patient's intake of these essential elements
is deficient.

If the prosthesis fits poorly, there may
be need to refit it or perhaps remake it
completely. If a refitting procedure or a
remake is decided upon, then provision
should be included in the therapy for af-
fording the foundation tissue an opportunity of returning to a state of health before the refitting is accomplished. This
may consist of treatment with one of the
tissue-conditioning materials, or perhaps
leaving the prosthesis out of the mouth
altogether for a short period of time (see
Chapter 16, The Use of Tissue Conditioners).

Epulis Fissuratum (Inflammatory Hyper-plasia)

This condition is found most commonly
under complete dentures, but it does
occur under removable partial dentures,
usually under an anterior flange. The soft
tissue in the mucobuccal fold area hyper-
trophies (Fig. 15.9) in response to irritation by the denture flange, which is
usually sharp and, in effect, has become
grossly overextended as a consequence of
the denture base becoming displaced. The
reason for this is that as the bone of the
residual ridge resorbs, it allows the denture to "settle," thus projecting the denture flange farther upward into the mucobuccal fold. The inflammation is

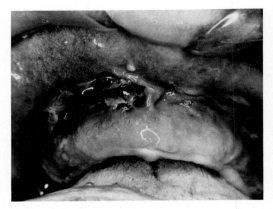

Fig. 15.9. Although the epulis fissuratum shown
here was caused by the flange of a complete denture,
the condition is sometimes found also beneath the
flange of a partial denture.

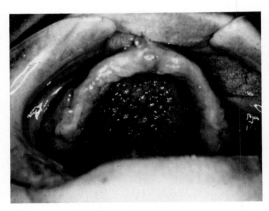

Fig. 15.10. Papillary hyperplasia of the palate
consists of multiple papillary projections of the
mucosa of the hard palate. It is found fairly often
beneath complete maxillary dentures (as shown here)
and occasionally underneath a partial denture that
covers this area of the palate.

usually low grade and chronic in type, and
the patient typically has no complaint
until he becomes aware of several elon-
gated rolls of hypertrophied tissue which
may overlie the denture border in the vestibule. Sometimes there is ulceration at
the bottom of the fold, or there may be no
discontinuity of the mucous membrane.

One approach to therapy is to leave the
denture out of the mouth until the abused
tissue has returned to a state of health. If
being without the prosthesis will impose a

genuine hardship on the patient, it may be possible, with the aid of one of the tissue treatment materials, for him to continue to wear the denture while healing takes place. Since a keystone of the treatment is elimination of the irritant, it will often be necessary to reduce drastically, or even to remove altogether, a flange from the denture.

Papillary Hyperplasia of the Palate (Papillomatosis)

Papillary hyperplasia can occur in any mouth in which the palate is covered with a prosthesis. As may be expected, it is found more commonly under the complete denture (Fig. 15.10), but it does occur on occasion under the partial denture. There is much clinical evidence that it is found most often under dentures that contain a relief chamber, and there is a strong correlation between 24-hour wear and papillary hyperplasia. The lesions consist of multiple papillary projections in the mucosa of the hard palate. Usually the inflammation is chronic, low grade in type, and the patient, while aware of the surface roughness in the palate, typically does not complain of discomfort. It has been postulated, by some highly regarded authorities, that this inflammatory lesion may be premalignant, although this view is not universally held. Notwithstanding a lack of clear evidence in this regard, the need for biopsy should not be overlooked.

The treatment of choice is somewhat controversial. Certainly, there is room for doubt of the efficacy of treatment by the conservative method. There is little question that the quickest and surest method of eradication of this lesion is by surgery.

Whatever the approach to treatment, the patient should be strongly urged to leave the denture out of the mouth for at least 8 of each 24-hour interval.

Denture Allergy

Allergy of the mucous membrane to the denture base material is extremely rare, and many men spend a lifetime in the practice of dentistry without ever encountering a bona fide case of an inflammatory contact reaction to the denture base material. Some investigators believe that certain individuals are sensitive to methyl-methacrylate and will react to it. Others believe that when a reaction does occur, it is caused by an acrylic resin that is not completely polymerized, and that the sensitivity is to the monomer and not to the cured methyl-methacrylate per se. It is noteworthy, in this regard, that free monomer is much more likely to occur in the self-polymerizing type of resin than with conventionally processed resin. The clinical symptoms of allergy are identical to those of denture sore mouth.

A rather simple test can be used to rule out allergy. A small wafer of the acrylic resin, which has been processed in the identical manner that was used to process the denture base, is placed on the skin in the medial aspect of the patient's forearm and covered with adhesive tape. A small disk or wafer of a different material, such as glass or metal, is strapped against the skin in a similar manner, and in the same general area of the forearm. The skin under the two wafers is inspected after 3 days. True allergy will be manifested by redness of the skin under the acrylic resin wafer and no reaction under the "control" material.

Bibliography

Bartels, H. A.: Significance of yeastlike organisms in denture sore mouth. Int. J. Orthodont. Oral Surg. *23:* 90–93, 1937.

Fisher, A. A.: Allergic sensitization of the skin and oral mucosa to acrylic denture materials. J. A. M. A. *156:* 238–242, 1954.

Fisher, A. K.: Inflammatory papillary hyperplasia of the palatal mucosa. Oral Surg. *5:* 191–198, 1952.

Markov, N. J.: Cytologic study of the effect of toothbrush physiotherapy on the mucosa of the edentulous ridge. J. Prosth. Dent. *18:* 122–125, 1967.

Miller, E. L.: Periodontics—Prosthodontics, their interrelationship. Jl. Alabama Dent. Ass. *53:* 23–30, 1969.

Newton, A. V.: Denture sore mouth. Brit. Dent. Jl. *112:* 357–360, 1962.

Sharp, G. S.: The etiology and treatment of the sore mouth. J. Prosth. Dent. *16:* 855–860, 1966.

Sharp, G. S.: Treatment of low tolerance to dentures. J. Prosth. Dent. *10:* 47–52, 1960.

Thoma, K. H.: Papillomatosis of the Palate. Oral Surg. *5:* 214–218, 1952.

Chapter 16

REFITTING PROCEDURES

This chapter deals with the refitting procedures that may be employed when the partial denture no longer fits accurately because of bone resorption and mucosal change beneath the denture base. The various procedures commonly employed to accomplish the refitting are described, and indications for the use of each are discussed. The resilient reline materials are evaluated, as are the tissue conditioning materials. The subject matter is organized in the following way.

Introduction
The Examination
Reline of the Denture
Rebase of the Denture
The Reconstruction Procedure
The Resilient Denture Liners
The Use of Tissue Conditioners

Introduction

There is abundant clinical evidence that normal, healthy alveolar bone which envelops natural teeth responds to the intrabony stress of the teeth in function by becoming stronger and more dense, provided the stress is within physiological limits. In contrast, when the teeth have been removed and the stress is applied, instead, to the external surface of the bone of the residual ridge through a denture base, the response of the bone may be resorption. Indeed, bone resorption accompanied by atrophy of the mucosal covering beneath the denture base is seen clinically so often as to be considered normal. When it occurs beneath the tooth-borne type of partial denture, the resorption typically results in the creation of spaces beneath the base which may be unsightly, unhygienic, or both. When the denture is a distal extension type of prosthesis, the denture base becomes displaced downward by rotating around the abutment teeth. Since resorption is so predictable, patients who are fitted with a dental prosthesis, especially the distal extension base type of partial denture, should be educated to expect change in the supporting tissues, just as the eyes change, and to anticipate the need for appropriate refitting procedures from time to time for as long as the prosthesis is worn.

Predicting the Need for Refitting

Any attempt to predict, with any degree of certainty, the period of time that a prosthesis can be worn before refitting will be necessary must be at best only a clinical estimate, because of the difficulty in assessing the numerous variables that play a role in bone resorption. Some of the more important of these factors are as follows:

1. The amount of time that has elapsed since the teeth were extracted from the denture-bearing areas. The ridge from which the teeth have been extracted for 6 months will be more stable and a less rapid rate of change can be expected than from the ridge which has been edentulous only 6 weeks.

2. The type of prosthesis. The partial denture which derives the greater share of its support from the residual ridge will need refitting more often than will the denture that is primarily tooth-supported, all else being equal.

3. The residual ridge of the mandible is much more prone to resorption, and the mandibular prosthesis will need attention sooner than will the maxillary partial den-

ture because of the greatly diminished load-bearing area of the former. Indeed, the maxillary partial denture may seldom need refitting because stress is distributed over a much greater area of support.

4. The host resistance factor, or more precisely, the "Bone Factor" described by Glickman.

The Effect of the Loss of Fit

Loss of fit of the distal extension base denture allows the denture to settle downward (tissue-ward), thus assuming a different posture relative to the remaining teeth (Figs. 16.1 and 16.2). As the occlusal plane is shifted to a less favorable inclination, centric occlusion is altered, the vertical dimension of occlusion is decreased, vertical overlap of the anterior teeth is increased, and the framework no longer fits the teeth in the way that it was designed to fit. As the denture continues to rotate about the fulcrum line (through the abutments), the posterior teeth reach a point where they may no longer intercuspate properly with their opponents, which tends to concentrate occlusal stresses in the anterior part of the mouth. A vicious cycle thus ensues of traumatic occlusion, bone resorption, and decreased vertical dimension, followed by more traumatic occlusion. If allowed to continue, a loss of tongue space, phonetic difficulty, and temporomandibular joint symptoms are common sequelae. It is noteworthy that the patient usually accommodates to the altered conditions from a functioning standpoint, being oftentimes unaware of the loss of fit until it has progressed beyond the point where remedial therapy would be most effective. However, an exception to this is the lingual bar type of denture, in which the loss of posterior support permits the lingual bar to rotate until it is in contact with the lingual mucosa (Fig. 16.3). This frequently results in a painful abrasion, which may be the patient's chief complaint when he presents for treatment.

The Types of Refitting Procedures

Rather than making the prosthesis over, it may oftentimes be returned to its orig-

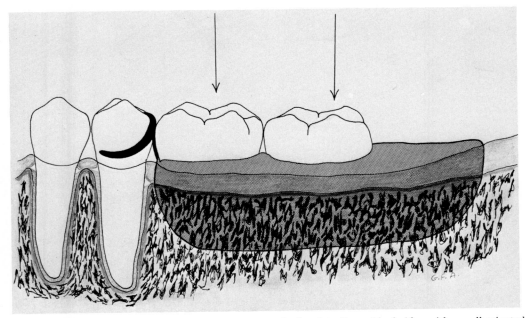

FIG. 16.1. This sketch depicts the denture base properly fitted to the residual ridge with a well oriented occlusal plane.

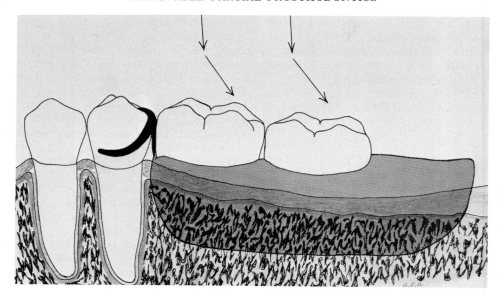

FIG. 16.2. This sketch portrays a loss of supporting structure beneath the denture, which permits the base to be depressed downward so that the occlusal plane is shifted to an unfavorable inclination.

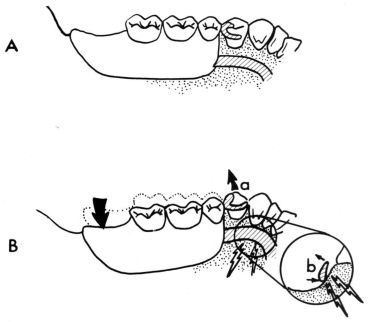

FIG. 16.3. The loss of supporting tissue beneath the distal extension base type of mandibular denture may permit the lingual bar to rotate to a point where it is in contact with the lingual mucosa. *A* depicts a well-fitting denture base, lingual bar, and clasp. In *B*, the loss of supporting structure has permitted the base to be depressed so that the occlusal level of the teeth has been altered (*dotted lines*), the clasp arms are rotated upward on the crown of the abutment tooth (*a*) and the inferior border of the lingual bar is rotated downward and inward to contact the mucosa (*b*).

inal state of usefulness by a simpler and less costly refitting procedure. The methods of refitting customarily employed are (1) the "reline," which consists in resurfacing the tissue side of the denture with new base material, (2) the "rebase," which is the refitting of the denture by complete replacement of the denture base material, without changing the occlusal relations of the teeth, and (3) the "reconstruction," which is a procedure whereby the denture is reassembled using the original framework with new teeth and new base material.

The Examination

Refitting of the prosthesis should not even be considered unless (1) the mouth is in a state of health, (2) the abutment teeth are stable and in good repair, and (3) the bone support is adequate. When these are the case and examination reveals that pressure applied to the base depresses it into the mucosa as it rotates around a fulcrum created by the occlusal rests, one of the refitting procedures may be considered. The judgment as to whether to employ one of the refitting operations or to remake the prosthesis completely should be based on the findings of a systematic examination. Each element of the prosthesis, framework, base, and teeth, should be examined critically to determine (1) its condition and (2) its fit (the "fit" of the teeth is the manner in which they intercuspate with their opponents).

The Framework. The condition and fit of the framework is the key to the feasibility of a refitting procedure. A denture with a broken clasp arm, for example, obviously cannot be restored to full usefulness by a refitting operation. Similarly, if occlusal rests are worn thin, or partially lost, as a result of grinding and/or wear, refitting should not be considered. If the framework is in good repair, however, the accuracy of its fit on the teeth should be determined. If it no longer fits the teeth accurately and cannot be made to do so with minor adjustments, the entire prosthesis should be made over from scratch, irrespective of other considerations. On the other hand, if all of the metal parts which contact the teeth are in intimate contact with proper tooth surfaces (occlusal rests in prepared recesses), it may be assumed that the framework is salvageable.

The Denture Base. If the acrylic resin base material has deteriorated or has been mended and patched to a point that is unsightly, the rebase is preferred over the reline. Similarly, if a previous reline has resulted in a visible junction between the new and the old material, or if discoloration of a previous reline material has occurred, a rebase is probably the method of choice.

The peripheral borders of the base should be carefully assessed. If there is inadequate coverage or improper extension, the rebase is favored over the reline, to accomplish the needed modification best.

The Denture Teeth. The condition of the denture teeth is a key consideration as to whether the denture should be refitted by either relining or rebasing, or whether the more lengthy reconstruction procedure would be the method of choice. If the teeth are plastic, the amount of wear which has taken place should be assessed (Fig. 16.4). Excessive wear would militate

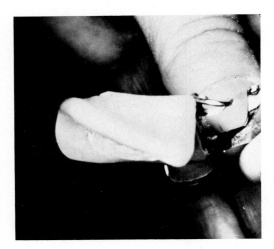

Fig. 16.4. If a partial denture which requires refitting has plastic teeth which are abraded, or porcelain teeth which are broken or have been lost, it should not be relined or rebased. The denture shown here has badly abraded plastic teeth. Since the metal framework fits the teeth well, it will be reconstructed.

for reconstruction. If the teeth are porcelain, there may be cracked or broken teeth, or some of the teeth may have been lost, and this, too, would be an indication for reconstruction in preference to a reline or rebase.

The Occlusion. An assessment should be made to determine the effect that a refitting operation will have on the occlusion, particularly on the occlusal plane. If tissue loss has been moderate, the occlusion can usually be restored by routine equilibration procedures in the mouth, following a reline or rebase operation. On the other hand, if the tissue loss has been extensive, the reline or rebase may elevate the occlusal plane to a vertical level which would require a prohibitive amount of adjustment to permit the teeth to articulate with their opponents. A factor which should not escape notice, in this connection, is the nature of the opposing occlusion. If natural teeth oppose the prosthesis, they may or may not have extruded as the denture base became depressed (Fig. 16.5). If the natural teeth

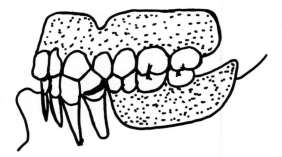

FIG. 16.6. This sketch depicts a complete denture opposing a distal extension base type of partial denture which requires refitting. Oftentimes, both dentures need to be refitted, in which case it is usually prudent to accomplish the refitting operation on one denture at a time.

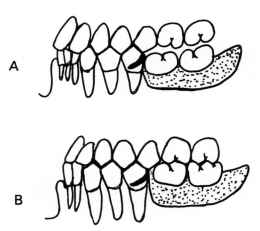

FIG. 16.5. If natural teeth oppose a distal extension base that is in need of refitting, the natural teeth may or may not follow the base as it is depressed downward. The natural teeth depicted in this sketch (A) have not extruded to any large degree, and the occlusal plane has not been excessively altered. Following a reline or rebase, the occlusion may be restored with routine equilibration procedures (B).

have extruded to any substantial degree, it means that the occlusal plane of the prosthesis could be raised only a slight amount without the need for excessive grinding of the denture teeth. If a prosthesis opposes the denture to be refitted (Fig. 16.6), it too may have shifted position because of resorption. This raises the question of whether (1) refitting one prosthesis will solve the problem, (2) both must be refitted or remade, or (3) a combination of procedures will best serve. There is no precise method of assessing the amount of change in the occlusion to be anticipated following the refitting. However, a reasonably accurate estimate can be made by placing utility wax in the denture base so that the base is elevated to a vertical level that returns the framework to its proper position on the teeth. If a great bulk of wax is needed to accomplish this, or if the patient is unable to close his mouth with the wax in place, it may be concluded that the alteration of the occlusal scheme will be too drastic with either a reline or a rebase. Therefore, reconstruction would be a better approach. If it appears from this test that the change will not be extensive, the reline or rebase may serve the purpose.

The Patient's Opinion as a Factor. When any refitting procedure is contemplated, it is important that the patient be questioned in order to obtain his views on the matter. If he was satisfied with his prosthesis until it no longer fit him, then a refitting procedure should be selected that will introduce a minimum of change to the prosthesis, over and above the refitting. On the other hand, if he liked it with some reservations and would welcome some modification, it is quite possible that the desired change can be incorporated into the prosthesis at the same time that it is refitted. Obviously, this could have a bearing on the choice of refitting method. If the patient is dissatisfied with some aspect of the prosthesis which cannot be readily altered by a refitting operation to bring about the desired change, then a complete remake may be in order.

Reline of the Denture

The reline operation is recommended when (1) there has been a moderate loss of fit, (2) the occlusion is correctable with simple equilibrating procedures following the refitting, (3) the framework design is good and it fits the teeth well, (4) the denture base is in good condition, (5) the teeth are not unduly worn, broken, or otherwise deteriorated, (6) the patient is content with the appearance, and (7) the denture peripheries are reasonably accurate and do not require extensive modification. (When the peripheral borders do require extensive modification the rebase is preferred over the reline.) The reline may be accomplished as a chairside one-step procedure by use of a self-polymerizing acrylic resin made especially for the purpose. It can also be done in the laboratory by means of conventional flasking procedures or by the use of a reline jig (Jectron Co., Toledo, Ohio).

There are two disadvantages to the reline procedure: (1) unless care is exercised, a junction line may be visible between the old and the new base material which may be distasteful to a fastidious individual, and (2) it is not always possible to match the color of the old and new acrylic resins perfectly. A telltale color difference between the two can also be a source of dissatisfaction to an exacting type of person.

The Chairside Reline

The one-step reline materials are acrylic resins to which have been added retarders and other modifiers so that the material can be added to the tissue surface of the denture and placed in the mouth to obtain a recording of the tissue. Afterwards, it hardens to become a part of the denture base. Since a chemical reaction begins to take place moments after the material is mixed, a considerable amount of exothermic heat is given off as it polymerizes. This has ominous implications in connection with intraoral use, and the manufacturer's directions should be followed to the letter to avoid causing the patient discomfort or even injury.

Besides the disadvantage of causing the patient possible discomfort because of the exothermic heat, the temporary reline materials have other disadvantages, chief of which is the fact that their use requires a one-step impression procedure. This entails a very real risk either (1) of getting the framework seated precisely in position on the teeth while creating a major alteration in the occlusion, or (2) of preserving the occlusion but failing to get the framework precisely seated on the teeth. A further disadvantage of chairside reliners stems from a lack of color stability exhibited by materials of some manufacturers.

All things considered, the temporary reliners do not qualify as reliable materials for long term mouth service. Their use should be limited, for the most part, to the tooth-borne type of prosthesis, and even then they should be considered a temporary expedient to tide the patient over a planned time interval until a more permanent type of treatment can be accomplished.

The Conventional Reline

The conventional reline is accomplished in the laboratory by either flasking or by means of a reline jig. Either regular or auto-polymerizing resin may be used to resurface the denture. When regular acrylic resin is used, a slow cure at not more than 160° F is recommended, since higher temperatures may cause the release of strains in the previously polymerized resin and warpage of the base.

Since the clinical procedure for both the reline and the rebase techniques is identical, the impression procedure for both is described under the rebase procedure.

Rebase of the Denture

The rebase operation is indicated when (1) there has been a moderate loss of fit, (2) the occlusion can be restored, following the refitting, by minor equilibration procedures, (3) the framework is of good design and fits the teeth well, and (4) the teeth are not excessively worn, broken, or otherwise deteriorated. The rebase is preferred over the reline when the base material has deteriorated or the flanges need substantial alteration. Oftentimes, acrylic resin bases that have been repaired several different times assume a mended, patchwork appearance which is distasteful to the patient. The rebase procedure, which replaces the old material with new, is indicated in this instance. Still another indication for a rebase procedure is when a self-polymerizing resin has been previously used as a reline and the material has become discolored. It bears repetition, however, that when the prosthesis has broken or has badly worn teeth, the reconstruction procedure is the method of choice in preference to the rebase.

The Rebase Impression

There are two objectives to be achieved in registering the rebase or the reline impression. One is to fill in the void between the denture base and the supporting structures caused by resorption of the residual ridge. The other is to extend the coverage of the base to its proper limits, consistent with the comfort of the patient. To accomplish the latter, all borders of the finished denture should, in addition to being properly extended, be round, smooth, and highly polished, so that the movable soft border tissues can function around and over them without becoming irritated or exerting a dislodging force against the denture. In order to create such a border in the denture, it must first

be incorporated into the borders of the impression. This is the purpose of the border molding procedure.

All undercuts, such as the one sometimes found in the mylohyoid ridge area, which might interfere with flasking operations should be removed. The peripheral borders of the base should be inspected for underextension and, if present, corrected with modeling composition. If the original base does not cover at least two-thirds of the retromolar pad, it should be extended with the modeling composition to do so. Similarly, it should be extended buccally to rest on the buccal shelf, if it does not already cover this primary stress bearing area. When the border molding is complete, the impression may be registered with fluid wax, metallic oxide paste (Fig. 16.7), or one of the rubber impression materials. The open mouth impression method should be employed, so that the framework can be correctly positioned on the teeth and maintained in this position throughout the impression procedure.

A cast is poured into the impression, leaving the framework exposed, so that it can be picked up in the top half of the flask during the flasking operation or so that it can be readily removed from the cast if a reline jig is employed.

If a zinc oxide-eugenol type of impression material is used, meticulous care must be taken to remove completely all traces of it from the base material during laboratory operations. Otherwise the eugenol can act as a retarder to interfere with polymerization of the resin. The margins of the denture should be scrupulously cleaned to minimize the possibility of creating an unsightly junction line beteen the new and the old materials.

The Hazards of Refitting

One should not lose sight of the fact that the reline and rebase operations are not free of hazard. Although the prosthesis is guided into place by the clasps and the guide planes as the impression is being registered, there is always the possibility of disturbing the occlusion by a drastic change in the occlusal plane in relation to the opposing arch of teeth. Another source

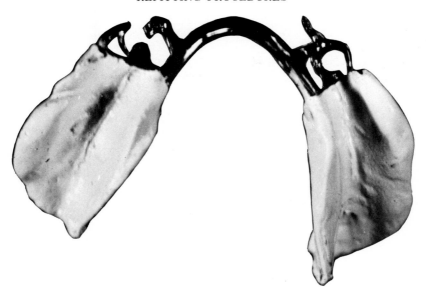

FIG. 16.7. This distal extension base denture has been border molded, and the impression obtained with a zinc oxide-eugenol impression material. Either a rebase or a reline procedure may be accomplished with such an impression.

of error in the rebase procedure is in allowing the individual teeth to shift during laboratory operations. In addition, the base can be distorted by an incorrect application of heat during the curing process, and there is always the possibility of breaking porcelain teeth in flasking. Finally, the metal framework is always vulnerable to distortion, during laboratory operations.

The Reconstruction Procedure

The reconstruction procedure consists in removing the acrylic resin and the teeth from the framework and processing a new base with new teeth onto it. Obviously, a well-fitting framework, in good repair, is a prerequisite for its use. There are two circumstances when it may be employed to advantage: (1) when the teeth have lost their ability to function, as a result of breakage, wear, or loss, and (2) when the occlusal plane has been irretrievably lost.

Impressions are made of both arches and casts poured in the usual manner. A functional impression and an altered cast procedure may be followed, if desired, after which jaw relation records are obtained. The framework is placed on the cast and the teeth are arranged to articulate with their opponents. Following a try-in, the prosthesis is processed, finished, and inserted in the usual manner.

The reconstruction procedure is a time-saver when compared with a complete remake of the denture and, of course, is more economical. It is especially indicated for the patient who has lost a great deal of bone over a short period of time, perhaps as a result of illness, with the result that a rebase or reline would create a drastic change in the occlusal scheme (Table 16.1).

The Resilient Denture Liners

An occasional patient will be encountered for whom a comfortable prosthesis simply cannot be constructed by conventional methods. Despite countless adjustments and carefully executed refitting procedures, followed by still more adjustments, discomfort and pain persist when the denture is worn. Such a patient typi-

Table 16.1.
A Summary of Refitting Procedures

Procedure	Adaptation to the Mucosa	Design and Fit of Framework	Occlusion	Condition of the Base Material	Condition of the Teeth	Miscellaneous Considerations
The reline	Lost, needs to be refitted to the mucosa	Must be well-designed and fit the teeth well	Restorable with simple equilibration procedures following the refit	Must be in good condition	Must be good	Patient approves the esthetics. Slightly different color of base and reline material is a possibility
The rebase	Lost, needs to be refitted to the mucosa	Must be well-designed and fit the teeth well	Same as above	May be deteriorated. Base will be replaced with new base material	Must be good. Teeth will not be replaced	Patient may object to a color difference which might occur with the reline
The reconstruction	Lost, needs to be refitted to the mucosa	Must be well-designed and fit the teeth well	New teeth will be reset	May be poor. New base material will be used	Worn, broken, or lost. New teeth will be used	Patient desires some change which can be accomplished with the reconstruction procedure

cally exhibits an inferior denture foundation, coupled with a lowered resistance of these structures to stress. Etiological factors accounting for the lowered host resistance are many and varied, advancing age and failing health being common ones. The fact that rapid bone loss often accompanies the female climacteric, especially when the latter is complicated by osteoporosis, is an important consideration. It may be noted, too, that the mandible is affected much more often than is the maxilla, since stress, which cannot be widely distributed because of the small bearing area of the former, is thus concentrated and magnified in its effect on the residual ridges. To compound the problem, the resorption of the residual ridge of the mandible often has the effect of bringing into prominence certain anatomical entities, such as the genial tubercles and the mylohyoid ridge, which may be exceedingly vulnerable to any pressure from the hard denture base.

When the prosthesis has been carefully planned and well designed, fits the bearing area, and has a harmonious occlusion, one may understandably be hard-pressed for a key to the solution. Certainly, every effort should be made to ensure that the patient ingests and assimilates a well-balanced diet containing adequate amounts of protein, minerals, and vitamins, and that any existing systemic condition is under the observation and control of a competent internist. Still, it is probable that there will always be a certain few individuals who, notwithstanding a concerted effort by both prosthetist and physician, possess such an extremely low tissue tolerance that they simply cannot wear a conventional prosthesis with success, and who will continue to seek relief from their discomfort. A resilient denture liner may, sometimes, be at least a partial solution to the problem.

Types of Resilient Liners. Resilient liners presently available for use are of three main types: (1) silicone rubber, (2) plasticized acrylic resin, and (3) elastomeric acrylic. The rationale for the use of a soft liner is that part of the energy, which is transferred to the denture during occlusal contacts, is expended in deforming the resilient lining material before it can be transmitted to the mucosa and bone as trauma. Theoretically at least, a soft material should be more comfortable to the mucosa than a hard one, and this seems to be borne out clinically.

Disadvantages of Resilient Liners. Although the potential of these materials must be conceded, it should be pointed out that certain problems have attended their use in the past, a tendency to acquire stains, bleaching in cleansing solutions, hardening with dimensional changes, failure to bond to the denture base, odor, and bad taste, to name the most common. Despite these possible drawbacks, the resilient reliners do have a place in the prosthodontic armamentarium, although their use should be limited to those patients who can be kept under observation over an extended period of time, so that both the prosthesis and the mouth tissues can be periodically evaluated.

The Use of Tissue Conditioners

The prosthodontist is often called upon to construct dentures for a patient who is wearing a prosthesis which fits so poorly, and intercuspates with the teeth in the opposing arch so badly, that it has created hyperemic, hypertrophic, chronically irritated tissue beneath it. Rather than perpetuate the condition of this abused tissue, some therapy should be instituted which will permit it to return to a state of health and normal contour before a refitting procedure is accomplished. There are three approaches to the problem: (1) complete tissue rest, (2) surgical intervention, and (3) use of a tissue treatment material.

Complete Tissue Rest

This method consists in simply leaving the prosthesis out of the mouth until the tissues have returned to a normal contour and a state of health. Although this is an effective method, as well as being the most economical, it often meets firm resistance from the patient. For this reason it is actually the least feasible approach for the majority of patients.

Surgical Intervention

Although effective and reasonably fast, surgical intervention has two serious drawbacks: (1) subjecting the patient to an unpleasant operation, followed by an uncomfortable healing period, and (2) introducing the risk of eliminating tissue that might be usable for support of the denture. Perhaps more to the point, clinical observation bears out the fact that it is seldom necessary, with the exception of papillary hyperplasia which may require surgery to eradicate completely the small papillary projections in the palate.

The Tissue Conditioning Material

The tissue conditioning material consists of a poly-ethyl-methacrylate powder, to which has been added plasticizers and retarders for the purpose of controlling (retarding) the polymerization of the resin. The powder is mixed with a liquid composed primarily of ethyl alcohol. Since the material does not become hard for several days (as the alcohol is slowly lost), the abused tissue is relieved of the root cause of irritation. Removal of the irritant gives it an opportunity to regain its normal contour and to return to a state of health. Normally, the material inside the denture is replaced at approximately 3-day intervals, so that it continues to provide a soft cushion between the irritated mucosa and the hard denture base. It is imperative that any sharp border or flange that could possibly contribute to the irritation of the tissues be eliminated entirely. This might involve reduction of a denture flange, or even its elimination altogether.

Many highly regarded authorities believe that the tissue treatment material should be employed routinely before refitting or remaking any oral prosthesis. This reasoning is based on the belief that when a denture has reached a point that it no longer fits its foundation it is evidence per se that the foundation tissue has been abused, and therefore that it has lost its normal contour. Accordingly, the tissue should be given the opportunity to return to a state of health before it is required to assume the burden of another prosthesis. It is hard indeed to fault the basic soundness of this logic.

Bibliography

Blatterfein, L.: Rebasing procedures for removable partial dentures. J. Prosth. Dent. 8: 441–467, 1958.

Glickman, I.: Clinical Periodontology, Ed. 2. W. B. Saunders Company, Philadelphia, 1958.

Osborne, J., and Lamme, G. A.: Partial Dentures, Ed. 2. Blackwell Scientific Publications, Oxford, 1959.

Steffel, V. L.: Relining removable partial dentures for fit and function. J. Prosth. Dent. 4: 496–509, 1954.

Weinman, J. P., and Sicher, H.: Bone and Bones, Ed. 2. The C. V. Mosby Company, St. Louis, 1955.

Wilson, J. H.: Relining the saddle supported by the mucosa and alveolar bone. J. Prosth. Dent. 3: 807–813, 1953.

Chapter 17

REPAIRS, ADDITIONS, AND
MODIFICATIONS

*This chapter is concerned with management of
the various mishaps which may befall the
removable partial denture to render it
unserviceable. Methods of adding a tooth or a
clasp to the prosthesis, following extraction of
a natural tooth, are also discussed. Subject
matter is arranged in the following manner.*
Introduction
Simple Repairs
Complex Repairs
The Bent or Distorted Prosthesis
Additions and Modifications

Introduction

Despite careful planning and competent
construction with materials of good
quality occasional breakage and distortion
of the prosthesis will inevitably occur to
render it unserviceable. Generally, the
root cause of the mishap is attributable to
one or more of the following causes, listed
here not necessarily in order of frequency:
(1) careless handling in the laboratory, (2)
inadequate mouth preparation, (3) poor
construction, (4) loss of fit, or (5) careless
manipulation by the patient.

Determining the Cause of Breakage

When breakage which is not a result of
careless handling does occur, it is important that a determination be made of the
cause so that, in addition to accomplishing the repair, corrective steps can be
taken to prevent its recurrence. If the
failure is due to loss of fit, to inadequate
mouth preparation, or to poor construction, the probabilities are that it will recur
unless the underlying cause is established

and eliminated. Unfortunately, there is
much evidence to suggest that repairs are
often made to dentures of all types
without regard to the underlying cause.
This practice is counterproductive since,
more often than not, such a prosthesis will
be foredoomed to repeated breakage, with
attendant expense and inconvenience to
the patient.

Many patients do not visit the dental
office except in response to pain or discomfort. When an unserviceable prosthesis prompts the visit, an opportunity is
afforded to examine the patient's mouth
so that, at the very least, he can be in-
formed of his current dental health status
in addition to having the prosthesis restored to function. To do less is to ignore
the very real possibility of placing a repaired prosthesis in a mouth which har-
bors recurrent decay, a loose abutment
tooth, or even frank pathosis. Certainly it
is undeniable that when an unserviceable
prosthesis is handed to the dentist, repaired, and handed back to the patient,
he will be no better off, from a dental
health standpoint, than he was before it
became unserviceable. Therefore, if the
prosthesis cannot be tried in the mouth
for evaluation prior to the repair procedure, because it is distorted or broken, an
evaluation should be accomplished,
without fail following the repair. This
draws attention to the fact that the repaired prosthesis should be delivered to
the patient in much the same manner as
would be followed in the insertion of an
entirely new prosthesis. In particular, the
occlusion should be examined to ensure
that the repair procedure has not intro-

duced any change in the relationships of opposing tooth surfaces.

Repair of the Prosthesis versus the Remake

When a removable partial denture suffers a damaging mishap and is unserviceable, the judgment to be made is: Can it or should it be repaired, or must it be entirely remade? In point of fact, it is possible to repair almost any broken prosthesis, provided all of the broken pieces are at hand. Moreover, even lost portions can be replaced with acrylic resin or, in the case of metal, be recast and soldered to the framework. However, the time and effort required to accomplish some combinations of repair-refitting procedures would be so extensive and so time consuming as to make them unfeasible from an economic standpoint. Thanks to the production-line methods employed by most commercial dental laboratories, the cost per unit of new work is usually quite reasonable, whereas the cost of the technical expertise required for hand-crafted, repair-type procedures may be disproportionately expensive. As a consequence, it is often more economical to remake the prosthesis than to carry out a complicated, time-consuming repair. Furthermore, the mouth which has borne a prosthesis for a considerable period of time will, more often than not, require treatment of one kind or another before a prosthesis should be worn at all, and a complete remake of the prosthesis will, as a rule, be indicated following accomplishment of the needed treatment.

Finally, it should be kept in mind that the reconstruction procedure (Chapter 16) is sometimes the most feasible solution to the broken partial prosthesis, provided the framework is in good repair.

Classification of Repair Procedures

Repair procedures for the removable partial denture may be classified, for convenience of discussion, as either simple or complex. A simple repair is one that can be accomplished without the need for an impression. A complex repair is one that requires an impression and cast (and frequently a countercast). A broken denture tooth or a cracked interchangeable facing are examples of simple repairs. The replacement of the missing part of a denture flange or a broken clasp are examples of the complex type.

Simple Repairs

Repairs involving only the teeth or the resin are usually of the simple type. In dealing with the repair of acrylic resin, it should be borne in mind that if methylmethacrylate has been out of the mouth (in a dry environment) for 24 hours or more it will be dehydrated and very likely distorted. Consequently, it is a good policy to soak such a prosthesis in water overnight, prior to accomplishing the repair procedure, if the procedure is one that might affect the adaptation of the resin to the mucosa.

Resin Repairs

Segments of acrylic resin which have been cracked or broken apart may be chemically bonded together again by means of self-polymerizing resin. The technique consists in reuniting the broken parts in proper alignment and holding them together with sticky wax while a stone cast is poured. A repair line is then prepared in the resin, to a width of 2 to 3 mm. on either side of the fracture line, and either tinfoil or a tinfoil substitute is applied to the stone cast at the fracture site. Autopolymerizing resin may be introduced into the repair site by one of two methods: (1) the polymer may be sprinkled into the fracture site followed by a drop of monomer, or (2) an inlay brush may be moistened with monomer, dipped into polymer to pick up some powder, and the damp mixture applied to the repair site. In either case, the material is added until the site is slightly overfilled, after which the denture is placed in the pressure bath for approximately 20 minutes at 30 pounds of pressure. When it is removed from the polymerizer it is smoothed and polished with suitable finishing instruments.

The Broken Denture Tooth

When the diatoric of a porcelain denture tooth becomes partly destroyed in the process of fitting it into a space of limited proportions, there may be insufficient mechanical anchorage to hold it securely in the acrylic resin and, as a result, it may fall out after a brief period of mouth service, or the porcelain may simply break at its thinnest point. The acrylic resin tooth, on the other hand, sometimes comes loose because it has failed to bond chemically to the resin of the base. The usual explanation for this is that a thin film of wax has been left on the teeth in the denture mold during boil-out, which acts as a separator to prevent bonding of the two resins to one another.

Replacement of a broken tooth in an acrylic resin base requires first that the remnants of the broken tooth be removed. The base material is then prepared for the new tooth by cutting a box-like preparation into the lingual surface of the resin. A tooth of the proper mold and shade is fitted into the space, and held in place between the adjoining teeth with sticky wax, while the new acrylic resin is introduced into the preparation. A tooth replaced in this manner must be adjusted in the mouth to intercuspate properly with the teeth in the opposing arch. Replacement of a lost or broken tooth which has been abutted to the mucosa of the ridge usually requires that an impression be made with the prosthesis in place. A cast is then poured, so that the replacement tooth can be refitted to the ridge of the cast and attached to the denture base with autopolymerizing acrylic resin.

The Broken Porcelain Facing

A broken porcelain facing is replaced by fitting a new one of the same mold and shade to the backing and to the mucosa with the prosthesis in place in the mouth. If chair time must be conserved, an impression can be made with the partial denture in place and the facing fitted to the stone cast in the laboratory. Final finishing touches can be accomplished in the mouth just prior to cementing the facing to the backing.

Removing the Facing From the Backing. It may be necessary on occasion to remove a porcelain facing from a framework so that a repair can be made to the framework, or it may be necessary to remove the remnants of a cracked or broken facing so that it can be replaced with a new one. In the first instance there is a danger of fracturing the porcelain. In the latter instance, the remnants may cling to the backing with an inordinate tenacity, resisting all efforts to pry them loose. If the framework is made of dental gold alloy, the porcelain may be loosened by heating the framework in either phosphoric or hydrochloric acid. The framework should be placed in a ceramic pickling dish, covered with the acid, and held over a flame until the cement disintegrates. If hydrochloric acid is used, it may be covered with a thin film of liquid petrolatum to control the noxious fumes. It should be noted, however, that the chromium-cobalt alloys are attacked by some acids. Hence, in dealing with alloys of this type the above procedure should be employed only with nitric acid, to which they are impervious.

The Broken Tube Tooth

The broken tube tooth can be replaced by waxing a replacement onto the framework, flasking the wax pattern, and packing the mold with a suitable shade of tooth-colored acrylic resin. The new tooth can then be cemented into place on the prosthesis. An alternate method for replacing a tube tooth is to hollow out a plastic denture tooth to fit the post while, at the same time, grinding and shaping the tooth to fit the metal boxing. A tooth prepared in this manner may be cemented onto the framework with a thin mix of acrylic resin of the proper shade.

Complex Repairs

Almost any repair or modification can be made to a removable partial denture, provided an accurate impression can be obtained with the prosthesis in its proper position in the mouth. It is imperative that the impression be registered without any movement of the base, since any shift in its position would have the calamitous effect of altering the relationship of the framework to the abutment tooth. It is important, therefore, that the impression tray not be permitted to contact the prosthesis, and that a soft impression material be employed. Alginate is ideal for the purpose. When a repair is to be made which does not involve the adaptation of the denture base to the ridge, all undercuts should be blocked out prior to pouring the cast, so that the prosthesis can be readily removed from it.

When an impression has been registered with the partial denture in place and a cast poured in stone, the prosthesis can be disassembled unit-by-unit, following which broken metal parts can be soldered together and missing parts replaced. All units can then be accurately reassembled, provided plaster matrices have been constructed beforehand. In disassembling the prosthesis, porcelain teeth can be removed from the resin by the careful application of heat with the alcohol torch, while resin teeth can be removed by cutting around them with a bur. The resin of the base is likewise removed from the framework by the judicious application of heat.

The Broken Clasp Arm

One of the most common types of breakage to occur to the removable partial denture is fracture of the retentive arm of the clasp. The repair procedure of choice for this mishap will depend on the type of clasp and the part of the clasp that is broken. Although breakage of the chromium-cobalt cast clasp is not common it does occasionally occur. When it does, it is almost always due to mishandling by either (1) the patient (dropping the prosthesis), (2) the technician (losing control of it in the lathe), or (3) the dentist (nicking it with the contouring pliers as he makes an adjustment).

Repair with Wrought Wire. In the case of a broken retentive arm of the circumferential type clasp, the simplest method of repair is to contour a wrought wire arm and to attach it to the denture

base with autopolymerizing resin (Figs. 17.1–17.4). While quick and relatively simple, this method is not always the neatest, and may not be the best one from all viewpoints.

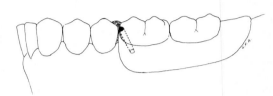

Fig. 17.1. The remnant of the broken clasp arm should be severed at its junction with the clasp body, and the area smoothed and polished. The denture is placed in the mouth, an impression is obtained with hydrocolloid, and a cast is poured in stone. When the cast has been separated from the impression, an opening is made in the resin of the lingual flange which passes through the base just below the occlusal surface of the denture tooth, immediately adjacent to the minor connector.

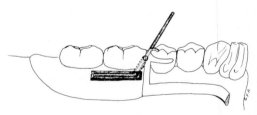

Fig. 17.2. A box-like preparation is made in the resin of the lingual flange to house an anchorage for the new clasp arm. Gold wrought wire of 18 gauge is contoured to enter the hole in the lingual side of the denture and emerge on the buccal aspect.

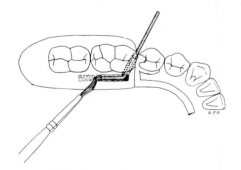

Fig. 17.3. The wire is anchored in the resin with autopolymerizing acrylic resin.

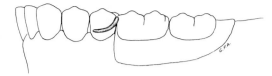

F<small>IG</small>. 17.4. The wire is adapted to the buccal surface of the tooth, and the repair site is smoothed and polished.

Refabrication of the Clasp. A more definitive method of dealing with the broken clasp is to remake the clasp entirely. When this method is followed, an impression is taken with the prosthesis in place, and a cast is poured. A buccal matrix is made of the denture base on the side to be repaired, and the teeth and base are removed from the framework. The new clasp is waxed and cast, and then attached to the framework with solder. Following this, the teeth are waxed back in their former positions by means of the matrix, and the base is processed in the usual manner. Although more time consuming, this method comes closest to returning the prosthesis to its original "like new" condition.

The Broken Reciprocal Clasp Arm. The reciprocal clasp arm seldom breaks. When it does, it is usually preferable to refabricate the entire clasp, as described in the preceding paragraph.

The Broken Bar Type Clasp. If the retentive tip of the bar type clasp is broken, it may be possible to reattach the broken segment (if it is available) to the approach arm with solder. However, the fracture site must be far enough removed from the acrylic resin of the base so that the soldering operation can be accomplished without having the heat endanger the resin. When this is the case, the soldering can be accomplished without disassembly of the prosthesis, provided the teeth and the base are well-protected with damp asbestos, or with soldering investment, while the weld is made with the electric soldering apparatus.

When the broken segment of the bar clasp is not available, or the fracture point is so close to the acrylic resin of the base

that it may be overheated by the soldering operation, complete disassembly of the prosthesis and remake of the clasp is usually the preferred approach. Although this type of repair can sometimes be accomplished by attaching a wrought wire arm in the resin of the base, it is generally not entirely satisfactory, since the retentive undercut on the abutment tooth is seldom properly located for the circumferential type of clasp arm to restore the clasp to its former state of usefullness.

The Broken Occlusal Rest

The most common cause of the broken occlusal rest is that the metal was too thin over the marginal ridge of the abutment tooth, the usual reason for this being that insufficient space was provided during the mouth preparation. The explanation for this is that the vertical height of the marginal ridge was not reduced sufficiently to accommodate a thickness of metal capable of withstanding the rigors of mouth service. Therefore, the procedure for effecting the repair of an occlusal rest from such a cause is first to provide the needed space by reducing the marginal ridge of the abutment tooth by the required amount. An impression is taken with the prosthesis in place, and a cast is poured in stone. A platinum foil matrix is then burnished to the rest recess, and a small section of gold wire is placed on the platinum matrix in contact with the body of the clasp. Following this, white gold solder is flowed onto the assembly to fuse the wire to the clasp, thus creating a rest which fits the newly prepared recess.

The Broken Major Connector

Breakage of the major connector is seldom encountered, with one exception, i.e., the lingual bar which breaks at its junction with the retention latticework. When this occurs, it is almost always a consequence of the finish line having been placed too deep in the wax pattern. This results in the metal being simply too thin at this point to withstand rigorous occlusal stresses, and it breaks from fatigue. A partial denture rendered unserviceable from this cause is best handled as a modified reconstruction procedure (see Chapter 16). A new segment is waxed, cast, and attached with solder to the framework (from which the resin and the teeth have been removed). The reconstruction is then completed in the usual manner.

The Bent or Distorted Prosthesis

Occasionally a removable partial denture becomes distorted so that it will no longer fit the teeth, as a result of having been caught and thrown by a revolving wheel in the polishing lathe, or of being dropped by the patient. If it is simply a bent clasp arm, it may be possible to correct it by the skillful application of force with the contouring pliers. On the other hand, if the entire framework seems to be out of alignment it must be regarded as a major problem, and if the patient is responsible for the mishap it would be prudent to inform him in advance that straightening procedures are difficult at best, and often not entirely successful.

The first step is to obtain an impression of the arch involved, since an attempt to carry out bending and straightening procedures in the mouth is a frustrating exercise in futility. It is to be expected that the resin bases will not accurately fit the stone cast, and so the cast should be relieved accordingly. The bending and straightening procedures are accomplished by alternately bending the bar and trying the framework on the cast. It may be logically assumed that a distorted lingual bar bends at its weakest point on impact. Theoretically, at least, if the proper amount of pressure is applied to the bar in an opposite direction the metal will again distort at the same point, so that it is returned to its original contour. With the help of an accurate stone cast, a reasonably satisfactory result can usually be accomplished. Sometimes it may be best to remove the resin bases, readapt the framework to the cast, and then reconstruct the denture.

Additions and Modifications

Replacing a Restoration under a Clasp

A missing, broken, or otherwise defective restoration in an abutment tooth under a clasp can usually be replaced to fit the clasp with reasonable accuracy, provided the prosthesis fits the mouth in all other respects (Fig. 17.5). If the restoration is to be an inlay, it may be waxed directly in the mouth, or it may be accomplished indirectly by taking an impression and making a cast. The indirect method is the only feasible method in the case of the full crown. It is accomplished as described in the next paragraph.

The tooth is prepared in the usual manner, and an impression of the tooth is obtained with either rubber base or agar

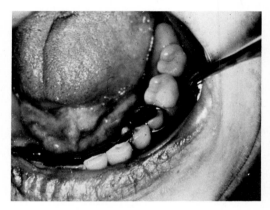

FIG. 17.5. The mandibular partial denture shown here fit the teeth and the denture-bearing areas, but the amalgam restoration in the second bicuspid under the clasp, as well as the one on the first bicuspid which supported an occlusal rest (an indirect retainer), were defective and in need of replacement.

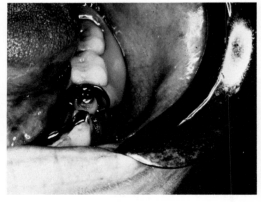

FIG. 17.6. The two bicuspids have been prepared for full cast crowns. The photograph shows the denture in place and the prepared teeth.

type hydrocolloid. The partial denture is placed in the mouth, and a second impression is made, again using rubber base or agar. Care should be taken not to exert any pressure on the denture with the tray, which might alter the relationship of the clasp to the tooth. The crown is waxed to proper contour and to the opposing occlusion, cast, and cemented into place (Fig. 17.6–17.10).

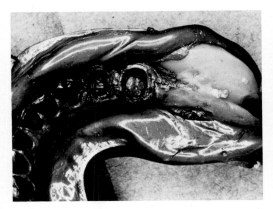

FIG. 17.7. An impression is taken of the entire arch, in rubber base material with the partial denture in place. It is important to select an impression tray that does not impinge on the prosthesis at any point, lest it displace it and thus destroy the relationship of the denture to the teeth. Working dies may be made by making a pour of stone into the two teeth to be restored. When this stone has hardened, the dies are removed and trimmed. Any undercuts which would interfere with easy removal of the denture from the cast should be blocked out with wax or modeling clay prior to pouring the working cast.

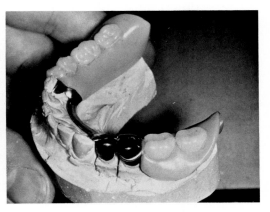

FIG. 17.9. Wax patterns are made for both teeth, to conform to the clasp arms and to the occlusal rests. A guiding plane should be incorporated, with the aid of the surveyor, in the distal surface of the wax pattern for the second bicuspid. The crowns are made to intercuspate with their opponents by means of the countercast. If an attempt is made to add a bulge of wax to the pattern for the purpose of creating a retentive undercut for the clasp terminal, it will probably be distorted or effaced by the clasp arm when the denture is removed from the cast. Therefore, the retentive undercut should not be incorporated into the wax pattern until after removal of the partial denture from the cast. The desired contour to create the retentive undercut is then added to the wax pattern, and the crowns are cast and finished.

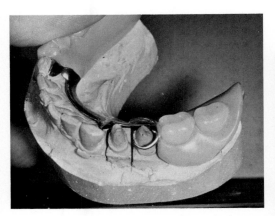

FIG. 17.8. A stone cast is poured into the impression. This photograph shows the partial denture in place on the cast with the two prepared teeth. The cast should be properly articulated with a countercast.

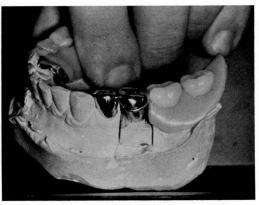

FIG. 17.10. Shown here are the finished crowns in place with the partial denture in position.

Loss of the Abutment Tooth

When an abutment tooth must be extracted, it is usually not feasible to press an adjacent tooth into service as an abutment. More often than not, an entirely different design and completely new construction would better serve the patient's needs. Certainly, the fact that the original abutment tooth was lost should suggest the possibility that the current status of the oral health may be less than optimal. However, it may, on occasion, be desirable to carry out the procedure as a temporary expedient, perhaps to tide the patient over the healing period of the extraction site.

The clasp which engaged the missing abutment tooth should first be removed from the denture, and any roughness caused by its removal smoothed. A rest recess and a guiding plane are prepared in the new abutment tooth. The prosthesis is seated in the mouth, an alginate impression is taken, and a stone cast poured. A clasp for the new abutment is waxed and cast, and the clasp is soldered to the framework or processed into the resin as dictated by the design of the denture. A prosthetic tooth is fitted into the space created by the missing tooth, and attached to the denture with auto-polymerizing acrylic resin.

The Loss of a Nonabutment Tooth

When a nonabutment natural tooth is lost, a replacement tooth can usually be added to the prosthesis rather simply if it can be attached to the resin of the base. If it must be added to the metal segment of the framework, however, it becomes a more complex procedure, since this usually entails providing some retentive device on the framework to which the tooth can be anchored. Generally, this will involve a soldering operation, and the feasibility of embarking on such a course, as opposed to remaking the denture, is open to question in many instances. Remake of the prosthesis, following a thorough examination and accomplishment of all needed treatment, is more to be recommended in the usual case.

Bibliography

Asgar, K., and Peyton, F. A.: Casting alloys to embedded wires. J. Prosth. Dent. **15:** 312–321, 1965.

Dental Laboratory Technicians' Manual, AFM 160-29, Department of the Air Force. U.S. Government Printing Office, Washington, D.C., 1959.

Chapter 18

PRECISION ATTACHMENTS AND STRESSBREAKERS

This chapter explains the basic principles of the precision attachment and analyzes their advantages, disadvantages, indications and contraindications. The concept of stressbreaking is examined and some of the shortcomings of these devices are pointed out. Subject matter is arranged in the following manner.

Introduction
Advantages of the Precision Attachment
Indications for Use of the Precision Attachment
Disadvantages of the Precision Attachment
Contraindications for Use of the Precision Attachment
The Precision Rest
The Stressbreaker
Indications for Use of the Stressbreaker
Disadvantages of the Stressbreaker

Introduction

The precision attachment is a special type of direct retainer used in partial denture construction. It consists of a closely fitting key/keyway mechanism, one part of which is attached to the abutment tooth and the other to the metal framework. Frequently used synonyms are: "internal attachment," "frictional attachment," "slotted attachment," "key/keyway attachment," and "parallel attachment." The precision attachment is sometimes said to be a connecting link between the fixed and the removable type of partial denture because it incorporates features common to both types of construction.

Precision and Semiprecision Attachments

Precision attachments may be prefabricated by a manufacturer or they may be fabricated in the dental laboratory. These two basically similar types of construction are customarily differentiated by terming the former "precision" and the latter "semiprecision" attachments.

The manufactured type of attachment is made of precious metal and, as the terminology implies, the fit of the two working elements is machined to very close tolerances, hence is more precise in construction than is the typical laboratory fabricated attachment. The male portion most often takes the shape of a "T" or "H" which fits an appropriately shaped slot. The female attachment is fitted into the restoration in the tooth either by casting the gold to it or by placing it in a prepared receptacle in the restoration, and attaching the two together with solder (Fig. 18.1).

The semiprecision attachment is also referred to as the "precision rest," the "milled rest," or the "internal rest." As a rule, this type of retainer takes the form of a dovetail-shaped keyway built into the proximal surface of a wax pattern of (usually) a gold crown. The stud or male portion is then fabricated as an integral part of the metal framework.

Intracoronal and Extracoronal Attachments

Precision attachments may be classified as "intracoronal" or "extracoronal." An intracoronal attachment is one that is

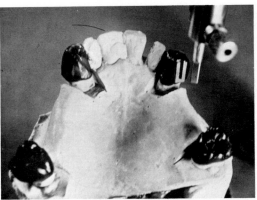

FIG. 18.1. The path of insertion has been selected, and the cast is locked into the cast holder in this horizontal plane. The female portion of a prefabricated type of precision attachment (Ney-Chayes, Ney Gold Company, Bloomfield, Conn.) has been fitted into the wax pattern with a paralleling mandrel in the surveyor spindle. The gold will be cast to envelope the receptacle. An alternate method is to attach the receptacle to the restoration with solder.

contained within the contours of the crown of the tooth, while the extracoronal type may be all or partly contained outside the confines of the crown. The usual reasons for employing the extracoronal type is either that the crown of the tooth is too small to accommodate all of the receptacle or that the pulp of the tooth is so large that it might be encroached upon by an attachment which was completely housed within the crown. The extracoronal type of retainer often has built into it a movable joint of one type or another (a stressbreaker) which permits the base to move independently of the retainer. (Stressbreakers are discussed in another part of this chapter.)

Advantages of the Precision Attachment

Two principal advantages are claimed for the use of the precision attachment. Foremost is the fact that the labial or buccal clasp arm can be eliminated altogether (Fig. 18.2). As expected, this makes for a spectacular improvement in the cosmetic excellence of a partial denture,

particularly one for the maxillary arch. The second advantage is not as dramatically demonstrable. It rests on the premise that the precision attachment is less stressful to the abutment tooth than is the conventional clasp. The basis for this reasoning is that, located as it is deep within the confines of the tooth, all stress is directed along the long axis of the tooth, thus being resisted by virtually all of the fibers of the periodontal ligament. Stress so directed is concentrated nearer to the center of rotation of the tooth than is the case with a conventional clasp, which is clearly more ideal from a standpoint of leverage. Moreover, reciprocity is assured so that there is no problem of "whiplash" effect, which the conventional clasp sometimes generates. Certainly, when four strategically located teeth (in all four quadrants of the mouth) are available, it must be conceded that masticatory stresses are almost ideally controlled with precision attachments.

Generally it can be said that the precision attachment type of retainer enjoys an enviable reputation as a means of retaining the partial denture. However, it should be pointed out that each step of the construction for a precision type retainer must, perforce, be very carefully planned prior to fabrication and, in addi-

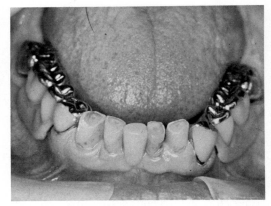

FIG. 18.2. A prime advantage of the precision attachment is the fact that the labial or buccal clasp arm can be eliminated, which may dramatically improve the esthetic result in some instances. The prosthesis shown here is retained by four precision attachments.

tion, the patient must be carefully selected. Moreover, the clinical preparation for the precision attachment is so exacting as to make it virtually impossible for important details of construction to be delegated to the laboratory technician. As a consequence, the precision type of construction is employed, by and large, by the most technically competent prosthodontists with the assistance of the most skilled and experienced laboratory technicians. Not surprisingly therefore, the success rate for this type of retainer is much above average. It may be fairly contended, however, that much of the success is due to careful planning and a high order of clinical competence, rather than to any inherent merit of a particular key/keyway device.

Indications for Use of the Precision Attachment

The prime indications for use of the precision attachment is for the all tooth-supported partial denture when (1) four large, well-formed abutments are available and (2) when clasp arms would otherwise be displayed in the anterior part of the mouth, which would be displeasing to the patient. Although in selected instances it may be employed, in preference to conventional retainers, to stabilize teeth which have been weakened by periodontal diseases, there are certainly limitations in this regard. Unless there are four abutments available to support the prosthesis it is doubtful that precision attachments will ensure any greater longevity than would properly designed clasps. Finally, the precision retainer can sometimes be used to advantage in the badly misaligned abutment tooth (e.g., the buccally inclined maxillary canine) to eliminate the need for the extensive cutting of tooth structure that is required for conventional clasping.

The precision attachment is customarily employed with a conventional lingual clasp arm; a type of construction which has much to recommend it. The clasp arm helps guide the attachment into place, thus making it less difficult for the patient to insert. As a consequence, wear of the key/keyway is reduced, since the greatest wear occurs during insertion and removal rather than during function.

Disadvantages of the Precision Attachment

There are disadvantages as well as limitations in the use of the precision type of retainer. For one thing, the tooth must be extensively cut to provide the requisite space to accommodate the keyway. For another, the bulge in the crown, created by the keyway, may deprive the underlying gingival tissue of its customary massage. Still another drawback is that the two parts of the laboratory type of attachment seldom fit with perfect precision, and the presence of even a minute crevice between the two parts raises the specter of uncleanliness of the keyway. Moreover, the attachment is subject to wear as a result of the friction between the metal parts, and this can create a maintenance problem. As wear occurs, the male portion fits ever more loosely in the keyway, thus eventually permitting excessive movement of the base and posing the threat of injury to the abutment. Interestingly enough, the patient is seldom aware of either the wear or the excessive movement because of the slow, gradual nature of its onset. Thus it may progress beyond the point where the damage is reversible before it is recognized and remedial treatment can be instituted. It deserves mention, however, that some types of precision attachments are designed so that they can be adjusted to increase the degree of frictional resistance to the key in the keyway. When this is the case, much of the wear can be compensated for by adjustment, provided it is accomplished at the time that it is needed.

The extracoronal type of retainer, while not requiring a large box-like preparation within the crown of the tooth, has numerous other disadvantages not shared by the intracoronal type. If the attachment extends outward from the tooth near the gingival border, there is a very real danger of gingival irritation followed by the usual inflammatory sequelae. Moreover, the extracoronal type of attachment must occupy the space immediately adjacent to the abutment tooth, which is precisely where a replacement tooth would ideally be positioned for maximum esthetic effect. A precision device which is visible in the mouth from a conversational distance will be ruinous to the appearance.

Limitations of the Precision Type of Attachment

Since the keyway must be of reasonable length to generate the required frictional resistance to unseating forces, the clinical crown of the abutment tooth must be of at least average height. Thus it follows that the precision type of attachment will not be successful when used with the tooth which has either a short or a very small crown. It should be noted, however, that clinical crown length may oftentimes be increased by means of gingivectomy or even alveoloplasty, provided an adequate crown/root ratio is maintained. Another factor limiting the use of the precision device is the size of the pulp, because of the danger of encroachment upon this sensitive organ.

Generally, fabrication of the denture with precision attachments requires the services of a skilled technician, although the laboratory steps can be accomplished by the dentist in his own office laboratory if he is so inclined. It is important to note also, that repair of the precision attachment is costly, and trained technicians, competent to perform repairs and maintenance, are not ordinarily available in geographic areas which are remote from population centers.

Because of its limitations, and the fact that it is inherently expensive to produce, it is doubtful that this type of construction will ever be available for routine, widespread use in dental practice.

Contraindications for Use of the Precision Attachment

The precision attachment should not be used in the distal extension base type of partial denture, particularly in the mandibular arch. The reason for this contraindication is that some movement of the distal extension base, supported as it is by a displaceable mucosa, is inevitable, and since the key/keyway mechanism allows no freedom of movement, other than in a vertical plane parallel to the long axis of the tooth, a great deal of masticatory stress will be transmitted directly to the abutment tooth as torque. This is almost certain to imperil the health of the periodontal apparatus (Fig. 18.3).

Exceptions to this prohibition are sometimes made in the maxilla, however, where the available soft tissue support is apt to be much greater and almost certainly of better quality, and where the display of a clasp arm may be a greater cosmetic impairment than it is in the mandibular arch. When the precision attachment must be employed with the distal extension base because of esthetic imperatives, excessive stress of the abutment tooth may be avoided, in some degree, by the use of two or more teeth splinted together as abutments, coupled with the employment of a stressbreaker.

Since the prosthesis with a precision attachment must be inserted along one precise path of insertion, the patient must possess at least an average degree of manual skill to manage the maneuver with facility. For this reason, the key/keyway type of construction generally is contraindicated for the senescent individual or for the one with an incapacitating handicap.

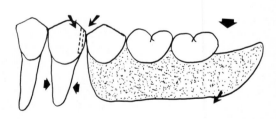

Fig. 18.3. Shown here schematically is the fact that the key/keyway mechanism allows no freedom of movement whatever, other than in a vertical plane parallel to the long axis of the tooth. If an attachment of this type is employed with a distal extension base, movement of the base in function will result in the transmission of more harmful torsional stresses to the abutment tooth than would be the case with a conventional extracoronal retainer (a clasp).

The Precision Rest

The precision rest consists of a narrow slot or keyway with vertical walls, which is built into a casting in an abutment tooth and into which is fitted a male attachment that has been made an integral part of the partial denture framework. A lingual clasp arm is customarily used with the precision rest, which helps to guide the attachment into place in the tooth. A slight lingual retentive undercut may be built into the lingual surface of the casting to augment the retention contributed by frictional contact between the walls of the keyway and the male portion.

The indications for use of the semiprecision type of retainer, together with the advantages, disadvantages, and limitations, are generally the same as for the manufactured type of key/keyway construction. The crown length of the abutment tooth must be of at least average height, so as to provide a keyway of sufficient vertical depth to provide the required degree of retention. Most of the keyway should be confined within the crown of the tooth and, since the pulp must be protected by an adequate thickness of secondary dentin, this virtually rules out the semiprecision type of construction for the younger age groups.

The semiprecision type of retainer has an advantage over the manufactured type in the fact that it is somewhat simpler to construct, hence is less time consuming and, as a consequence, not as costly. A disadvantage is that the parts do not fit together with the same degree of machined precision.

The Stressbreaker

It seems clear that the partial denture base that is unsupported at one end may move on its displaceable foundation when masticatory loads are applied, and certainly the prospect of this movement transmitting torsional stress to the abutment through the direct retainer has ominous implications from a standpoint of abutment tooth health and longevity. This has led to the concept that the abutment tooth should be relieved of this load and the burden placed on the residual ridge instead. The transfer of stress is accomplished either by the employment of a specially designed device (Fig. 18.4) interposed between the denture base and the clasp, or of a framework design which permits movement of the base independently of the clasp (Figs. 18.5 and 18.6). The direction and extent of the movement which the base is permitted to make depend upon the design and construction of the particular stressbreaker device being employed. The multitude of designs for stressbreakers which have been devised by a host of dentists and laboratory technicians illustrate a variety of concepts as to just how the stress should be dissipated. Commonly used designs are a hinge and a ball-and-socket as well as the flexibility of the metal of the framework itself (Fig. 18.7). If the device is of a hinge design (Fig. 18.8), the base is permitted movement in a vertical plane only. The movement may be unrestricted, or it may be controlled within definite limits by a stop arrangement built into the device. The hinge type of device spares the tooth virtually all of the stress which results from vertical movement of the base, but it

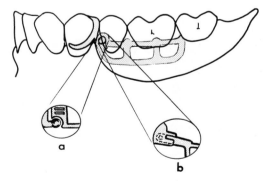

Fig. 18.4. A stressbreaker is a specially constructed device which is interposed between the denture base and the clasp, or a design of the framework, that permits movement of the base independently of the clasp. Shown here schematically at *a* is a ball-and-socket type of stressbreaker which permits the base to move in all planes. A hinge type of device is depicted at *b* which permits movement of the base in a vertical plane only.

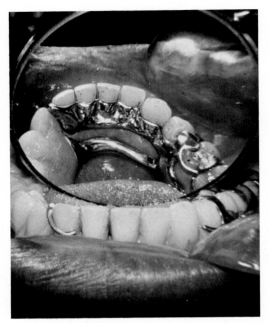

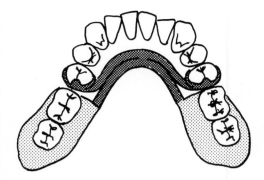

FIG. 18.7. Shown here is a schematic representation of a split bar type of stressbreaker. The two segments of the bar are attached only in a narrow area at the midline. Although the two distal extension bases are free to move, the magnitude of the stress transmitted to the abutment is dissipated to a large degree by the flexibility of the alloy.

FIG. 18.5. The stressbreaker shown here depends on the flexibility of the alloy in the area of the framework where the two segments join. Note that the clasp on the lateral incisor does not connect directly to the denture base, so that movement of the distal extension can take place without the transmission of stress directly to this abutment. The indirect retainer (the lingual apron) will not be as effective a stabilizer of the distal extension base as would be the case with conventional construction.

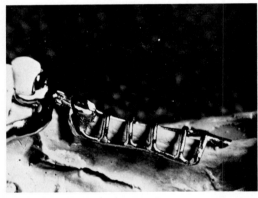

FIG. 18.8. Shown here is a hinge type of stressbreaker in which the denture base is permitted to move in a vertical plane only. This particular type of stressbreaker (the Hingelock, Swing-Lock Division of Idea Development Co., Dallas, Tex.) features a vertical stop incorporated into the keyway, which limits the amount of downward movement of the base.

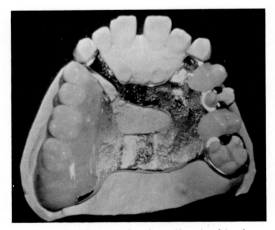

FIG. 18.6. The stressbreaker effect in this photograph is supplied by the flexibility of the alloy of the framework where the two segments join.

is still subjected to all of the lateral and torsional stress. If the device works on the ball-and-socket principle, movement of the base is allowed in all planes, and the tooth is relieved of virtually all stress. Obviously, all stress not borne by the teeth must be borne by the residual ridges.

Indications for Use of the Stressbreaker

Since the stressbreaker does, in fact, relieve the abutment tooth of the forces generated by the masticatory load, the stress then unavoidably must be borne by the residual ridge. It follows, therefore, that a prime indication for the application of this principle would be the mouth wherein an abutment tooth is inherently weak (a lateral incisor), and the patient possesses both well formed residual ridges and a positive bone factor. Although this is a combination not commonly encountered clinically, it does occur. Perhaps the prime exemplar is the patient who has retained only one mandibular cuspid and three or perhaps four incisors, so that one of the incisors must be pressed into service as an abutment (Fig. 18.9).

Another indication for use of the stressbreaker is the case in which the precision attachment must be employed for cosmetic reasons in the mandibular arch with the distal extension base.

Disadvantages of the Stressbreaker

It may be fairly contended that the stressbreaker principle is open to serious question. Clearly, there are major flaws in a partial denture design that places the major share of the masticatory load on the residual ridge, particularly in the mandibular arch where this structure is not designed for load bearing. The residual ridge, in the bicuspid region in particular, is typically narrow and made up primarily of cancellous bone, so that from an architectural standpoint it is simply not built to withstand stress. Consequently, a stressbreaker placed on a cuspid or first bicuspid allows excessive movement of the denture base, with the result that stress is concentrated in an area which very likely will not have the capacity to withstand it. As a result, the bone of the residual ridge will quickly resorb.

Stressbreaking devices generally allow too much movement, the stress is not uniformly distributed, and the benefits of both cross-arch stabilization and indirect retention are lost. Thus, the residual

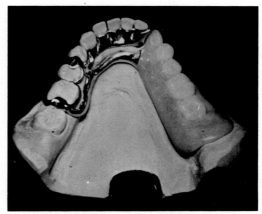

Fig. 18.9. Shown here is a combination of semiedentulousness where the stressbreaker can be used to advantage. The lateral incisor is an inherently weak abutment, but the residual ridge is large and well formed, hence better able to withstand stress than is the lateral incisor.

ridges are much more apt to be overburdened without the support and stabilization which the abutment teeth, auxillary rests, and indirect retainers contribute to a partial denture of conventional construction.

It should be noted, too, that some designs of stressbreakers can interfere with the cosmetic excellence of the prosthesis by creating bulk in precisely the area that should be occupied by the replacement tooth or teeth for maximum esthetic effect. In addition, the bulky contour may cause food entrapment, which is likely to be an annoyance to the patient. Finally, the stressbreaker is more costly to make, more disposed to get out of adjustment, and more difficult to adjust and repair than is the conventional retainer.

Bibliography

McCall, J. O., and Hugel, J. M.: *Movable-Removable Bridgework.* Dental Items of Interest Publishing Company, Brooklyn, 1950.

Preiskel, H.: *Precision Attachments in Dentistry.* The C. V. Mosby Company, St. Louis, 1968.

Schuyler, C. H.: Analysis of the use and relative value of the precision attachment and the clasp in partial denture planning. J. Prosth. Dent. *3:* 711–714, 1953.

Schuyler, C. H.: The partial denture as a means of stabilizing abutment teeth. J. Amer. Dent. Ass. *28:* 1121–1125, 1941.

Chapter 19

THE INTERIM PROSTHESIS AND THE TREATMENT PROSTHESIS

This chapter deals with the prosthesis that replaces an anterior tooth or teeth and is worn for a short, planned period of time—the interim prosthesis. Also discussed is the treatment prosthesis that is constructed and worn as an aid in accomplishing a specific objective, as a part of the overall treatment. The subject matter is arranged in the following manner.

Introduction
The Interim Prosthesis
The Design and Fabrication of the Interim Prosthesis
The Treatment Prosthesis

Introduction

The term "temporary prosthesis" is well established in dentistry, and is both descriptive and widely employed. However, its use in discussions with the patient should be discouraged, since it is apt to cause misunderstanding. The term "temporary" may lead him to believe that, following a short period of wear of a temporary prosthesis, he will be fitted with a permanent one. The implications of the term "permanent prosthesis" are too well known to need elaboration here, the concept of a permanent prosthesis having long been acknowledged as a root cause of misunderstanding between dentist and patient. Accordingly, in communicating with the patient it is recommended that the term "temporary" be discarded in favor of adjectival designations based on the function which the prosthesis is meant to perform.

Applying the adjectival nomenclature to the temporary prosthesis, it is apparent that the ones most frequently employed in practice can be classified logically into two principal types: One, the "interim" prosthesis, is employed to provide the patient with a tide-over cosmetic facade for the time interval between the extraction of an anterior tooth (or teeth) and the construction and insertion of the definitive prosthesis. The second is the "treatment" prosthesis which is designed to aid in the accomplishment of a specific phase of the therapeutic continuum. Both types will be discarded and replaced by a more permanent type of construction when they have fulfilled their intended function.

The Interim Prosthesis

The prime purpose of the interim prosthesis is to restore appearance until a prosthesis of more definitive design can be constructed. In some instances, the maintenance of space may be a secondary objective. The interim prosthesis may be employed in a variety of circumstances; when (1) healing is progressing following an extraction or a traumatic injury, (2) a prosthesis is desirable during the time that prolonged treatment is being accomplished (e.g., periodontal or endodontic therapy), (3) the patient cannot spare the time at the moment for the extensive preparatory treatment which may be required for definitive treatment, (4) the pulp chambers are so large that a fixed prosthesis is not feasible, and (5) the clinical crowns have not fully erupted and are so short that clasping by conventional means has little chance of succeeding.

The interim type of prosthesis is made

for both the maxilla and the mandible, albeit much more frequently in the case of the former, since the space created by a missing maxillary tooth is so much more conspicuous, hence cosmetically more incapacitating, than is the case in the mandibular arch. Another reason is the fact that the maxillary anterior teeth, by virtue of their more exposed, forward position in the face, are much more vulnerable to traumatic accident than are the mandibular teeth.

Generally, the interim partial denture is employed to replace one or two anterior teeth (Fig. 19.1) although, in some circumstances, it may replace as many as four. Posterior teeth should not, as a rule, be replaced, since this tends to encourage the patient to exert stresses on the prosthesis that it is not intended or designed to withstand and that may be damaging to the supporting structures.

Factors in Retention

The prosthesis may be retained in the mouth either by means of clasps or by exploiting natural retentive factors which are present in different mouths in varying degrees. One of the most effective of these potential sources of retention is the lingual surface of a posterior tooth (Fig. 19.2).

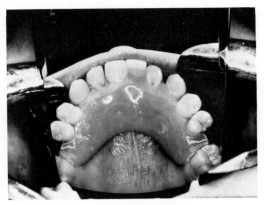

FIG. 19.2. A prime source of retention for the interim prosthesis is frictional contact with the lingual surfaces of the posterior teeth. The prosthesis in this photograph replaces the left central incisor. Note that the missing posterior teeth have not been replaced.

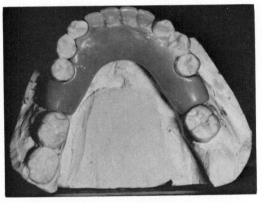

FIG. 19.3. Posterior edentulous spaces, when tooth bounded, provide a very effective means of retention for the claspless interim partial denture. The prosthesis shown here replaces four mandibular incisors. Note that the proximal surfaces of the teeth adjoining the edentulous spaces have been exploited for the retention which they can provide.

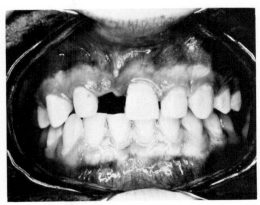

FIG. 19.1. The interim partial denture is most commonly employed to replace one or two anterior teeth. The prime purpose is to restore appearance until a prosthesis of a more definitive design can be constructed.

Frictional resistance between the denture and the tooth surface can be an effective retaining force provided (1) the teeth have clinical crowns of at least average height, and (2) the interproximal embrasures are such that a portion of the proximal surfaces of adjoining teeth are accessible to being contacted by the denture base. Posterior edentulous spaces, particularly if tooth bounded (Fig. 19.3), afford an excellent opportunity to extend the base of the denture into intimate contact with the proximal surfaces of the teeth which adjoin the space, thus contributing considerable frictional resistance to dislodgment.

Interfacial tension between the denture base and the mucosa is another source of retention. Its efficacy depends on intimate contact of the base with the mucosa, coupled with a normal supply of thin saliva. The degree of retention so derived is directly proportional to the amount of areal coverage.

The contour of the palatal vault is another factor in retention, a deep vault being more retentive than a shallow one. The character of the palatal mucosa is also significant, a thick resilient mucosa being more retentive than a thin hard one, while a prominent median raphe is a negative retention factor.

The occlusion may likewise play an important role in retention, particularly the relationship of opposing anterior teeth. A deep vertical overlap is a distinct liability to the stability of the prosthesis, especially if the mandibular incisors must contact the prosthesis in centric position because of stringent space limitations.

The presence or absence of a labial flange also has a bearing on the retention. A well fitting flange can contribute importantly to the retentive properties.

Finally, not to be overlooked, is the role played by the tongue and the patient's oral, neuromuscular mechanism, which are perforce inseparably linked. Indeed, this is perhaps the most potent single natural retentive factor of them all. If it is favorable, it can counterbalance a host of negative factors. The patient who is motivated by a desire to wear the prosthesis and who possesses average neuromuscular control will wear it with success irrespective of almost any other consideration.

The Pros and Cons of Clasping

It is generally preferable not to employ clasps to retain the interim denture unless natural retentive factors are exceedingly unfavorable. The reason for this is that clasps themselves can introduce problems in the design and wear of the prosthesis. For example, one problem frequently encountered with clasps is the necessity of crossing the occlusal surfaces of the posterior teeth from the lingual to the buccal side when interocclusal space is restricted. Moreover, clasps are prone to get out of adjustment and a bent clasp can do irreparable damage to the mouth in a short period of time, oftentimes unbeknown to the patient. Furthermore, adolescents, in particular, tend to be careless in their handling of the denture, thus exposing it unnecessarily to distortion and breakage, and clasps are exceedingly vulnerable to deformation.

In making a decision as to the advisability of employing clasps, the mental attitude of the patient should be given consideration. If he is the type who may be expected to adjust slowly or poorly to a prosthesis, it might be prudent to design the denture with clasps. Following a short period of wear, the clasps might be bent out to a point that they are out of contact with the surface of the abutment teeth so that they contribute little or nothing to the retention. If the patient manages satisfactorily with this arrangement, the clasps might then be removed from the denture altogether. Another approach to clasping is to make the prosthesis without clasps, with the understanding that they will be added if the patient deems it necessary following a short trial period of wear. If it is subsequently decided that clasps should be added, an impression is made with the denture in place and a cast poured, after which the clasps are contoured and processed into the base with autopolymerizing acrylic resin. From a practical standpoint, it is typical to find that the patient will seldom elect to have the clasps added, because during the trial period he will have developed the requisite neuromuscular skill to manage the denture without clasps.

Types of Clasps

Clasps may be made either of gold wrought wire or of stainless steel orthodontic wire. Eighteen-gauge wire is the most commonly used size, and the simple circlet clasp is the design most often employed. Occlusal rests may be used if there is adequate interocclusal space to accommodate them. Also worthy of mention, prefabricated clasps of stainless steel are marketed which are well suited for use with the interim type of removable prosthesis.

The Interproximal Retention Point

When retention cannot be obtained from the lingual surfaces of the teeth because the crowns are too short, and other retentive factors are likewise unfavorable, the interproximal retention point may be employed to aid in the retention of the prosthesis. Retention points are made as follows: small holes are prepared in the interproximal embrasures of the cast, between several teeth on either side of the arch, to accommodate an 18-gauge wire. One end of a steel or gold alloy wire is placed in each hole to a depth of ½ mm., and the opposite end is fashioned into a loop to extend onto the palate where it will be anchored into the palatal resin. When the denture has been processed, the ends of the wire are adjusted to fit into the embrasures in the mouth. As a final step, the interproximal points should be rounded and polished.

Another indication for employment of the interproximal point is the case in which there is insufficient interocclusal space to allow for a conventional clasp to cross the occlusal surfaces from the lingual to the buccal side.

The Hazard of Swallowing or Aspirating the Prosthesis

The possibility of swallowing or aspirating a small oral prosthesis should not be overlooked. For this reason, it may be contended that clasps should be employed routinely in the fabrication of the interim prosthesis, so that should an accident occur, the radiopaque metal would render the appliance visible in the x-ray during a radiographic search of the trachea or alimentary tract. It is worthy of note, in this regard, that a radiopaque acrylic resin (Coe Laboratories, Chicago, Ill.) is available on the market, which would make the use of clasps unnecessary for this purpose.

The Design and Fabrication of the Interim Prosthesis

The extent of areal coverage as well as the configuration of the base depends primarily on the natural retentive factors that are available. If most factors are favorable, i.e., high vault, cooperative patient, good saliva, and employment of a labial flange, the areal coverage may be limited to a small horseshoe configuration. Similarly, the horseshoe configuration usually will suffice when clasps are to be employed. On the other hand, if most retentive factors are unfavorable it may be prudent to extend the coverage over the entire palate and to incorporate a post dam seal on the posterior border.

Preparation of the Cast

When the horseshoe design is to be used, the posterior border should be slightly beaded to provide a seal, while the area adjacent to the teeth should be relieved to protect the free gingival margins from pressure. The beading is accomplished by lightly scraping the cast. Relief is provided by flowing a thin film of baseplate wax onto each gingival crevice, to a depth of approximately ½ mm. If additional retention from the lingual surfaces of the teeth is deemed necessary (because other retentive factors are not favorable), the lingual surfaces of the stone teeth may be sanded slightly with a standpaper disk.

Arranging the Tooth or Teeth

The replacement teeth of the interim prosthesis should be aligned with the labial surfaces of the natural teeth, so as to present an optimally natural appearance. If this requires that the teeth be brought forward from the residual ridge, a labial flange should be employed. When a labial flange is employed, the gingival borders of the replacement teeth should be aligned to harmonize with those of the natural teeth, so as to present a pleasingly natural appearance.

Abuting the Tooth or Teeth. If the replacement teeth are to be abutted directly to the ridge, the stone of the cast should be relieved liberally to a depth of at least 1 mm. in the area to be occupied by the ridge lap (Fig. 19.4). If the teeth are to appear natural in the mouth, they must be intimately adapted to the mucosa. The only way to ensure that there will be a closely fitting contact is to remove an adequate amount of stone from the cast prior to positioning the teeth. If the amount of stone removed proves to be slightly in excess of need, as evidenced by a blanching of the mucosa at the time of insertion, it is a simple matter to decrease the pressure by lightly disking the ridge lap of a tooth with a rubber disk. When the teeth have been arranged properly on the cast, they may be retained in position while the base is formed by attaching them with sticky wax to adjoining teeth, or a labial plaster matrix may be made to hold them in place.

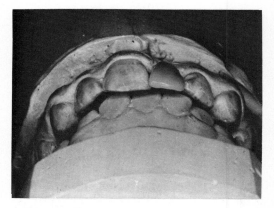

FIG. 19.5. In constructing an interim removable partial denture for the mouth with a deep overbite, it will sometimes be necessary to reduce the incisal level of the opposing mandibular teeth. Enough reduction should be accomplished to provide sufficient interridge space for a thickness of acrylic resin which will withstand the stresses of function without fracture.

Occlusion. If possible, the artificial anterior teeth should be cleared of contact with their antagonists in all excursive movements within the patient's functional range. Unfortunately, this is not always possible without detracting from the esthetic value, particularly when dealing with an occlusion in which there is a deep vertical overlap of the anterior teeth. When the vertical overlap severely restricts the space for a replacement tooth, it may be necessary to reduce the height of the mandibular incisors (Fig. 19.5), and to reinforce the tooth with clasp wire (Figs. 19.6 and 19.7).

Fabrication of the Base

If clasps are to be employed, they should be contoured and placed in position on the teeth with the tangs extending onto the palatal portion of the cast (Fig. 19.8). The clasps may be held in position against the teeth with sticky wax. A dam of modeling clay or utility wax is placed around the outline of the base (Fig. 19.9), and the base is formed by applying alternate layers of polymer and monomer. The base is then cured for 20 minutes in the polymerizer at 30 pounds of pressure.

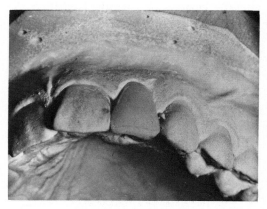

FIG. 19.4. The replacement teeth of the interim prosthesis should be aligned with the labial surfaces of the adjoining natural teeth so as to create an optimally pleasing natural appearance. When the replacement teeth are to be abutted directly to the residual ridge (not placed in a denture flange), the stone of the cast should be relieved liberally in the area to be occupied by the ridge lap, so that the tooth will fit snugly against the mucosa. The cast shown here has been relieved to a depth of 1 mm. to ensure an intimate adaptation of the ridge lap to the mucosa.

Insertion and Counseling the Patient

Over and above the routine recommendations and directions which should be given to any patient who is preparing to wear an oral prosthesis for the first time, it should be emphasized that the temporary prosthesis is a tide-over appliance. As such, it is not meant to supplant natural teeth completely, but only to hide the fact that natural teeth have been lost in a conspicuous area of the mouth. If it serves to disguise this fact, it will have achieved its intended purpose. It would be well also to point out to the patient that he cannot

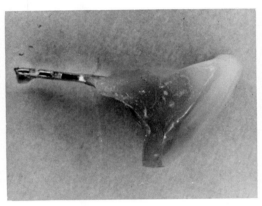

FIG. 19.6. When the space between the mandibular incisors and the maxillary ridge is extremely limited, it may be advisable to reinforce the acrylic resin tooth with a gold or stainless steel wire, as shown here. The wire will impart additional strength so that the tooth is not as apt to be sheared off in service.

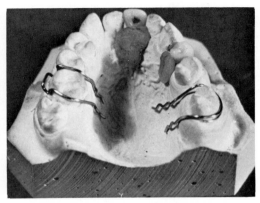

FIG. 19.8. If clasps are to be employed to retain the prosthesis, they should be contoured to fit the teeth and be provided with loops or twists to help anchor them in the acrylic resin of the base. Prior to forming the denture base, the clasps are placed in position on the teeth, with the tangs extending onto the palatal portion of the cast. The clasps may be secured in this position by means of sticky wax applied to the clasp arms on the buccal or occlusal surface of the tooth.

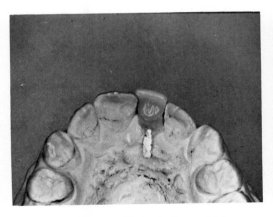

FIG. 19.7. The mandibular incisors which oppose these maxillary teeth barely clear the palatal mucosa, despite having been reduced substantially in height. Therefore, the plastic replacement tooth has been reinforced with a gold alloy wire to impart added strength.

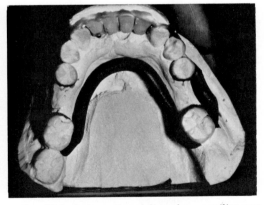

FIG. 19.9. A dam of modeling clay or utility wax is placed around the periphery of the area that is to be occupied by the base. The base is formed by applying by the sprinkle method autopolymerizing resin and curing it in the autopolymerizer, or by waxing a pattern and accomplishing a flasking procedure.

expect to bite into an apple, the way he did with his natural teeth, without dislodging the prosthesis. Instead, he must learn to force the apple down over the lower natural teeth to minimize the hazard of an embarrassing dislodgment. It should be emphasized too that the prosthesis must *not* be worn at night. In addition to the ill effects to the mucosa induced by 24-hour wear, there is a danger of swallowing or aspirating the prosthesis during sleep. For the same reasons, the prosthesis should be removed while he is engaged in any contact sport. The prosthesis must be kept scrupulously clean, and the oral cavity should be monitored for early signs of irritation or inflammation.

The Treatment Prosthesis

The treatment prosthesis is a type of temporary partial denture that is designed and constructed specifically to aid in the achievement of a definite treatment objective, as an integral part of the overall treatment plan. The most commonly employed types of treatment prostheses are discussed in succeeding paragraphs, according to the function which each performs.

Maintaining Interarch Space

When a tuberosity is surgically trimmed for the purpose of creating space for a removable partial denture, a treatment type partial might be employed to cover the area of the surgery. The purpose of such a splint is to prevent slumping of the wound, with a resultant diminution in the amount of interridge space. When this technique is employed, the denture base is often lined with a tissue treatment material to act as a soothing surgical dressing.

Maintaining a Predetermined Vertical Dimension of Occlusion

When extensive restorative work is being accomplished, the desired vertical dimension of occlusion can be established with a temporary prosthesis. As the restorations are finished and cemented into place, segments can be eliminated from

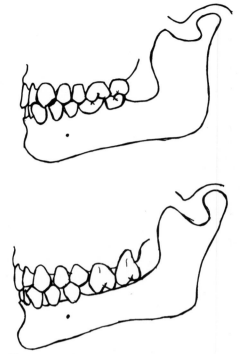

FIG. 19.10. Oftentimes early loss of posterior teeth permits opposing teeth to overerupt into the edentulous space to a point that there is inadequate space for a prosthesis. It may be possible, in selected instances, to retrieve a portion of this space with a treatment prosthesis. The *top sketch* depicts a normal occlusal plane. The *bottom sketch* shows a collapsed occlusion following loss of the mandibular molars and extrusion of the maxillary teeth.

the treatment prosthesis in a tooth-by-tooth fashion as they become superfluous.

Treating TMJ Symptoms

When the etiology of temporomandibular joint (TMJ) symptoms is suspected of having a basis in an altered (decreased) vertical dimension of occlusion, the level of the occlusion may be altered experimentally by attaching occlusion rims and acrylic resin overlays to a partial denture metal framework. The resin may be readily altered to increase or decrease the height of the occlusion in consonance with clinical signs and subjective symptoms. When the symptoms have been satisfactorily alleviated, a more permanent type of prosthesis, either fixed or removable, may be constructed to function at the newly established vertical dimension of occlusion.

Creating Interridge Space

A bite plane type of treatment partial denture may be used to intrude groups of teeth while, at the same time, permitting other groups to extrude, for the purpose of retrieving urgently needed interridge space as well as improving the configuration of the occlusal plane. The most commonly encountered type of collapsed occlusion is the instance in which the early loss of the mandibular molars has permitted the maxillary molars to overerupt to a point where they contact an edentulous area of the mandibular ridge (Fig. 19.10). Under the circumstances there is, of course, no room for a denture base. Space may sometimes be retrieved, in selected patients in the younger age groups, by making a partial denture framework to fit the lower teeth and attaching acrylic resin bases to it. The bases are adjusted so that only the maxillary posterior teeth are in contact with it in centric position. If the patient wears this 24 hours a day, except while eating, the maxillary teeth will usually intrude the slight amount necessary to provide sufficient space to accommodate a denture base on the mandibular ridge.

Another type of closed intermaxillary space which must occasionally be dealt with is the edentulous anterior maxillary space in which the lower anterior teeth have erupted to a point where they contact the mucosa of the maxillary ridge, thus preempting the space needed for a prosthesis. Again, in the younger patient, a bite plane treatment partial can be constructed so that the lower anterior teeth contact the bite plane, thus intruding them while, at the same time, allowing the posterior teeth of each arch to overerupt slightly. When combined with moderate reduction of the incisal edges of the teeth, the net effect will be to create enough interridge space to permit the placement of a partial denture.

Bibliography

Osborne, J., and Lammie, G. A.: *Partial Dentures.* Blackwell Scientific Publications, Oxford, 1952.

Stileman, R. D. W.: Spoon dentures. Brit. Dent. Jl. *91:* 294–297, 1951.

Chapter 20

PARTIAL DENTURE MATERIALS

The subject of this chapter is the physical properties of the various materials that are commonly employed to fabricate the removable partial denture, with particular emphasis on the alloys used for the framework. In addition, it contains a comparison of the physical properties of the gold alloys with those of the chromium-cobalt alloys which are of clinical significance. The subject matter is presented in the following way.

Introduction

Because of the enormous diversity of partial denture designs and types of construction, there is a requirement for fabricating materials which possess a wide range of physical properties. Fortunately, these needs have been met by the dental manufacturers, who offer a variety of different materials for forming each of the structural units, i.e., the framework, the base, and the teeth. Examples abound of the options which are available to the designer of a prosthesis. The base can be constructed of a plastic, chromium-cobalt alloy, or gold alloy, each of which contributes a different combination of characteristics to the prosthesis. If plastic is the material selected, a further choice can be made of a polymethyl-methacrylate, polyvinyl acrylic, or polystyrene. Teeth may be selected of acrylic resin, porcelain, metal, or a combination of metal and acrylic resin. The framework may be constructed of gold alloy, chromium-cobalt alloy, or a combination of the two. Finally, either alloy can be employed in either its cast form or its wrought form, or in a combination of the two. So important is the contribution made by the component materials that the success of an oral prosthesis may well hinge directly on the combination of materials chosen for its fabrication. One who is acquainted with the advantages, disadvantages, and limitations of the various materials is in a position to exploit the advantages of one while avoiding the weaknesses of another.

The Role of the Dentist in Prescribing Materials

There is no escaping the fact that the clinician alone is in a position to make an assessment of the behavior of the various materials under the stress of mouth service. While it is true that the technician may be thoroughly familiar with the working properties of each material, he has little or no opportunity to observe or compare the manner in which it reacts to the rigors of use and abuse to which it is subjected by a cross section of partial denture wearers. Thus it follows that the dentist should prescribe the combination of materials that is to be used to fabricate the prosthesis, rather than to delegate this responsibility to another person. To do this competently, he must have a sound knowledge of the advantages, disadvantages, and limitations of each of the materials that are available for this purpose.

Denture Base Materials

Three groups of plastic denture base materials are marketed for use in constructing the denture base. These are (1) the polymethyl-methacrylates, (2) the polyvinyl acrylics, and (3) the polystyrenes. There is little difference clinically among these three insofar as the properties of color, dimensional stability, tissue compatibility, strength, and acceptance by the patient are concerned.

Although as a group the plastic resins are far from ideal as materials with which to fabricate the denture base, they are generally conceded to be the most nearly ideal of any material presently available. If the denture is to be processed in the dental office, the polymethyl-methacrylate (acrylic resin) has an important advantage over the others, in that it can be processed rather easily with relatively uncomplicated, inexpensive equipment. An additional plus factor possessed by acrylic resin is that a denture can be individually characterized by the addition of tints and fibers to the mold, and this can be an important advantage under some circumstances.

Denture Tooth Materials

Teeth are manufactured and marketed of acrylic resin, porcelain, and a combination of acrylic resin and metal. The acrylic resin tooth, more commonly referred to as the "plastic" tooth, is used more often than any other for the removable partial denture because of its unique physical properties, although the porcelain tooth is also frequently employed. Certainly, there are circumstances which call for the physical properties of each and, in truth, all types of artificial teeth may find a place in partial denture construction.

Both porcelain and acrylic resin teeth have strengths, weaknesses, and limitations. The salient characteristics of each type of tooth, particularly as they pertain to its use with the removable partial denture, are ennumerated below.

Characteristics of Acrylic Resin Teeth

1. Acrylic resin teeth are tough, durable, and highly resistant to breakage.
2. The plastic material absorbs some masticatory stress, and may thereby contribute to preservation of the residual ridge.
3. The resin of the tooth bonds chemically to the plastic base, and thus prevents "percolation" of fluids between base and tooth.
4. The fact that the resin bonds chemically to the plastic base probably results in a stronger, more durable base, since it is a homogeneous unit.
5. The plastic is lighter in weight, which might be a worthwhile advantage in some maxillary dentures.
6. Resistance to masticatory abrasion is extremely poor. Not only do posterior teeth wear, changing the vertical dimension of occlusion, but the labial surfaces of the anterior teeth wear also. The esthetic qualities built into the denture may thus be slowly lost as a result of it.
7. The rebasing procedure is somewhat more difficult to accomplish with the denture which has plastic teeth.
8. Wax up of the denture in the laboratory, as well as polishing, is more difficult.
9. There is the possibility that plastic teeth will absorb stain under some conditions.

Characteristics of Porcelain Teeth

1. Wear resistance is excellent.
2. Porcelain cuts and grinds more efficiently than does plastic.
3. Because the labial surface of porcelain anterior teeth is not subject to wear, they will retain their appearance for the life of the denture.
4. Porcelain is friable, and hence more prone to breakage.
5. Percolation around the necks of porcelain teeth can occur.
6. Porcelain teeth are more apt to cause a clicking noise in the mouths of patients who do not possess good neuromuscular control.
7. Porcelain, because of its hardness, may be more traumatic to the residual ridge.

Alloys Used for the Partial Denture Framework

Two groups of alloys are in common use for fabrication of the partial denture framework: (1) the gold alloys (Table 20.1), and (2) the chromium-cobalt alloys (Table 20.2). The chromium-cobalt alloys enjoy a much greater use in dentistry; indeed it has been estimated that 90% of all partial dentures are made of one or the other of the commercial brands of chromium dental alloys. It must be conceded, however, that by any objective standard neither alloy can be shown to possess superior properties for dental use. The reasons for this paradox may be traced to the sequence of events that has transpired, beginning with the introduction of the one-piece partial denture casting in the 1920's and followed by the first application of the chromium-cobalt alloys for dental use a few years later.

TABLE 20.1.

The Make-Up of a Typical Saddle, Bar, and Clasp Gold Alloy (Type IV)

Component Metal	Approximate Percentage	Contribution to the Alloy
	%	
Gold	60–71	Gold color, tarnish resistance, ductility
Silver	4.5–20	Ductility, whitens
Copper	11–16	Adds strength, hardens, reduces melting point, reduces tarnish resistance
Palladium	0–5	Raises melting point, hardens, strengthens, whitens
Platinum	0–3.5	Hardens, strengthens, raises corrosion resistance, raises melting point
Zinc	1–2	Oxide scavenger

This table shows the component metals of a typical gold alloy suitable for use for fabricating a partial denture framework. The percentages of each metal are approximations meant only to convey the comparative amounts of each constituent metal to be found in a typical alloy.

TABLE 20.2.

Make-Up of a Typical Chromium-Cobalt Dental Alloy

Component Metal	Approximate Percentage	Contribution to the Alloy
	%	
Chromium	26–30	Tarnish and corrosion resistance
Cobalt	27–30	Hardness, strength
Nickel	35–40	Ductility
Molybdenum	4–6	Hardness, strength
Beryllium	1–3	Strength, reduces melting point, finer grain structure

This table shows the component metals which make up the typical chromium-cobalt alloy suitable for fabricating the partial denture framework. The percentage of each metal is an approximation, meant only to convey the relative amounts of the constituent metals to be found in a typical alloy.

Viewed in historical context, it is apparent that the rise in popularity of the chromium-cobalt alloys occupies a reciprocal cause-and-effect relationship with the rapid evolution of the commercial dental laboratory industry in the United States during the decades since the 1930's. This, in turn, is closely intertwined with the revolutionary changes that have taken place in dental practice during this same period. For a clearer understanding of the circumstances which paved the way for these events, they should be viewed against a backdrop of the social revolution that has taken place in American society during the same period, particularly the tremendous elevation of its living standards.

Historical Background

Throughout the second decade of the twentieth century virtually all removable partial dentures were made either by fabricating individual clasps of wrought wire, or by casting them and then soldering them to a wrought lingual bar or processing them into a vulcanite denture base. It is significant that a high percentage of these prostheses were made by the dentist himself, in his own laboratory, which traditionally occupied a room adjoining his office. An example of the type of partial denture construction typical of the time was the removable prosthesis which Dr. Norman Nesbett of Boston introduced to the profession in 1918. His method consisted of casting the clasps for each tooth individually and then attaching them by means of solder to a cast gold boxing which enclosed the replacement tooth or teeth.

The Nesbett method exemplified the approach to prosthodontics which was characteristic of the period. Since the typical oral prosthesis was a product of the craftsmanship of the individual dentist, it was well suited to the office-laboratory type of operation. The fabrication of a partial denture required meticulous assembling operations in the mouth, interspersed with painstaking soldering operations in his laboratory. It was customary for the dentist, who devoted a portion of his practice to prosthodontics, to spend a substantial amount of time in his laboratory where he performed tasks that, at a later time, were to be largely delegated to auxiliaries.

Introduction of the One-Piece Casting

In 1925 Dr. Polk E. Akers published a paper describing his technique for casting a removable partial denture framework in one piece. Although the method which he recommended was not immediately adopted by dentists in great numbers, the technique must be regarded, in retrospect, as a momentous technical breakthrough, and over the period of the next few years it became widely accepted.

The significance of Dr. Aker's contribution, in the evolution of both dental practice and the commercial dental laboratory, was that the procedure for fabricating the one-piece cast framework could be much more readily adapted to the production line methods of the commercial laboratory than to the smaller confines and more limited equipment of the average dental office laboratory.

Introduction of the Nonprecious Metal Dental Casting

In 1920, Fredrick Hauptmyer, Chief of the Krupp Dental Clinic in Essen, Germany, described the process which his staff employed in fabricating oral appliances for workers in the Krupp Industries. The material employed in the fabrication of the framework was an alloy of the "18-8" type (18% chromium and 8% nickel). The rest of the alloy was made up of iron. This may explain the fact that the chromium-cobalt alloys are sometimes referred to as "steels" which is, of course, a misnomer. Steel is made up largely of iron and carbon (a carbon steel), or iron, chromium, and nickel (a stainless steel). In contrast, the chromium-cobalt alloys contain only traces of iron as an impurity, the amount being so small as to be insignificant.

The success which heralded the use of a nonprecious alloy for intraoral use did not go unnoticed. There is presumptive evidence, at least, that it acted as an inspirational wellspring for the concept of employing the chromium-cobalt alloys in cast form for dental use, a method that was introduced to the profession just a few years later.

The Use of Chromium-Cobalt for the Framework

In 1929 Erdle and Prange developed a technique, as well as the materials, for casting a chromium-cobalt-tungsten type of alloy to which they gave the name "Vitallium." Alloys of this type are classified metallurgically as "Stellite" alloys, which are defined as extremely hard, highly corrosion resistant alloys made up principally of chromium-cobalt and tungsten. In the early 1930's another chromium-cobalt alloy was patented and marketed under the name of "Ticonium," and during the next decade a considerable number of different chromium-cobalt type dental alloys were formulated and marketed under various trade names. At the midpoint of the twentieth century, there were in the neighborhood of 25 different brands of chromium-cobalt dental alloys marketed in the United States, although most were distributed only regionally. While a number of these alloys are presently available to the profession through franchised commercial laboratories in various parts of the country, a still greater number have fallen by the wayside and are no longer marketed.

Ticonium and Vitallium are, by any yardstick, the largest companies in the business of producing chromium-cobalt alloys for intraoral use. Both companies have franchised laboratories in virtually all large cities of the United States, as well as in many foreign countries. Not surprisingly, the question of which of these two giants of the industry markets the better alloy is a subject of considerable interest. Most practitioners who have had an opportunity to observe the physical characteristics of both alloys favor one or the other, for reasons invariably based altogether on personal judgment. Certainly, no valid research has been published to document any clear superiority of either one over the other, and indeed, both alloys have proven themselves thoroughly reliable clinically over a period of many years. Rather than attempting to select the superior alloy for one's patients, a better approach would be to select the commercial laboratory which enjoys the most favorable reputation for integrity and which demonstrates the highest caliber of craftsmanship. Having selected a laboratory by these criteria, one should then become familiar with the physical properties and working characteristics of whichever alloy they are franchised to process. Clearly, the technical skill and craftsmanship of the technicians, combined with high standards of quality control, are of greater import than is any slight difference in physical properties of the two alloys.

The Economics of Gold versus Chromium-Cobalt

The chromium-cobalt alloys have traditionally been offered to the dental profession through the commercial laboratory by means of a franchise arrangement between the manufacturer and the dental laboratory. A laboratory which has a Ticonium franchise, for example, obtains from the parent company the specially designed equipment, as well as the materials needed to process the alloy, together with a continuing supply of the alloy itself. The price of the alloy to the laboratory is customarily considerably less than the price of an equal quantity of dental gold alloy. In fact, cost differential per unit of metal is perhaps the greatest ostensible difference between the gold and chromium alloys and might, at first glance, appear to be a major factor in the greater popularity of the chromium. On closer analysis, however, it is quite apparent that to explain the much greater use of chromium-cobalt on a basis of cost alone is a misleading oversimplification.

It must be conceded, however, that, from the viewpoint of the commercial dental laboratory, the base metal would be a more profitable item to promote, other things being equal. There would be an understandable incentive to concentrate on developing an efficient production line for processing the particular brand of chromium alloy to which the laboratory had access by virtue of the franchise arrangement. Because of the differences in techniques, equipment, and materials required to process gold and chromium-cobalt, the two alloys cannot be intermixed in a production line, and it is rarely if ever commercially feasible for a laboratory to operate a separate production line for each alloy. Hence, the most economically sound method of operation for the franchised laboratory is to concentrate its attention on an efficient production line for the franchised metal. An obvious corollary would be a tendency to encourage the use of a particular brand of "white metal," and indeed to promote it aggressively to the dentist.

It is worthy of mention too that the laboratories who were awarded the franchises during this era of rapid growth were, by and large, the better established, more successful ones in each geographic area. Typically, this type of laboratory already had on its payroll the most highly skilled technicians in the locality, and as expected, the partial dentures which they produced were quite apt to be superior to the ones produced in gold by the average smaller, less competitive laboratories in the area. The net effect was to reflect credit, albeit unmerited, on the chromium type of alloy itself at the expense of the gold alloy.

During the 1930's and 1940's the commercial dental laboratories passed through a period when it was customary for the franchised laboratories to offer the profession a framework fabricated of either gold alloy or chromium-cobalt alloy, with little or no price differential between the two. The pendulum had begun to swing, however. At some point in time during this two-decade interval, the ratio of partial dentures made of gold to those made of chromium-cobalt gradually shifted from a preponderance of gold alloy to the present higher percentage of chromium-cobalt. The rapidly changing economic environment of the country was making itself felt in dental practice as well as in the laboratory industry.

The Impact of World War II

The evolution of dental practice was given tremendous impetus by the events during and following World War II, and it was accompanied by a corresponding upsurge in growth of the commercial laboratory industry. Literally millions of young men and women in the armed services were the recipients of definitive dental treatment, many for the first time in their lives. The great majority were so favorably impressed with the obvious benefits of oral health, that following demobilization these newly created civilians adopted regular dental care as a way of life. This comparatively affluent component of postwar society now demanded regular dental attention not only for themselves but for the members of their families as well. A predictable result was that every able-bodied dentist had as large and busy a practice as he was capable and willing to care for. The pent up need for dental treatment, occasioned by postponement of

regular care for the civilian component of society during the war, was another factor in the unprecedented demand for service. A natural corollary of the tremendous demand for the dentist's services was that he was forced more and more to rely on dental auxiliaries, so that he could devote his full energies to patient treatment. Since fabrication of the partial denture framework is a phase of dental practice well suited to delegation to a subprofessional, the typical practitioner tended to rely more and more on the commercial laboratory for this service. The dental laboratory industry rose to the challenge by offering an ever wider range of services to the profession, as well as an ongoing improvement in the caliber of craftsmanship. In assigning priorities to the various phases of his practice, the average dentist became increasingly preoccupied with the purely professional aspects of a busy clinical practice, and was inclined to depend more and more for laboratory assistance on a reliable commercial laboratory. This provided strong incentives for the laboratory to deliver a prosthesis that fit the mouth, could be worn with comfort, and was reasonably durable. The kind or type of alloy used to fabricate the framework became a matter of secondary importance, so long as the prosthesis provided the patient with satisfactory, trouble-free service. Certainly it must be conceded that the chromium-cobalt type alloys have this capability when properly designed and processed.

As the laboratories attained an ever higher degree of excellence in the processing of the chromium-cobalt alloy, they necessarily became more and more highly specialized, to a point where the entire partial denture operation was geared to the volume production of a framework made of the chromium-cobalt alloy for which they had the franchise. Chromium-cobalt could be quickly and efficiently fabricated at relatively moderate cost per unit by means of assembly line techniques while, in contrast, a gold framework must be processed as virtually a one-man, individually crafted operation, with the attendant inefficient use of time and higher cost to the laboratory. As a result of these economic imperatives, the typical franchised laboratory bases its prices on a fixed cost per unit for a framework cast of chromium-cobalt alloy and adds to that price a fixed surcharge for one fabricated of gold alloy. Another system of pricing in fairly common use is to add the cost of the gold used to make the casting to the price that would be charged if the framework were cast of chromium-cobalt. Either pricing method places the gold in an uncompetitive position from a standpoint of economics and discourages its use among customers of the franchised laboratories. The long term effect of these evolutionary events has been that most of the partial dentures produced are made of one of the chromium-cobalt alloys. Those made of gold alloy are, for the most part, made in the smaller laboratories of the large cities, or in the smaller communities where there is no franchised chromium-cobalt laboratory. A very few are made in the private laboratories of individual dentists.

In summary, both gold and chrome-cobalt alloys are eminently suited for fabrication of the partial denture framework. Due to economic imperatives, however, the great majority of partial dentures are fabricated of chromium-cobalt alloy.

A Comparison of Gold Alloy versus Chromium-Cobalt Alloy as a Material for the Framework

The physical properties of the two groups of alloys will be compared in the following paragraphs within a frame of reference of clinical application.

The Inherent Value of Gold

The fact that gold is a noble metal and that it always retains a scrap value is sometimes considered an advantage by the layman, since the chromium-cobalt alloys have virtually no scrap value at all. This reasoning will not bear logical analysis, however, because neither of these attributes makes the gold any more suitable for use in the prosthesis. Actually, the scrap value of the gold in dollars and cents is only a fraction of its cost to the

patient. Any such preoccupation by the patient with the cost of dental materials should be discouraged, since he is paying not for materials but for professional service.

Color

The color of a partial denture alloy per se neither adds nor detracts from its intrinsic value as the basic structure for an oral prosthesis. However, it can be a significant factor from a psychological standpoint. Traditionally, the yellow golds have always been equated with affluence in ancient as well as modern day cultures, representing an emotional attachment deeply rooted in history. Although gold may have lost some of its former prestige in the eyes of the average American, it is still generally preferred over a white or silver metal such as a chromium-cobalt alloy. When metal must be displayed in the anterior part of the mouth, this factor may become a matter of pivotal importance. If the design of a partial denture is such that the individual must display a metal clasp, and if he is given an opportunity to express a choice, most individuals will indicate a preference for gold. It is worth noting, in this regard, that a gold wrought wire of characteristic yellow-gold color can be attached to a chromium-cobalt framework for a labial or buccal clasp arm when there is no way to avoid its display.

Corrosion and Tarnish Resistance

The resistance of an alloy to staining or corrosion is extremely important for an alloy that must be exposed to oral fluids, which typically vary over a comparatively wide range of acidity and alkalinity. By virtue of the physical properties of their constituent metals, the chromium-cobalt alloys are extremely resistant to surface attack by the oral fluids. The gold alloys may be rated satisfactory in this respect, although tarnish and discoloration of gold alloys are by no means unknown clinically. Individual body chemistry, in particular that of the saliva, is thought to play an important role in the resistance (or lack of it) to tarnish, which probably accounts for the fact that a gold alloy will tarnish rather quickly in one mouth while maintaining indefinitely its brilliance and luster in another. Also worthy of note is the fact that diet may also be a factor. In a comparison of the two alloys, the chromium alloys must be conceded to be superior to golds in tarnish resistance.

Specific Gravity

Specific gravity is the weight of a unit of a material compared with an equal volume of water at the same temperature. The specific gravity of the chromium-cobalt alloys is approximately half that of gold alloys. This can be an important consideration in planning the design of a partial denture where maximum support is needed but minimum bulk is desired. It should be pointed out that another physical property plays an important part in any discussion of strength versus bulk, i.e., modulus of elasticity (discussed in a succeeding paragraph). However, considering specific gravity alone for the moment, the chromium alloys possess a distinct advantage over the golds in a maxillary prosthesis, because of their lighter weight. On the other hand, the higher specific gravity of the golds might be considered an advantage for the mandibular denture in instances where the greater weight might be thought to contribute a stabilizing effect.

Hardness

Hardness is a measure of an alloy's resistance to indentation, marring, or scratching. The hardness of gold alloys is measured on the Brinell scale of hardness, while that of the chromium-cobalt alloys is given as a Rockwell hardness number. While conversion between these two scales is not entirely satisfactory in terms of precise comparisons, it is generally conceded that the chromium-cobalt alloys have a hardness number approximately one-third greater than that of the type "IV" casting gold alloys.

Hardness has significance in assessing a partial denture alloy from the following aspects: (1) its resistance to marring or scratching, (2) its potential harmful effects on the abutment tooth, (3) its effect when the metal is used as a biting surface, and (4) the ease with which it can be polished following an adjustment.

Resistance to Scratching. A rough, marred, or scratched surface is much more susceptible to surface staining, as well as to the adherence of debris. Therefore, a high degree of hardness of an alloy can be counted an advantage. Both alloys are satisfactory in this regard.

Potential Harmful Effects on the Abutment Tooth. It must be recognized that an overly hard surface might conceivably scratch, or otherwise damage, the enamel of the abutment tooth or the surface of a metal restoration. The hardness of neither gold nor chromium-cobalt is harmful to enamel, and neither will scratch a gold or porcelain restoration. It is clinically significant, however, that both gold and chromium-cobalt will scratch and mar silver amalgam if placed in direct contact with it.

Use of the Alloy as a Biting Surface. When occlusal overlays make up an integral part of the framework or when a small edentulous space is restored with a metal tooth, the extreme hardness of the chromium-cobalt alloy, as a biting surface for the opposing teeth, must be counted a disadvantage. The relatively softer gold alloy would provide a more physiologically compatible biting surface, although it most be conceded that the weight factor would be disadvantageous. Finally, the gold would wear rather than the opposing tooth, whereas the opposite is true of the chromium-cobalt alloy.

Ease of Polishing. Still another aspect worthy of consideration is the fact that the hardness of the chromium-cobalt alloys makes them more difficult to smooth and polish following adjustments. Special abrasives and ultrahigh speed equipment (capable of turning a minimum of 20,000 rpm) are, in fact, required to accomplish the task properly. The fact that gold alloy can be smoothed and polished with equipment and materials readily available in the dental office must be considered a distinct advantage of the gold over the chromium-cobalt alloy.

In summary, hardness is an important physical property in a partial denture alloy. Both chromium-cobalt and gold have it in adequate amounts, although under some circumstances the relatively softer gold may be superior to the chromium-cobalt.

The Modulus of Elasticity

The modulus of elasticity is a measure of the stiffness of an alloy: one with a high modulus of elasticity being stiff, and one with a lower modulus being more flexible. Typical figures for the modulus of elasticity may range between 15×10^6 pounds per square inch for a gold alloy, to 32×10^6 for one of the chromium-cobalt alloys. From a clinical standpoint, this means that a cast clasp made of a gold alloy will be approximately twice as flexible as one of identical size, shape, and length made of a chromium-cobalt alloy. A flexible alloy will absorb more stress than one of little flexibility; and, therefore, it will transmit less stress to the abutment tooth. From a standpoint of flexibility of the retentive clasp arm, the gold must be acknowledged superior. However, it should not escape notice that the stiffer alloy would have a marked advantage in clasping a tooth surface which afforded only a bare minimum of usable undercut.

Flexibility may be considered a two-edged sword in a partial denture alloy—to be desired in a retentive clasp arm but to be avoided in a major connector. Certainly, the higher modulus of elasticity of the chrome must be counted a distinct advantage in the load bearing units of the framework, since they can be made thinner, hence less bulky, while still retaining the required degree of rigidity and strength. The property of high modulus of elasticity, coupled with lower specific gravity, makes chrome alloy superior in any circumstance where lightness and strength are needed together with minimum bulk (Fig. 20.1 and 20.2).

In summary, the higher modulus of elasticity of the chromium-cobalt alloy is a distinct advantage for fabricating the framework, with the exception of the retentive clasp terminal. This highlights the

advantage of the combination clasp in which the superiority of each of the two alloys is exploited: the lightness and strength of the chromium-cobalt combined with the resiliency and toughness of the gold alloy.

Yield Strength

The yield strength of an alloy is a measure of the stress to which it may be subjected without causing permanent de-

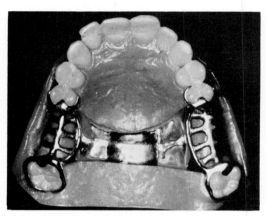

FIG. 20.1. The property of high modulus of elasticity, coupled with lower specific gravity, makes the chromium-cobalt alloy superior in any circumstance where lightness and strength are needed together with a minimum of bulk. This photograph shows a casting made of gold alloy. Note that it is somewhat more massive than the chromium-cobalt alloy framework shown in Figure 20.2.

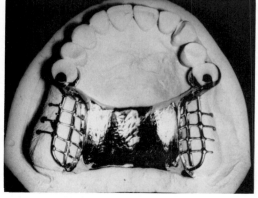

FIG. 20.2. The framework shown here is made of chromium-cobalt alloy. Note that it is somewhat smaller in bulk than the gold casting shown in Figure 20.1.

formation. The properties of proportional limit and elastic limit, while technically not the same as the yield strength, are very closely related from a standpoint of clinical performance of an alloy. A dental alloy with a low yield strength will possess also a low proportional limit as well as a low elastic limit and will not be suited for use in an oral prosthesis. Gold alloys and chromium-cobalt alloys for partial dentures have essentially similar properties of yield strength, which can be described fairly as completely adequate. Certainly, both have proven themselves eminently satisfactory in this regard, as attested by huge numbers of clinical successes. Failure of an alloy in service can almost always be attributed to laboratory error, faulty clinical judgment, or mishandling, rather than to any inherent weakness of the alloy itself.

Percentage Elongation

Percentage elongation is a measure of the ductility of an alloy, and relates to the degree of adjustment to which it may be subjected. In clinical terms, it can be regarded as the opposite of brittleness. Generally, the gold alloys are much more amenable to bending and rebending than are the chromium-cobalt alloys although, certainly, the chromium-cobalt alloys may be recontoured to a reasonable degree, provided the task is approached with a knowledge of their physical properties, and the bending force is applied with discretion. Since a properly heat-treated gold alloy clasp can be bent and reshaped with virtually no risk of breakage, the gold alloys must be accorded a rating superior to the chromium-cobalt alloys in this property.

Galvanic Potential

All metals can be placed on a scale of varying degrees of electromotive potential. Gold, platinum, and silver are high on the scale, whereas chromium, cobalt, tungsten, and nickel are lower. When two dissimilar metals are connected by means of an electrolyte (in the oral cavity the saliva), an electrical current may be set up between the two. This discovery was made by an Italian physician named Galvani, hence the term "galvanism." The strength of this electrical current, termed the electromotive force, as well as the effect that it produces in the mouth will depend, among other things, on the difference in electromotive potential of the two alloys. If the difference in electromotive potential is substantial, the patient may feel overt shock when they are brought into contact by an intervening film of saliva. If the difference is slight, the result may be slow deterioration of one or both of the metals by corrosion. Perhaps because of differences in salivary chemistry (pH is definitely a factor), some individuals are extremely susceptible to pain, discomfort, and damage to the oral structures from galvanism, while others whose oral cavities contain the same combinations of different alloys appear to be immune to the phenomenon. Fortunately, the alloy of the partial denture rarely creates a problem as a cause of galvanism, although it should not go unnoticed that the possibility does exist. If the two alloys are to be compared on the basis of potential problems as a result of galvanism, the chromium type alloy must be given the higher rating.

Availability of Service

An attribute more difficult to delineate, although certainly not lacking in import, might be termed the "repairability" of an alloy. If the prosthesis becomes bent, broken, or distorted in service, how difficult will it be for the patient to have it returned to a state of full usefulness? Any oral prosthesis, no matter how carefully designed and skillfully fabricated, is subject to deformation or breakage under certain circumstances. For this reason, a partial denture alloy should ideally be repairable in any well equipped dental office in any part of the world. In comparing the two alloys in this regard, the gold alloys must be accorded an unchallenged superiority. The reason for this is that fabrication or repair of the chromium dental alloys requires special materials and equipment not found in the average dental office, in addition to specially trained tech-

nicians found only in a franchised laboratory. Not only are the services of franchised laboratories not available in many
parts of the world, but they are not
readily accessible in areas of the United
States which happen to be located at a
considerable distance from the larger
cities. Thus, the alloy of choice is gold for
any person who resides in, or travels frequently to, an area of the globe where the
services of a franchised dental laboratory
are not available. Clearly, in an age when
global travel is commonplace, the repairability factor must be given due consideration in the best interests of the patient.

Ethical and Philosophical Considerations

A more nebulous, as well as frequently
overlooked, item of comparison between
the gold and chromium alloys relates to
certain ethical and philosophical considerations. Many conscientious practitioners
of dentistry feel that the franchise arrangement, by which the chromium-cobalt
alloys are proffered to the profession, in
effect deprives him of an important control of his practice. When he contracts
with a technician, not in his employ, for
fabrication of a prosthesis, he must temporarily surrender control of this link in
the treatment chain. The disadvantages of
such a working arrangement are all too
apparent. The dentist feels an ethical, as
well as a moral, obligation to provide
whatever care is needed by his patient to
the limit of his ability, and understandably looks askance at a modus operandi
which, in effect, transfers control of the
treatment to a third party. A classic example of the disadvantages of this shift of
control occurred in one large midwestern
city when virtually all of the commercial
dental laboratories ceased operations because of a labor-management dispute. The
prosthodontic activities of many dentists
were severely curtailed, if not virtually
stopped, during the many weeks required
to resolve labor-management differences.
This brings into focus not only the complete lack of control exercised by the
dental profession over the commercial
laboratory, but of even greater importance, demonstrates the fallacy of the

dentist becoming overly dependent on the
commercial laboratory. Closely related is
the question of the advisability of depending exclusively on the chromium-
cobalt alloys for fabrication of the partial
denture (Table 20.3, Summary Comparison).

Surgical Implants

Both Vitallium and Ticonium have for
many years been used for surgical implants. Vitallium is used more extensively
for this purpose than is Ticonium, having
been implanted successfully in virtually
every part of the human body. The principal use of the alloy in implantation is, of
course, in orthopedics. When used as an
implant, the chromium-cobalt formula is
modified by increasing the amount of mo-
lybdenum and decreasing the carbon. Both
alloys have been used for denture implants
with notable success. Although denture

TABLE 20.3.

A Summary Comparison of Physical Properties of Type IV Gold Alloy, and Chromium-Cobalt Alloy

Property	Gold Alloy	Chromium-Cobalt Alloy
Color	Superior	usually ade-quate
Corrosion resist-ance	usually ade-quate	outstanding
Weight (Specific Gravity)	specific gravity 16	specific gravity 8
Hardness	adequate	much harder but generally adequate
Modulus of elas-ticity	approximately half that of chromium-cobalt	approximately twice that of gold
Yield strength	completely ade-quate	completely ade-quate
Adjustability, repairability (percentage elongation)	superior	less than ideal
Galvanic poten-tial	usually low	very low
Availability of service	superior	poor

implant failures are certainly not unknown, none has ever been attributed to any shortcoming of the alloy itself, which certainly attests to its compatibility with the tissues of the body.

Heat Treatment of Partial Denture Alloys

Gold Alloy

Proper heat treatment or heat handling of gold alloy, either cast or wrought, is an integral part of the fabrication of a framework. Indeed, neglecting to heat treat is to invite almost certain failure. Desirable physical properties can be increased by an appreciable amount when proper methods are followed, and there is little doubt that improper heat handling is responsible for much of the breakage and failure of partial denture gold alloy in service. The term "heat treatment," in the broad sense, refers to the softening process (annealing), as well as the hardening process, although in more common parlance the term "heat treatment" is usually restricted to the hardening or tempering of the alloy. In general, when gold alloys are heated to 1300° F. (cherry-red) and then quenched in water, the alloy will be in its softest state. All physical properties will be decreased, with the exception of ductility and malleability which will be increased. Although the clasps are easiest to adjust in this softened state, the partial denture would not be strong enough for mouth service. If the alloy is heated to 840° F., allowed to cool slowly to 480° F., and quenched in water, it will be in its hardest state. All properties are thus increased, with the exception of ductility and malleability which are decreased. This is the condition that a partial denture prosthesis should be in for mouth service.

Chromium-Cobalt Alloy

The chromium-cobalt type of alloy cannot be alternately hardened and softened by the application of heat as is the case with the gold alloys. However, a precise heat treatment, which brings out the optimal properties of the alloy, is built into the technique of fabrication. Proper treatment of the metal by heat is accomplished by bench cooling the flask after casting, until it reaches a temperature at which it can comfortably be held in the hands. If a hot flask (shortly after casting the molten metal into the mold) were to be plunged into water, the metal would be rendered brittle and unfit for mouth service. Heat treatment is normally the responsibility of the laboratory and, in the normal course of events, the dentist need not be concerned with this phase of fabrication.

Bibliography

Akers, P. E.: A new and simplified method of partial denture prosthesis. J. Amer. Dent. Ass. *12:* 711–715, 1925.

Dental Laboratory Technician's Manual, AFM 160-29, Department of the Air Force. U.S. Government Printing Office, Washington, D.C., 1959.

Nesbett, N. B.: A simple form of removable bridgework with cast clasps. Dent. Cosmos *60:* 204–209, 1918.

Paffenbarger, G. C.: Bonding porcelain teeth to acrylic resin bases. J. Amer. Dent. Ass. *74:* 1018–1023, 1967.

Paffenbarger, G. C., Caul, H. J., and Dickson, G.: Base metal alloys for oral restoration. J. Amer. Dent. Ass. *30:* 852, 1943.

Phillips, R. W., and Leonard, L. J.: Study of enamel abrasion as related to partial denture clasps. J. Pros. Dent. *6:* 657–671, 1956.

Skinner, E. W., and Phillips, R. W.: *The Science of Dental Materials*. W. B. Saunders Company, Philadelphia, 1967.

Taylor, D. F., Leibfritz, W. A., and Adler, A. G.: Physical properties of chromium-cobalt dental alloys. J. Amer. Dent. Ass. *56:* 343–351, 1958.

Chapter 21

SYSTEMS FOR CLASSIFYING
THE PARTIALLY EDENTULOUS
ARCH

This chapter addresses itself to the subject of classification of the partially edentulous dental arch. Twelve of the systems that have been proposed to the profession by various writers are mentioned, and another, the Kennedy system, is described in some detail because it is the most widely used. The various systems are arranged in chronological order, and the subject matter is presented in the following manner.

Introduction
Historical Background
Synopses of the Systems

Introduction

There are more than 65,000 possible combinations of standing teeth and edentulous spaces which may be encountered in the human dental arch. It is not surprising, therefore, that a speaker or writer sometimes finds it cumbersome to convey, to the mind's eye of a listener or reader, a precise word picture of a particular dental arch that he wishes to discuss. Dental writers and educators have long felt that a system of classifying the partially edentulous arch would be an enormous aid in overcoming this semantic barrier, so that a given combination of spaces and teeth could conveniently be referred to by a class, rather than by a wordy description. Most scientific disciplines do, in fact, make use of classification systems to bring order out of a highly complex, seemingly heterogeneous, mixture—the

grouping of plants and animals (taxonomy) being a classic example. In dentistry, the classification of occlusions by Angle and of cavities by Black are used universally. Indeed, it is hard to envision a discussion concerning orthodontics or operative dentistry without them.

Two principal benefits might accrue from the universal adoption of such a system for prosthodontics. (1) It would open channels of communication between speaker and listener, otherwise obscured by ambiguity. A universally understood system of classification would enable the speaker or writer to communicate with much greater facility in describing an oral cavity in which missing teeth were to be replaced by a partial removable prosthesis. (2) It would contribute materially to the systemization of the art of partial denture design. A design that proved successful for a given combination of edentulous spaces and standing teeth could be employed, with perhaps minor modifications, for another mouth with a similar combination of spaces and teeth. Thus, basic design principles could be formulated which might be applied to other arches of the same classification.

Historical Background

The fact that there is no universally employed classification system in widespread use throughout the profession is not because none has been conceived and recommended. On the contrary, the dental literature abounds with proposed systems for classifying the partially edentulous arch, beginning with the one conceived by Cummer which is the earliest on record. Although most of these have obvious merit, and all have had supporters, none has been without critics and detractors too, with the result that no one system has enjoyed anything like unanimous acceptance. As a result, the subject has become so muddled and confused that if one employs the terminology of a particular classification to describe a dental arch, he must append the system to which he has reference, to be sure that he is understood.

The following paragraphs mention briefly the systems of classification which have been offered to the profession by various writers, beginning with the one advocated by Cummer in 1920. The Kennedy system is described in some detail, since it is the one most universally used throughout the United States.

Synopses of the Systems

Cummer's System

The first system to receive recognition from the profession was one proposed by Dr. W. E. Cummer in 1921. By mathematical computations Cummer calculated that some 65,534 possible combinations of teeth, present and missing, can occur in each jaw. Because of the anatomical differences between the maxilla and mandible, it would seem logical to double the figure, until it is remembered that a pattern of teeth and edentulous spaces appearing on one side of a dental arch is a mirror image of one occurring on the contralateral side. Cummer believed that the possible combinations and their classifications had a particular relevance to partial denture design and that, therefore, a good classification system would simplify immensely the development of sound and universally applicable design principles. He believed too that all partially edentulous dental arches could be classified into one of four classes. Although the Cummer system was never widely used, it did unquestionably influence thinking on the subject and has undoubtedly provided an

inspirational wellspring for many of the classification systems that have been proposed since the article first appeared in print. Cummer's proposal must be considered one of the classic essays on the subject.

The Kennedy System

Just a few years later (1923), Dr. Edward Kennedy proposed an entirely different method of classification from the one advocated by Cummer. Kennedy foresaw the benefits which could be derived from the adoption of a system which would create a common language, thus facilitating the exchange of opinion and knowledge between members of the profession. His system makes it possible to place any partially edentulous arch into one of four groups, with a few subdivisions (modifications) under each group. The system is based on the relationships of the edentulous spaces to the abutment teeth. The four classes and their modifications are illustrated in Figures 21.1 through 21.4. There are no modifications of Class IV, because if more than one space is present in a dental arch it would fall into one of the other classifications. The Kennedy method of classification is the best known of all systems that have been proposed through the years, and is more widely used than any other. It also enjoys the distinction of forming the basis for at least two other systems which have been advocated in more recent years by writers in the partial denture field (Applegate-Kennedy system and Swenson system).

Bailyn's System

In 1928 Dr. Charles M. Bailyn introduced a classification system based on whether the prosthesis is tooth borne, tissue borne, or a combination of the two. While Bailyn acknowledged that the systems of both Cummer and Kennedy were helpful, he believed that the profession still needed a system in which mere mention of the class would evoke the rules of procedure for prosthesis design. Although he felt that his system fulfilled this requirement, it did not gain a wide following.

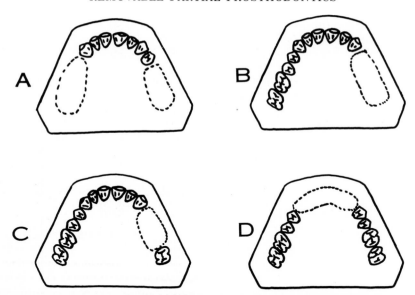

FIG. 21.1. The Kennedy Classification System: *A*, Class I, bilateral edentulous areas posterior to the remaining teeth. *B*, Class II, a unilateral edentulous area posterior to the remaining teeth. *C*, Class III, a unilateral edentulous area with teeth anterior and posterior to it. *D*, Class IV, an edentulous area anterior to the remaining teeth.

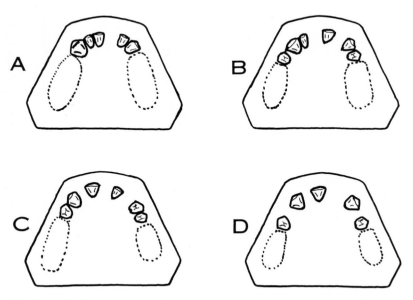

FIG. 21.2. The Kennedy Classification System: modifications of Class I. *A*, Modification I, an edentulous space in addition to one(s) calling for the original classification. *B*, Modification II, two edentulous spaces in addition to the basic class. *C*, Modification III, three edentulous spaces in addition to the basic class. *D*, Modification IV, four edentulous spaces in addition to the basic class.

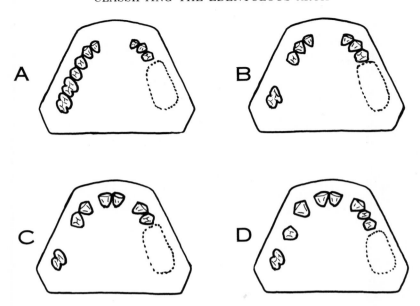

FIG. 21.3. The Kennedy Classification System: modifications of Class II. *A*, Modification I, one edentulous space in addition to the basic classification. *B*, Modification II, two edentulous spaces in addition to the basic class. *C*, Modification III, three edentulous spaces in addition to the basic class. *D*, Modification IV, four edentulous spaces in addition to the basic class.

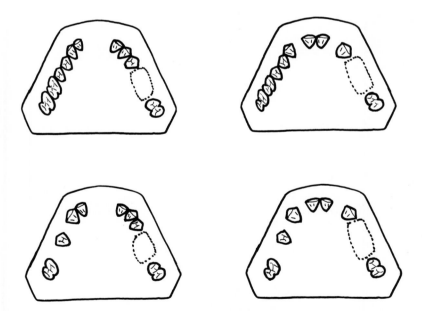

FIG. 21.4. The Kennedy Classification System: modifications of the Class III. *A*, Modification I, one edentulous space in addition to the basic class. *B*, Modification II, two edentulous spaces in addition to the basic class. *C*, Modification III, three edentulous spaces in addition to the basic class. *D*, Modification IV, four edentulous spaces in addition to the basic class.

Neurohr's System

Dr. Ferdinand Neurohr, in his textbook "Partial Dentures" published in 1939, devoted an entire chapter to the subject of classification of the partially edentulous jaw. He described the difficulties in communication which he frequently experienced as a lecturer and clinician when a member of the audience requested an opinion in regard to proper treatment of a specific partial denture case. Although Neurohr sought to simplify the classification process, the system which he proposed is actually one of the most complex to be found in the dental literature.

Mauk's System

In 1941 Dr. Edwin H. Mauk offered the profession a system of classification which evolved following a study of 1000 casts of partially edentulous arches. While Mauk conceded that his system was somewhat lacking in statistical and mathematical completeness, he believed that it could be used to identify the type of cases which it would be feasible to treat by means of removable partial dentures. His system is based on (1) the number, length, and position of the spaces, and (2) the number and position of the remaining teeth. The Mauk System did not receive wide recognition.

Godfrey's System

In 1951 Dr. R. J. Godfrey described the classification system which was taught and used at the University of Toronto at that time. The system is based on the location and extent of the edentulous spaces where teeth are to be replaced on the bases. A feature of Dr. Godfrey's system is that there are no subdivisions or modifications to the main classes. The system did not attain widespread use.

Beckett's System

In 1953 Dr. Leonard S. Beckett of the University of Sydney (Australia) proposed a system which, like the one proposed by Bailyn, is based on whether the saddle is tooth borne, tissue borne, or a combination of the two. The three basic classifications were: Class I, bases which are tooth borne; Class II, bases which are mucosa borne; and Class III, inadequate abutments to support the base. Dr. Beckett's system did not attract wide attention or usage in this country.

Friedman's System

Dr. Joel Friedman introduced a system in 1953 which he based on three essential segment types. The letter "A" designates an anterior space, i.e., one or more of the six anterior teeth. The letter "B" designates a bounded posterior space. The letter "C" refers to a cantilever situation or a posterior free end space. Friedman's proposal is referred to in several articles to be found in the literature on the subject of classification. However, it did not attract a large following and is not widely used.

The Austin-Lidge System

Austin and Lidge offered a system based on missing teeth or edentulous spaces. In this system the letter "A" is used to designate an anterior space or spaces, "P" for posterior spaces, and "Bi" to designate a bilateral condition. Various combinations of standing teeth and spaces can thus be designated such as A2P1, or A1P2, and so on. The system did not become widely known or adopted.

Skinner's System

In 1957 Dr. C. N. Skinner offered the profession a system of classification based on the relationship of the abutment teeth to the supporting residual ridge. He reasoned that since the value of a removable partial denture is directly related to the quality and degree of support which it receives from abutment teeth and the residual ridge, a classification system should be based on these factors. Therefore, he felt that these same elements should be guiding factors in the design and structuring of the prosthesis. The system advocated by Skinner is not widely used.

The Applegate-Kennedy System

Dr. Oliver C. Applegate emphasized the urgent need for a system of classification which would gain universal acceptance and wide usage. He felt that a system based solely on the number and location of the remaining teeth is less meaningful than one that takes into account the capability of the teeth which bound the edentulous space to act as abutments. Accordingly, the classification should be decided after final determination of the abutments which are to be employed in the design. Applegate contends that the system which he proposed is so closely interrelated with recognized design principles that the classification of a dental arch by his method thus becomes almost automatically the basis for the proper design of that prosthesis.

Swenson's System

The Swenson system is based on the Kennedy system. The four primary classes are very similar to those of Kennedy, whereas the modifications are more drastically dissimiler. The system did not attract a large following.

Avant's System

In 1966 Dr. W. E. Avant proposed a classification based on the requirements that a system should satisfy in order to meet with universal acceptance. According to Avant, such a system should enable one to (1) visualize the type of partially edentulous arch represented, (2) differentiate between potential tooth borne and extension base partial dentures, (3) get a general idea of the type of partial denture design to be used, and (4) know the general location of the teeth being replaced.

In the Avant system the dental arch is divided into three segments or groups of teeth, two posterior and one anterior. With this as a basis, all partially edentulous dental arches can be classified into one of five groups.

Bibliography

Angle, E. H.: Classification of malocclusion. Dent. Cosmos *41:* 248–264, 1899.

Applegate, O. C.: *Essentials of Removable Partial Denture Prosthesis.* Ed. 3. W. B. Saunders Company, Philadelphia, 1965.

Austin, K. P., and Lidge, E. F.: *Partial Dentures.* The C. V. Mosby Company, St. Louis, 1957.

Avant, W. E.: A universal classification for removable partial denture situations. J. Prosth. Dent. *16:* 533–539, 1966.

Bailyn, C. M.: Tissue support in partial denture construction. Dent. Cosmos *70:* 988–997, 1928.

Beckett, L. S.: The influence of saddle classification on the design of partial removable restorations. J. Prosth. Dent. *3:* 506–516, 1953.

Black, G. V. and Blackwell, R. E.: Operative Dentistry, Ed. 9, Vol. 2. Medico-Dental Publishing Co., Milwaukee, 1955.

Cummer, W. E.: Possible combinations of teeth present and missing in partial restorations. Oral Health *10:* 421–430, 1920.

Friedman, J.: The ABC classification of partial denture segments. J. Prosth. Dent. *3:* 517–524, 1953.

Godfrey, R. J.: A classification of removable partial dentures. J. Amer. Coll. Dent. *18:* 5–13, 1951.

Kennedy, E.: *Partial Denture Construction,* Ed. 2. Dental Items of Interest Publishing Company, Brooklyn, 1951.

Mauk, E. H.: Classification of mutilated dental arches requiring treatment by removable partial dentures. J. Amer. Dent. Ass. *29:* 2121–2131, 1942.

Miller, E. L.: Systems for classifying partially dentulous arches. J. Prosth. Dent. *24:* 25–40, 1970.

Neurohr, F.: *Partial Dentures.* Lea & Febiger, Philadelphia, 1939.

Skinner, C. N.: A classification of removable partial dentures based upon the principles of anatomy and physiology. J. Prosth. Dent. *9:* 240–246, 1959.

Terkla, L. G., and Laney, W. R.: *Partial Dentures,* Ed. 3. The C. V. Mosby Company, St. Louis, 1963.

Chapter 22

A PHOTOGRAPHIC SUMMARY OF CLINICAL PROCEDURES

This chapter presents a pictorial summary of the salient clinical steps which may be followed in the construction of a removable partial denture. The photographs depict one workable sequence of procedures which demonstrate a variety of clinical techniques. The various steps are presented in the order listed.

The Impression
The Study Cast
Establishing Occlusal Relations
The Facebow Transfer
Analysis, Survey, and Design of the Study Cast
Formulation of the Treatment Plan
Mouth Preparation
The Final Impression, The Master Cast
Definitive Design of the Framework
The Functional Impression, The Altered Cast
Functionally Generated Pathways
Articulation of the Prosthetic Teeth

Processing and Finishing the Denture
Insertion and Counseling

Introduction

The particular techniques here portrayed were not chosen because they represent a modus operandi favored for all partial denture construction, but rather because this particular sequence of steps demonstrates a variety of commonly employed clinical methods. The most suitable combination of techniques for construction of a given removable partial denture will vary according to the unique features of each mouth, the type of prosthesis or combination of prostheses being constructed, and the characteristics of the individual patient.

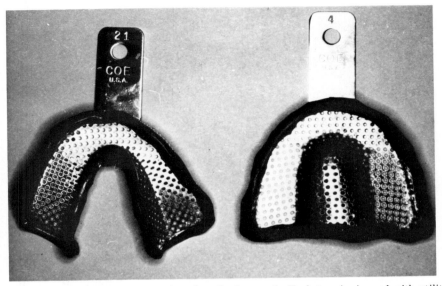

FIG. 22.1. Stock impression trays are selected to fit the mouth. Each tray is rimmed with utility wax to improve the fit.

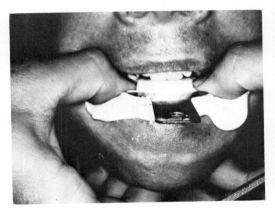

FIG. 22.2. The mandibular impression is customarily obtained first because it is usually better tolerated by a patient who is experiencing the impression procedure for the first time.

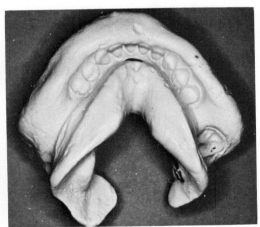

FIG. 22.3. The impression is inspected under a good light for flaws and defects which might disqualify it for use for a planning cast. Saliva should be blown out of the depths of the impression with a gentle stream of air to facilitate the inspection.

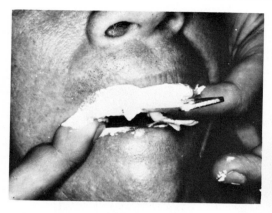

Fig. 22.4. The patient should be in an upright position with the occlusal plane approximately parallel with the floor for the maxillary impression which is obtained next.

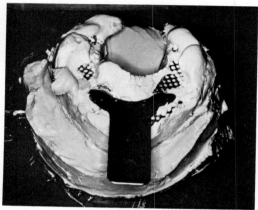

Fig. 22.6. The mandibular cast is poured by the two-step method. The impression is filled with stone and set aside until the stone has reached an initial set. When it has reached this point a patty of soft stone approximately 4 x 4 x 1 inch thick is formed and the impression is inverted onto it.

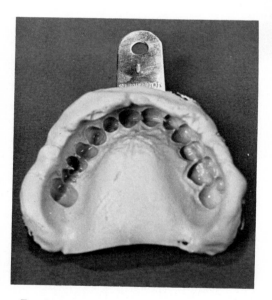

Fig. 22.5. The maxillary impression is inspected for defects.

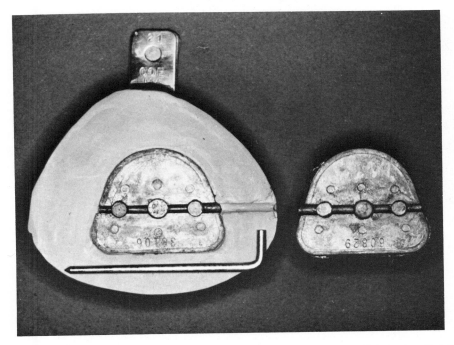

FIG. 22.7. A split remounting plate may be embedded in the base of the cast if desired so that it may be easily and quickly removed from the articulator, placed on the surveyor for analysis, and then returned to the articulator.

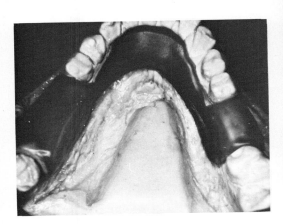

FIG. 22.8. A shellac (or gutta-percha) baseplate is adapted to the mandibular cast.

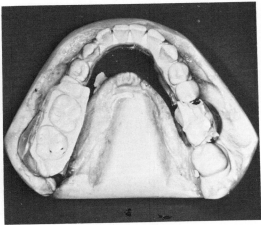

FIG. 22.9. Wax occlusion rims are attached and adjusted in the mouth to support a soft bite registration material such as zinc oxide paste, and centric occlusion is registered.

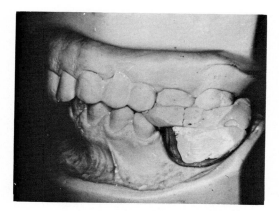

FIG. 22.10. The two casts are related to each other in centric occlusion by means of the checkbite.

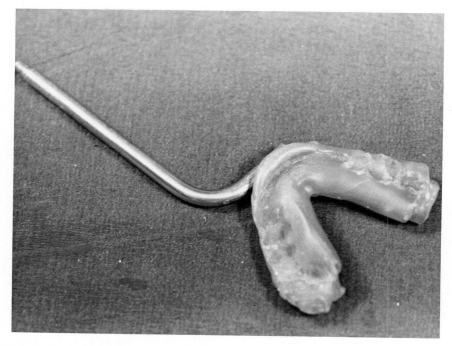

FIG. 22.11. A clutch of baseplate wax (or of modeling composition) is attached to the bitefork, and an index of the occlusal surfaces of the maxillary teeth is made in the softened wax.

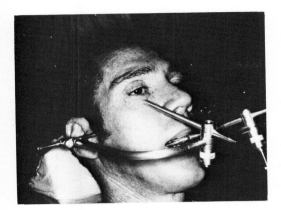

FIG. 22.12. The wax clutch is positioned on the maxillary teeth and attached to the facebow preparatory to transfer to the articulator.

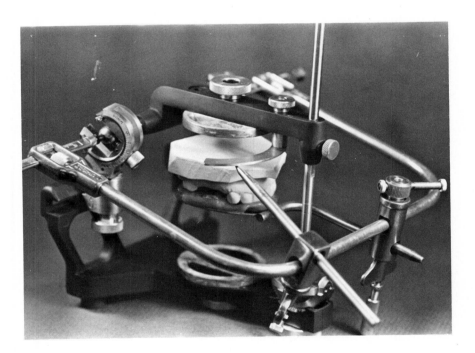

FIG. 22.13. The maxillary cast is transferred to the articulator.

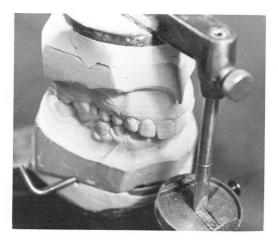

FIG. 22.14. The casts are attached to the articulator with plaster. Note the key for the split remounting plate extending from the junction of the mandibular cast and its plaster mounting.

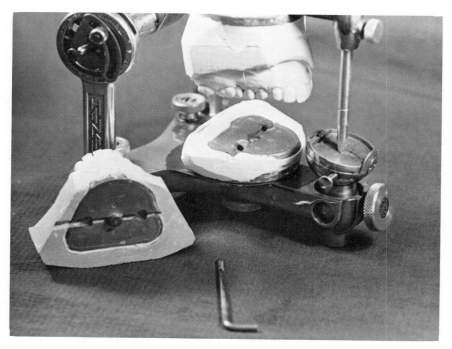

FIG. 22.15. The lower cast has been removed from its mounting on the articulator. It can be easily mounted on the cast holder of the surveyor while the surveying procedure is accomplished, then quickly removed and returned to its former position on the articulator.

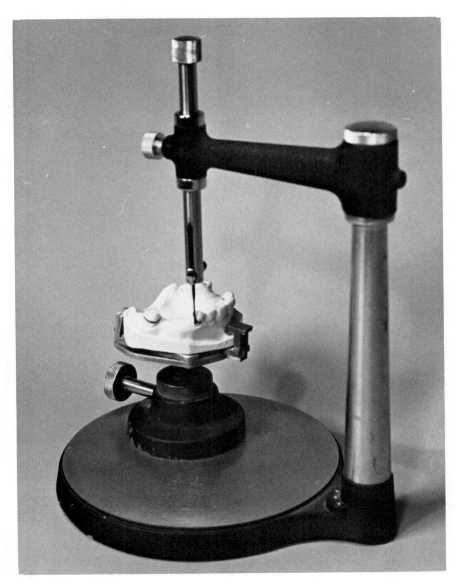

FIG. 22.16. The path of insertion is established, and the design of the partial denture is decided upon following analysis of the study cast.

UNIVERSITY OF ALABAMA
SCHOOL OF DENTISTRY

DIAGNOSIS AND TREATMENT PLAN

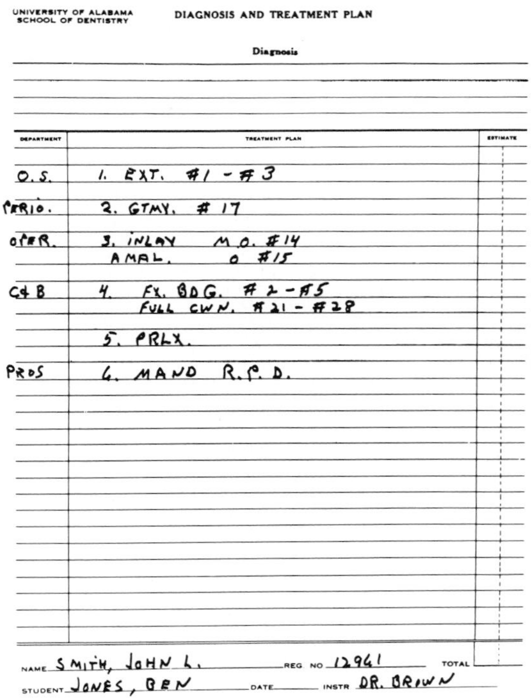

Diagnosis

DEPARTMENT	TREATMENT PLAN	ESTIMATE
O.S.	1. EXT. #1 - #3	
PERIO.	2. GTMY. # 17	
OPER.	3. INLAY M.O. #14	
	AMAL. O #15	
C&B	4. FX. BDG. # 2 - #5	
	FULL CWN. # 21 - #28	
	5. PRLX.	
PROS	6. MAND R.P.D.	

NAME SMITH, JOHN L. REG NO 12961 TOTAL
STUDENT JONES, BEN DATE INSTR DR. BROWN

FIG. 22.17. The treatment plan is formulated, listing all of the treatment that is to be accomplished in the sequence that it is to be performed.

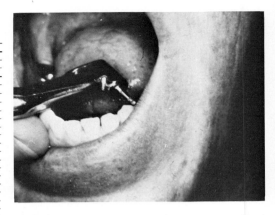

FIG. 22.19. All necessary treatment is completed and tooth alterations are accomplished.

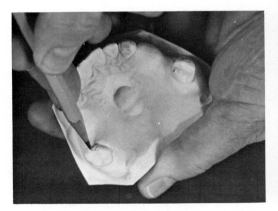

FIG. 22.18. The study cast can be used as a blueprint upon which to make notations of the tooth alterations (rest preparations, guiding planes, and reductions in contour) that are to be performed on the teeth.

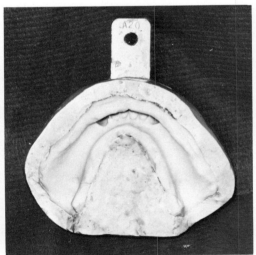

FIG. 22.20. The final mandibular impression is obtained in alginate type hydrocolloid. It is embedded in "complaster" so that it can be boxed preparatory to pouring the master cast.

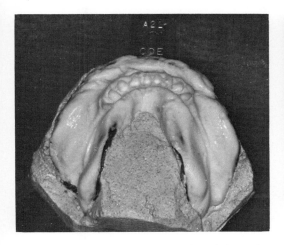

FIG. 22.21. The complaster is shaped into the configuration desired of the cast. Boxing wax is wrapped around it and sealed to the complaster with hot wax to form a matrix for the gypsum material.

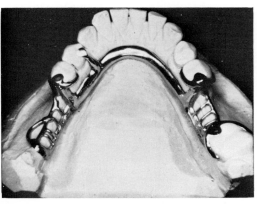

FIG. 22.23. The metal framework is returned from the laboratory on the master cast. The tissue side of the framework should be carefully inspected under good light and magnification for blebs or artifacts. If any are present, they should be removed before it is tried in the mouth.

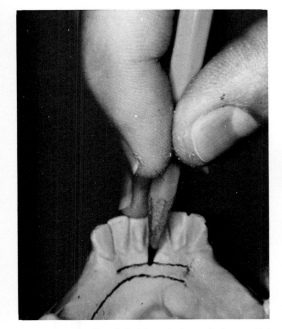

FIG. 22.22. The definitive design of the partial denture is sketched on the *study cast* (*not the master cast*). The laboratory authorization is prepared to include any special instructions to the laboratory technician that will aid him in accomplishing the tasks for which he is responsible.

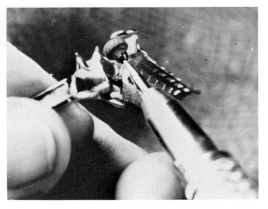

FIG. 22.24. The metal framework is fitted to the mouth in two separate steps: (1) fitting the framework to the teeth and (2) adjusting it to the opposing occlusion.

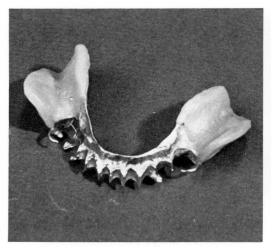

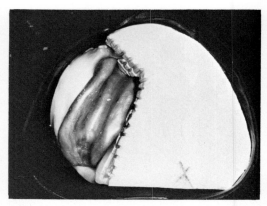

FIG. 22.27. The framework is placed in position on the master cast and the impression boxed with wax.

FIG. 22.25. When the denture has a distal extension base, an impression base of acrylic resin is attached to the retention latticework of the framework. The borders of the impression base are adapted to the peripheral tissues by border molding with modeling composition. A functional impression is then obtained in low fusing wax, rubber, or zinc oxide paste.

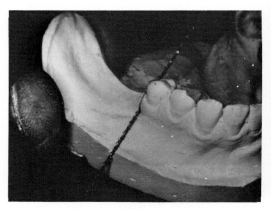

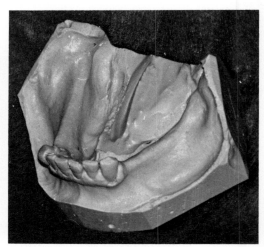

FIG. 22.26. The portion of the master cast that is destined to support the distal extension base is separated from the cast with a plaster saw.

FIG. 22.28. The impression is poured in stone (of a different color than the cast) to produce the altered master cast.

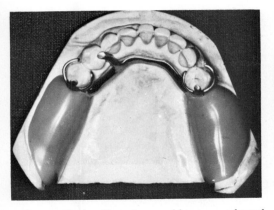

FIG. 22.29. Acrylic resin record bases are adapted to the edentulous portions of the cast and attached to the retention latticework of the framework.

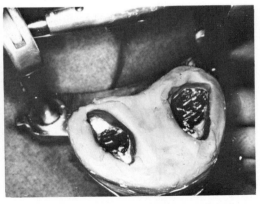

FIG. 22.31. The functionally generated pathways are enveloped in wax or modeling clay to form a matrix, and the mandibular cast is mounted on an articulator or jig. If an articulator is employed, the condyles should be locked in centric position so that movement of the articulator is restricted to opening and closing movements.

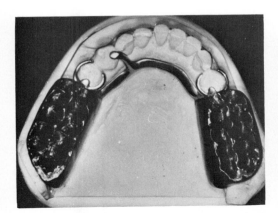

FIG. 22.30. Occlusion rims of hard inlay wax are attached to the record bases. The patient is instructed to chew and make simulated functional movements so as to create pathways in the wax with the natural teeth which oppose the edentulous space(s).

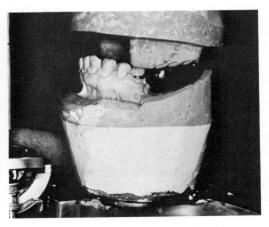

FIG. 22.32. The pathways are reproduced in stone and attached to the upper member of the articulator or jig.

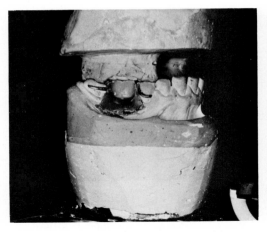

Fig. 22.33. Prosthetic teeth are arranged to articulate with the opposing stone pathways.

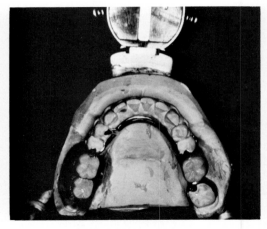

Fig. 22.35. When the teeth have been arranged to
articulate with the stone pathways the denture is
waxed and processed in the usual manner.

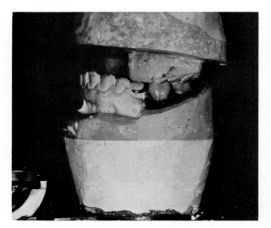

Fig. 22.34. Intercuspation is refined by marking
the prosthetic teeth with a marking medium such as
articulating paper or typewriter ribbon and grinding
the occlusal surfaces as indicated by the marks.

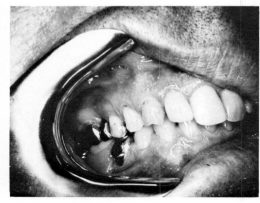

Fig. 22.36. The denture is inserted in the mouth.
Final adjustments are made to the bases and to the
occlusion.

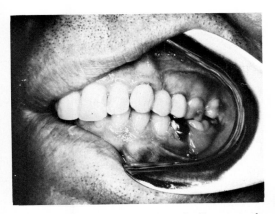

FIG. 22.37. Following any needed adjustments the denture is given a final polish, being sure to restore the surface smoothness of any teeth that have been altered by grinding.

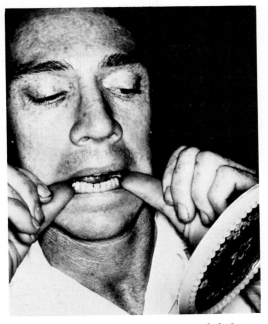

FIG. 22.38. The patient is instructed before a mirror in the proper manner of inserting and removing the prosthesis and is given individualized instruction in home care to best cope with the problems posed by his particular mouth and his prosthesis.

Chapter 23

DENTAL LABORATORY RELATIONS

This chapter is concerned with the working relationship between dentist and laboratory technician as each accomplishes his part of the fabrication of the prosthesis. The subject is discussed under the following topic headings.

Introduction
Reasons for a Lack of Accord
Establishing a Good Working Relationship
Responsibilities of the Dentist
Responsibilities of the Technician
Establishing Rapport
Legal, Ethical, and Moral Imperatives

Introduction

One consequence of the accelerating pace of modern day living and the increasingly heavy work load of the average dentist is that it has become a hallmark of good practice management to delegate an ever greater number of subprofessional tasks to auxiliary personnel. Since so many of the procedures in the construction of an oral prosthesis are performed in the dental laboratory, this phase of dental practice lends itself especially well to a partnership type of working arrangement. Because of the intermingled nature of the various steps performed by dentist and laboratory technician, the association between the two is, perforce, one of mutual interdependence. The quality of the output of each is quite literally dependent upon that of the other. Since each partner is so utterly dependent on the workmanship and integrity of the other, it is apparent that the alliance, if it is to be successful, needs to be a harmonious one, based on mutual respect and trust. Unfortunately, this happy state of

affairs does not always exist, and when the association is not a harmonious one, one of the predictable consequences is a lowering of quality of the prosthetic service provided for the patient.

Reasons for a Lack of Accord

The reasons for a lack of close accord are enormously diverse but, like most contentious matters, the root cause is misunderstanding. There is an abundance of evidence to indicate that a part of the blame must be shared by each side.

The failure on the part of some in the dental profession to understand fully the laboratory technician's rightful status as a partner on the dental health team is epitomized by two groups who hold extremist, although widely divergent, views concerning the role that he should play. One group regards the technician as a poorly educated, inadequately trained, menial, whose integrity often is open to question and whose every move must be closely supervised. The other group regards him as a father figure to whom can be delegated virtually all of the responsibility for construction of the prosthesis (once the impressions have been made), and to whom all problems associated with the prosthesis can be referred for solution. Obviously, both of these misconceptions are wide of the mark and, certainly, neither attitude can form the basis for a working relationship that is optimally effective and mutually gratifying.

Establishing a Good Working Relationship

A good working relationship must be based on a common understanding of the overall objectives, an awareness of the

338

rightful role that each must play in attaining the goals, and an appreciation of the particular problems peculiar to each sphere of activity. Ideally, to this will be added a sincere respect for the competence, sincerity, and basic honesty of the other partner. With this as a basis, operating guidelines for the partnership can be established within a framework of (1) legal imperatives, (2) ethical considerations, and (3) principles of sound business management.

Legal Imperatives

There are no federal statutes governing the operation of the commercial dental laboratory, or the working agreements between the dentist and technician. This authority is vested, instead, in the individual states. Most states have laws which stipulate a certain code of behavior for both parties. Generally, the laws stipulate that (1) the technician cannot render any service directly for the patient, and (2) he can legally perform only work authorized by the dentist. As a means of implementing this arrangement most states require that the technician perform laboratory services only when he has been authorized to do so by means of a written order from the dentist. The authorizing document is referred to, in some states, as a "prescription," and in others as a "work authorization." Whatever the appellation, its primary purpose is to protect the patient from being victimized by a person not qualified or licensed to practice dentistry. Both members of the partnership, therefore, have a responsibility to comply with both the letter and the spirit of the law by properly employing the required form.

Ethics

Section 6 of the Code of Ethics of the American Dental Association states: "The dentist has an obligation to protect the health of his patient by not delegating to a person less qualified any service or operation which requires the professional competence of a dentist. The dentist has a further obligation of supervising the work of all auxiliary personnel in the interests of rendering the best service to the patient."

It should be clear from the foregoing that the dentist must bear the ultimate responsibility for the patient's treatment. Although the contribution made by the laboratory technician is a significant one, he is responsible only to the dentist, never to the patient.

Applying Business Principles

A fundamental of good management is that each member of a partnership be assigned well defined responsibilities. Accordingly, there should be no reasonable doubt as to the tasks that each member of the dental health team is responsible for and, in the case of the laboratory technician, the manner in which each procedure is to be accomplished.

Responsibilities of the Dentist

The dentist must plan the prosthesis in its entirety. He must foresee the need for all preparatory mouth treatment, and ensure that it is properly accomplished. It is his responsibility to see that sufficient space is available for each structural element of the prosthesis, as well as for conditions which make possible the restoration of an acceptable occlusal plane. He must ensure that abutment teeth are properly contoured with guiding planes, retentive undercuts, and rest recesses to accommodate the types of clasps which he prescribes. In addition to prescribing the materials for the metal framework and the denture base, he must specify the composition, mold, and shade of the replacement teeth that are to be used. His is the responsibility to fit the finished prosthesis to the mouth, and to instruct the patient in its care. Finally, he must perform the necessary postinsertion adjustments and stand by to accomplish the periodic maintenance and refitting.

Responsibilities of the Technician

The technician, for his part, is responsible for the fabrication of the prosthesis with materials of the highest quality, in compliance with the directions provided on the work authorization form (or prescription), and supplemented by the blueprint drawn on the planning cast by the dentist. In addition, he is responsible for accomplishing many of the intermediate steps in accordance with the dentist's instructions as the treatment progresses through the various stages of fabrication.

Establishing Rapport

The purpose of the team approach is to utilize best the special talents of two highly trained specialists in rendering for the patient a prosthetic service of the highest quality. If the team is to achieve this objective consistently, the association not only must be a profitable one but also it must reward each participant with a sense of fulfillment. Generally, it may be said that establishing and maintaining a working relationship on this plane will require that the dentist take the initiative in assuming his rightful role of leadership and in insisting that the technician, in turn, understand and accept the responsibilities that are rightfully his.

Getting Acquainted

The dentist should, by all means, visit the laboratory that he has chosen for a partner, so that he can become personally acquainted with the staff and can familiarize himself with their methods of operation. Much worthwhile information can thus be exchanged for the edification of both parties; information that can contribute immeasurably to the success of the combined effort. The dentist will want to know the types and the scope of the services that the laboratory is staffed and equipped to offer. He will want to know about the time schedules required for completing the different laboratory procedures, as well as the fees that will be charged, and he will want to know the most expeditious means of transporting the work between the laboratory and the dental office.

The laboratory, for its part, needs to know the techniques that the dentist will employ in the various phases of prosthodontics, so that they can best gear the laboratory support to complement them.

The Work Authorization

The purpose of the document by which the dentist authorizes the laboratory work is (1) to provide the laboratory with clear, concise, readily understandable instructions concerning the work to be done and (2) to protect the patient from the illegal practice of dentistry. The form used for this purpose should, of course, be designed to comply with state laws. The format of the document should be such that most information dealing with the specifics of design and construction can be conveyed by means of checkmarks, so as to be readily understandable while requiring only a minimum of writing.

The importance of the proper use of this document to the dental profession, the dental laboratory industry, and the public can hardly be overemphasized.

Legal, Ethical, and Moral Imperatives

The prime purpose of the ethical code and the legal statutes is to safeguard the health and well being of the public. The dentist who does not honor this public trust by assuming his full responsibilities is derelict. Should such irresponsibility become widespread, there will be pressure from the public to change the laws so that this phase of dental practice can be rendered by another group; a group which, although not qualified by education, training, or experience, is, nonetheless, ready and willing to shoulder this responsibility and to accept the rewards which go with it.

Bibliography

Brown, E. T.: The dentist, the laboratory technician, and the prescription law. J. Prosth. Dent. *15:* 1132–1138, 1965.

Gehl, D. H.: Investment in the future. J. Prosth. Dent. *18:* 190–201, 1967.

Henderson, D.: Writing work authorizations for removable partial dentures. J. Prosth. Dent. *16:* 696–707, 1966.

Glossary

PROSTHODONTIC TERMS ESPECIALLY RELEVANT TO REMOVABLE PARTIAL PROSTHODONTICS

A mutually understood terminology is essential to clear understanding between the dentist and his assistant, his laboratory technician, and his hygienist, as well as with his professional colleagues. Certainly, it is an absolutely vital link between teacher and student. The purpose of this glossary is to provide the student with a ready reference which will assist him in acquiring a working vocabulary of technical terms in the shortest possible time. As the ancient Chinese proverb puts it, "The beginning of wisdom is the calling of things by their right names."

A

ablate—To remove by cutting. To eliminate by surgery.

abrasion—The wearing, grinding, or rubbing away of a substance by friction.

absorption—The soaking up of one substance by another. *Example:* A stone cast, placed in water, absorbs the water.

abut—To position the surface of one object directly against another object or surface.

abutment—The tooth which acts as an anchor for the partial denture. The tooth upon which the clasp or retainer is placed to retain, support, and stabilize the removable partial denture.

accelerator—An agent which speeds up a chemical reaction.

acrylic resin—The plastic resin widely em-

ployed to form the base of the denture. Chemically, methyl-methacrylate.

acquired centric occlusion—Refers to a relationship of the maxillary and mandibular teeth into which the patient tends to close from long standing habit. It often does not coincide with centric relation.

adhesion—The physical attraction between unlike molecules. Exemplified by two glass cement slabs, separated by a thin film of water, which tend to adhere to one another.

adjustment—The alteration of a prosthesis to make it more comfortable or so that it will function more efficiently.

alginate—A salt of alginic acid. An irreversible hydrocolloid impression material made up of salts of alginic acid together with various fillers and modifiers.

altered cast—*See* cast.

alveolar bone—The bone which surrounds and supports the natural teeth.

alveolar ridge—The ridge of bone formed collectively by the sockets of the teeth.

alveolus—The bony socket which envelops the root(s) of the teeth.

amorphous—Refers to the internal structure of a substance. An amorphous substance is distinguishable from a crystalline structure by the fact that the molecules of the latter are organized in a regular fashion in space (a space lattice), whereas the molecules of an amorphous substance are distributed in random fashion. Most dental waxes are amorphous, while metals and alloys are crystalline in structure.

anatomic crown—The part of the tooth that is covered with enamel.

anatomic tooth—An artifical posterior tooth which is designed to conform generally with the anatomy of the natural molars and bicuspids.

anatomical articulator—An instrument which can be adjusted to simulate closely the movements of the mandible.

angular cheilosis—The occurrence of fissures at the corners of the mouth caused by a vitamin (riboflavin) deficiency and exacerbated by a closed vertical dimension. Same as perleche or cheilosis.

anneal—The process of softening a metal by the controlled application of heat. An annealed gold alloy is soft and ductile.

anti-Monson curve—An occlusal plane which is convex upward instead of the conventional concave configuration.

approach arm—The minor connector that unites a bar type clasp with the framework.

aptyalism—Hyposecretion of saliva. It can result following ingestion of certain drugs, or from dehydration associated with fever or from diabetes. It may occur in the elderly without a systemic basis.

arch form—The contour of the dental arch, often classified as square, tapering, or ovoid.

arrow point tracer—The device used to scribe the gothic arch or arrow point tracing.

arrow point tracing—The lines created on a marking plate by a pointed scriber which represent the movements of the mandible. The point of the arrow indicates the most retruded, unstrained position of the mandible from which lateral movement can be made.

articulate—To bring together by means of a joint.

    articulate casts—To bring together the maxillary and mandibular casts. To mount the two casts on an articulator with the teeth properly intercuspated.

    articulate teeth—To arrange the maxillary and mandibular artificial teeth so that they intercuspate properly with one another.

articulator—A mechanical joint which holds the maxillary and mandibular casts in proper relationship to one another.

artificial denture—*See* denture.

artificial stone—Gypsum which has been calcined more slowly than plaster, so that the grains are much less porous. As a result, the stone is much harder and more durable than is plaster.

atrophy—A diminution in size of an organ or cell which has previously attained its natural size. It may be physiological or pathological.

attrition—A wearing away by friction.

autopolymer—A type of methyl-methacrylate which reaches a polymerized state as a result of the action of a chemical catalyst rather than heat.

autopolymerizing resin—*See* resin.

axial surface—A tooth surface that lies in a plane that is parallel to the long axis of the tooth.

axis—An imaginary line passing through a body, around which the body may rotate or have a theoretical potential of rotating.

B

back-action clasp—*See* clasp.

backing—The metal plate constructed to fit and retain the slot or pins of the porcelain or plastic facing. It may be manufactured or fabricated in the laboratory.

Baker B metal—A low-fusing metal sometimes employed in the dental laboratory.

balanced occlusion—*See* occlusion.

bar—A major connector employed to unite the two sides of a prosthesis.

bar clasp—*See* clasp.

basal seat—The area of oral mucosa which is covered by the base of the denture.

baseplate—The temporary denture form employed to obtain the interocclusal records and to hold the artificial teeth for try-in.

Bennett movement—The lateral bodily shift of the working side condyle as the mandible moves in a lateral excursion.

Bergstrom point—Bergstrom believed that the hinge axis of the condyle can be located on the skin of the face by measuring 10 mm. anterior to the center of a spherical insert for the external auditory meatus and 7 mm. below the Frankfort horizontal plane.

BHN—*See* Brinell hardness number under hardness.

biomechanics—The combination of biologic and mechanical laws and their interrelationship.

biometrics—The application of statistical methods to biological phenomena.

biscuit bite (mushbite)—A wax record of the supposed relationship of the jaws made by interposing a bulk of softened wax between the teeth or the edentulous ridges and instructing the patient to close into centric occlusion.

bite—The relationship of the jaws in centric occlusion.

bite block—The wax or compound rim that is attached to the baseplate which is used to record interocclusal relationships, and into which the artificial teeth are arranged for try-in.

bitefork (transfer fork)—The part of the facebow which is used to attach the occlusion rim or the wax record to the facebow.

bite rim (occlusion rim)—Same as bite block.

blockout—The process of eliminating undesirable undercuts from the master cast prior to duplication.

blockout tool—A tool used in the surveyor to shape the blockout wax around the abutment tooth.

body (of the clasp)—The part of the circumferential clasp formed by the junction of the occlusal rest, the shoulders, and the minor connector.

Boley gauge—A vernier type instrument calibrated in millimeters which is used for various dental measurements.

bolus—The comminuted mass of food and saliva prepared for swallowing.

Bonwill triangle—An equilateral triangle with the base corners in the center of each condyle and the apex at the mesial edge of the lower central incisors. Bonwill believed the average length of the sides to be 4 inches.

border molding—The shaping of the impression material by the tissues which function against and around the peripheral borders of the denture base.

border seal—Contact of the denture border with the adjacent soft tissue in such a manner as to exclude air from the interface of the two substances.

boxing—The matrix of wax which is wrapped around the impression for the purpose of confining the gypsum material while the cast is poured.

bracing—Resistance to horizontal or lateral force.

bracing arm—The reciprocal arm of the clasp.

bridge—A fixed partial denture.

broken stress bridge—Same as semi-rigid bridge.

Brinell hardness number—*See* hardness.

bruxism—The rubbing or grinding of the teeth together. It is usually done at night but may be practiced at any time.

bruxist—One who habitually grinds the teeth together.

buccal corridor—Same as buccal vestibule.

buccal flange—The portion of the denture base that lies adjacent to the cheek.

buccal notch—The V-shaped notch in the impression or in the denture flange formed by or for the buccal frenum.

buccal vestibule—*See* vestibule.

buccinator muscle—The cheek muscle.

butt—To position or fit the surfaces of an object directly against the surface of another object. Same as abut.

butterfly clasp—*See* clasp.

butterfly partial denture—*See* denture.

C

Camper's line—The imaginary line which connects the inferior border of the ala of the nose with the superior border of the tragus of the ear.

cancellous bone—A type of bone which contains many air spaces.

cantilever bridge—A fixed partial denture which has only one abutment. Sometimes referred to as a wing bridge.

carbon marker—A graphite point which fits the surveyor spindle, used to mark the survey line on the abutment tooth of the cast being surveyed.

carnauba wax—A type of wax obtained from the South American palm tree. It is a constituent of some dental waxes and impression materials.

cartilage—The gristle or white nonelastic connective tissue attached to the articular surfaces of bone.

case—A generic term sometimes used to refer to a patient for whom a prosthesis is being made, or at other times to the prosthesis itself.

cast—A positive replica of an object.

altered cast—A cast made from the master cast upon which the areas of residual ridge have been recorded by means of a functional impression technique.

corrected cast—Same as altered cast.

diagnostic cast—The cast upon which the planning and design of the prosthesis are accomplished. Same as study or planning cast.

duplicate cast—A cast made from an impression of another cast, usually (but not necessarily) used to designate the refractory cast.

investment cast—A cast made by duplicating the master cast in refractory material after it has been blocked out and relieved.

master cast—The accurate replica of the mouth, obtained after all required treatment and mouth preparation have been completed. It represents the mouth as it is to be fitted by the prosthesis.

planning cast—Same as diagnostic or study cast.

processing cast—The cast which is made by the laboratory from the master cast, upon which the denture bases are processed on the framework so that master cast is preserved. The processed denture can then be returned to the dentist on the master cast.

refractory cast—A cast duplicated from the master cast in investment material that will withstand the heat of the oven during burnout and casting. Same as investment cast.

study cast—The preliminary cast upon which the analysis and planning for the removable partial denture is accomplished. Same as diagnostic or planning cast.

casting—A metallic object made by forcing molten metal into a gypsum mold.

catalyst—A chemical substance capable of starting a chemical reaction without entering into the reaction itself.

centimeter—The one-hundredth part of a meter; about two-fifths of an inch

central bearing point—The upright part of the central bearing device which concentrates the forces generated between the upper and lower jaws at a point near the center of the two jaws.

central fossa—The shallow, rounded depression found on the molars in the approximate middle of the occlusal surface.

central sprue—The principal sprue.

centric checkbite—A positional record taken in wax, plaster, or zinc oxide paste which is used to position the casts accurately in centric relation.

centric occlusion—*See* occlusion.

centric relation—The relationship of the mandible to the maxilla when it is in its most retruded, unstrained position, at an established vertical dimension from which it can make lateral movement.

characterization (of the denture)—The individualization of the denture by adding color or altering contour for the purpose of making it more natural and lifelike.

Chayes attachment—A precision attachment designed by Dr. Herman Chayes and manufactured by the J. M. Ney Co.

checkbite—A positional record taken in wax, plaster, or zinc oxide paste used to position the casts accurately to one another.

cheilosis—Fissuring of the skin at the angles of the mouth with inflammation. It is considered a symptom of riboflavin deficiency and may be aggravated by a closed vertical dimension of occlusion.

cingulum rest—*See* rest.

circumferential clasp—*See* clasp.

clasp—An extracoronal direct retainer employed to retain, support, and stabilize the removable partial denture.

back-action clasp—A circumferential type of clasp designed so that the minor connector attaches at the terminal instead of at the body of the clasp.

bar clasp—A clasp design in which the retentive terminal approaches the undercut area of the abutment tooth from a cervical direction. Also called Roach clasp.

butterfly clasp—A synonym for an embrasure clasp.

circumferential clasp—A clasp designed so that the retentive clasp arm approaches the undercut from an occlusal direction.

combination clasp—A cast circumferential type clasp in which the retentive arm is made of wrought wire.

continuous lingual clasp—Same as Kennedy bar or double lingual bar. It is actually not a clasp but a major connector.

DeVan clasp—A clasp design in which the retentive arm approaches the undercut from a cervical direction and engages the proximal surface of the tooth.

double Aker's clasp—An embrasure clasp.

E clasp—A bar type clasp the configuration of which corresponds roughly to the letter "E."

embrasure clasp—A clasp which is, in effect, two circlet clasps joined at the body. The body crosses the occlusal embrasure of adjoining teeth, and the clasp arms extend mesially and distally to encircle both teeth. Same as double Aker's clasp.

hairpin clasp—Same as reverse loop clasp.

infrabulge clasp—A clasp designed so that the retentive terminal approaches the undercut from a cervical direction.

L clasp—A bar type clasp the configuration of which corresponds roughly to the letter "L."

mesiodistal clasp—A circumferential type of clasp which engages the mesial and distal surfaces of an anterior tooth from the lingual aspect.

reverse approach circlet clasp—A simple circlet clasp which engages the tooth from mesial to distal surface instead of the more conventional distal to mesial.

reverse loop clasp—A circumferential type clasp in which the retentive arm begins in the shoulder in the conventional manner but then descends and doubles back to engage an undercut on the same side of the abutment tooth.

ring clasp—A circumferential type clasp, similar to the back-action clasp, which has an additional strut or auxilliary brace extending from the framework to the clasp arm approximately midway in its length.

Roach clasp—Same as bar type clasp. The retentive terminal approaches the undercut from a cervical direction.

simple circlet clasp—Same as Aker's clasp.

T bar clasp—A bar type clasp in which the retentive element is shaped much like the letter "T."

vertical projection clasp—Same as bar type clasp.

Y clasp—A bar type clasp shaped to conform roughly to the letter "Y."

clasp arm—The part of the clasp which originates in the body and partially encircles the abutment tooth.

clinical crown—That portion of the crown of the tooth which is exposed above the enveloping mucosa.

cold curing acrylic resin—A methyl-methacrylate that polymerizes without being subjected to heat.

combination clasp—*See* clasp.

comminute—To grind and shred food prior to swallowing.

commissure (of the lips)—The point of union of the upper and lower lips.

compact bone—Bone in which the marrow spaces are fewer and smaller; hence the bone is more dense than is cancellous bone.

compensating curve—The antero-posterior curve that is incorporated into the alignment of the occluding surfaces and incisal edges of artificial teeth, which simulates the curve of Spee in the natural dentition.

complaster—A combination of approximately equal parts of plaster and coarse pumice, used to form a matrix for the impression so that it can be easily boxed for pouring of the cast.

condylar guidance—The part of the articulator which provides the path for the condyle of the articulator so that it can simulate, to greater or lesser degree, the movements of the natural condyle in the temporomandibular fossa.

condyle (mandibular)—The rounded process of the mandibular ramus which articulates with the temporomandibular fossa of the temporal bone.

continuous lingual clasp—*See* clasp.

coronal plane—A plane that is parallel to a line which divides the body into two equal halves: an anterior and a posterior.

corrected cast—*See* cast.

cul-de-sac (blind pouch)—The labial and buccal vestibules.

cuspid protected occlusion—Contact between the maxillary and mandibular cuspids only in lateral excursions of the mandible as distinguished from contacts by groups of posterior teeth.

D

Dalbo attachment—A type of precision attachment.

D-E hinge—A type of stressbreaker attachment.

deflective occlusal contact—A contact between occluding tooth surfaces which tends to shunt the mandible laterally from its normal path of closure into centric occlusion.

delayed denture—*See* denture.

dentimeter—An instrument used to measure the circumference of a tooth.

dentulous—With teeth.

denture—A set of teeth.

artifical denture—An artificial replacement for one or more missing natural teeth.

butterfly partial denture—A synonym for a prosthesis which is usually temporary, claspless, and made of acrylic resin, which replaces anterior teeth only.

delayed denture—A conventional denture as opposed to an immediate denture.

duplicate denture—A second denture made as

near like the first denture as possible, and usually intended to be used as a substitute for the first denture.

immediate denture—A denture that is constructed prior to extraction of the teeth that are to be replaced and is inserted immediately following extraction of the teeth.

implant denture—A denture that depends for its retention on a metal substructure which is closely adapted to the bone. The substructure has several projections which protrude through the mucosa to support and retain the denture.

interim denture—A dental prosthesis made to be used for a short, planned period of time as a cosmetic facade.

provisional denture—A term used to designate a temporary prosthesis made as an interim measure to help the patient become accumstomed to an artificial replacement. Same as temporary denture.

removable partial denture—A prosthesis that replaces one or more, but less than all of the teeth, which can be inserted and removed by the patient at will. Usually it is retained by either clasps or by precision attachments.

temporary denture—A prosthesis employed to provide the patient with a tideover cosmetic facade until missing anterior teeth can be restored with a more definitive type of replacement.

transitional denture—A removable partial denture which is meant to serve a short period of time preparatory to removal of the remaining teeth and construction of a complete denture.

treatment partial denture—A temporary removable partial denture, the main purpose of which is to aid in accomplishing some phase of the overall treatment.

unilateral partial denture—A partial denture that is confined to only one side of the arch.

denture brush—A brush especially designed to facilitate the cleansing of the denture. May be designed for a complete denture or for a removable partial denture.

design—The structural makeup of the removable partial denture. The configuration of the framework.

desiccate—To dry.

DeVan clasp—*See* clasp.

developmental groove—A groove in a tooth caused by the merging together of two lobes of the tooth during its development.

diagnosis—The art of identifying a disease from its signs and symptoms. An investigation or analysis of the cause or nature of a condition, situation, or problem. A state-

ment or conclusion concerning the nature or cause of some phenomenon.

diagnostic cast—*See* cast.

diastema—A space between adjacent teeth.

diatoric—The slot or hole designed in artificial porcelain teeth for the purpose of retaining them in the resin of the denture base.

die—A positive replica of an object, such as a tooth, in some hard substance such as stone or metal.

direct retainer—*See* retainer.

distal—Away from the midline.

disto-occlusion—The type of occlusion in which the mandible is in distal relation to the maxilla.

distoversion—Displacement of a tooth in a distal direction from its usual position in the dental arch.

double Aker's clasp—*See* clasp.

double casting—The process of casting an addition to an already fabricated metal prosthesis.

double lingual bar—The auxiliary bar which lies on the cingula of the mandibular anterior teeth. Same as Kennedy bar or continuous lingual clasp.

drag—The lower, model side of the denture flask.

drift—The migration of a tooth away from its normal position in the arch.

ductility—The property of a metal or alloy which permits it to be drawn into a wire without breaking.

duplicate cast—A cast which has been made from an impression of another cast.

duplicate denture—*See* denture.

durometer—An instrument for measuring the hardness of a substance.

dysfunction—Impaired function.

E

E clasp—*See* clasp.

eccentric—Deviating from centric.

edentulous—Without teeth.

elastic limit—The maximum stress to which a metal may be exposed and still return to its original dimension.

electromyography—The detection and recording of the electric currents that are produced in muscle tissue as a result of its activity. It has been used to establish the vertical dimension of rest position.

embrasure clasp—*See* clasp.

encirclement—The envelopment of a tooth by a clasp around more than half of the circumference of its crown.

equilibrate (occlusion)—The process of altering the contours of the teeth for the purpose of placing the occluding surfaces more in harmony with one another.

erosion—Superficial destruction or wearing away of tooth substance by chemical means, most often the labial and buccal surfaces.

esthetics (aesthetics)—Pertaining to beauty of form and color. The pleasing aspects of a dental composition. Generically, the appearance of a prosthesis in the mouth.

etching—The demineralization of enamel evidenced by a roughening of the surface.

etiology—The factors which are responsible for the existence of a disease or condition.

extraoral tracer—A Gothic arch tracing device which extends outside the mouth.

extrusion—The eruption of a tooth beyond its normal position in the occlusal plane. Overeruption.

F

facebow—A caliper-like instrument used to transfer the relationship of the maxilla and the condyle from the mouth to an articulator.

facet—A flattened area on a tooth caused by wear.

facing—A thin wafer of porcelain or plastic that closely fits a metal backing which is attached to the prosthesis. The facing may be attached to the backing by a key/keyway device or by pins.

female attachment—Female part (of the precision attachment); the hollow part (slot or channel) into which the male part fits.

festoon (verb)—The act of carving the denture wax or resin to simulate natural contours.

festooning or festoons (noun)—The carving created in the denture or the denture wax up to simulate nature.

final impression—*See* impression.

fineness—The proportion of pure gold in a gold alloy, expressed in parts per thousand. *Example:* an alloy of 500 fine is one-half pure gold.

finish line—The special preparation of the metal framework to create a smooth junction in areas where the acrylic resin and the metal come together.

flange—The section of the denture base which extends from the teeth to the peripheral border.

flash—The overflow of base material which results from overfilling the denture mold during the packing process.

flask—The metal container in which the wax pattern for a restoration (denture, crown, etc.) is invested.

> **casting flask**—One used to invest a wax pattern that is to be cast in metal.
>
> **denture flask**—A sectional container in which the denture is invested during its fabrication.

flat plane tooth—A nonanatomic denture tooth. One without cusps.

fornix (of the vestibule)—The reflection of the cheek onto the alveolar process in the depth of the vestibule. Same as mucobuccal fold.

fovea palatina—Small indentations in the area of the junction of the hard and soft palates formed by a coalescence of mucous glands.

Fox plate—A device used to establish the occlusal plane with the occlusion rims.

framework—The metal skeleton of the partial denture.

Frankfort plane—A line extending between the porion (the roof of the external auditory meatus) and the orbitale (the deepest point in the margin of the orbit).

free gingival margin—The gingival tissue which immediately surrounds the tooth and which lies occlusally or incisally to the floor of the gingival sulcus.

freeway space—The space between the occlusal surfaces of the maxillary and the mandibular teeth when the mandible is in rest position.

French posterior—A type of nonanatomic tooth named for its designer.

friable—Brittle.

fulcrum—The support upon which a lever rests when a force is applied.

fulcrum line—The imaginary line which passes through the abutment teeth, around which the denture would rotate were it not prevented from doing so.

functional chew-in—A technique in which the patient chews on a wax occlusion rim to produce a record of movement of the opposing teeth.

functional impression—*See* impression.

functionally generated path—The pattern

formed in an occlusion rim by the natural teeth of the opposing arch, which represents the functional movements of the mandible.

functional impression—An impression method in which functional pressures are simulated as the impression is being registered.

functional occlusion—*See* occlusion.

Functional posterior—An artificial tooth of the semianatomic type. It is distinguished by having the appearance of a worn natural tooth.

G

gelation—Solidification of a liquid substance in which a gel is formed, acting as a matrix between the undissolved particles.

generated path—A record of mandibular movement made by the teeth of one arch occluding with a wax or compound occlusion rim in the opposing arch.

genial tubercle—Small elevations on the lingual surface of the mandible at the midline into which the geniohyoid muscles insert.

geriatrics—The branch of medicine which deals with the medical problems of the aged.

gerodontics—The branch of dentistry which deals with the dental problems of the aged.

gingival bar—The truss arm which lies on the residual ridge, connecting two teeth on opposite sides of the arch. The bar is usually attached to crowns on the teeth by means of solder. Also called a splint bar.

gingival crevice—The trough formed between the tooth and the mucosa by the attachment of the gingiva to the tooth.

glaze—The surface gloss imparted to porcelain by the final firing at high heat.

glenoid fossa—The depression in the temporal bone which provides the articular surface for the mandibular condyle.

gnathion—A reference point on the anterior surface of the mandible at the midline. Closely related to, but not the same, as pogonion and menton.

gnathology—The study of the masticatory system.

Gothic arch—The tracing scribed by movement of the mandible with a tracing device which resembles an arrow point. Also likened to the sharp, pointed arch, typical of a style of Gothic architecture.

grain—The basic unit for weighing gold alloy. There are 24 grains in a troy pennyweight,

20 pennyweights in a troy ounce.

grain growth—The merging of smaller grains into larger grains which takes place during prolonged heating of a metal.

grind-in—The process of eliminating occlusal disharmonies by grinding the occlusal and incisal surfaces of the denture teeth. May be accomplished on the articulator, in the mouth, or in both.

Grittman articulator—A type of dental articulator named for its inventor.

group function—The contacts between groups of opposing posterior teeth in functional excursions of the mandible, as distinguished from a cuspid protected occlusion in which only the cuspids are in contact.

guide plane—The prepared axial surfaces of the teeth against which the removable partial denture glides as it is inserted and removed from the mouth.

gutta-percha baseplate—A baseplate manufactured of a latex type material that is adapted to the cast by heating and pressing it into place.

Gysi Simplex articulator—A type of articulator with nonadjustable condylar and incisal guides to permit average movement.

Gysi Trubyte articulator—An adjustable type of articulator named for its inventor.

H

hairpin clasp—*See* clasp.

Hall tooth (Hall's inverted cusp tooth)—A type of nonanatomic tooth named for its inventor.

Hamular notch—The fissure formed at the junction of the maxilla and the hamular process of the sphenoid bone. Same as pterygomaxillary notch.

Hanau articulator—An adjustable type of articulator named for its inventor.

hardness—Resistance to indentation or scratching.

Brinell hardness number—A measure of the hardness of the softer metals such as gold, silver, and copper. Often abbreviated BHN.

Knoop hardness number—An index of the hardness of a material. Employed for brittle materials such as porcelain and enamel.

Rockwell hardness number—A measure of the hardness of a metal or alloy. Used with metals that are too hard to be measured with the Brinell needle. *Example:* the chromium-cobalt alloys.

Vickers hardness test—A test of the hardness of an object. Made by measuring the indentation made by a pyramidal-shaped diamond point under various loads.

Hardy tooth—A type of posterior plastic tooth with a metal insert, named for the dentist who conceived the idea and introduced it to the profession. Also serpentine tooth.

heat soaking—The process of allowing the invested wax pattern to remain in the oven at the burnout temperature for a prescribed period of time, in order to remove all of the carbon residue and to expand the mold properly.

heat treatment—In a broad sense, the annealing (softening) and the controlled cooling (hardening) of a metal or alloy. The term is often employed to refer to the hardening process alone.

heel (of the denture)—The posterior extremity of a denture. The heels correspond to the retromolar pad area of the lower and to the tuberosity area of the upper denture.

height of contour—The greatest circumference of the crown of a tooth in a given horizontal plane.

high heat investment—*See* investment.

high lip line—The approximate level of the upper lip (usually established on the occlusion rim) when the patient smiles.

hinge axis—An imaginary line extending through both condyles, around which the mandible can rotate without lateral, or forward movement.

hinge movement—The component of the opening and closing movement of the mandible completely devoid of translatory motion.

horizontal overlap—The overlapping in a horizontal plane of the maxillary teeth over the mandibular teeth.

horizontal plane—A plane that is parallel with the horizon and perpendicular to the saggital plane.

Hydrocal—Trade name for a form of gypsum (artificial stone) that is especially calcined to make it harder and more durable than plaster.

hydrocolloid—An elastic type impression material, made up of salts of alginic acid together with various fillers and modifiers.

irreversible hydrocolloid (alginate)—An impression material that gels by a chemical reaction and cannot be returned to its original form.

reversible hydrocolloid (agar)—An elastic type impression material that can be softened to a near liquified state by heat, hardened by cooling, and then resoftened by again applying heat. The process can be repeated indefinitely.

hydroscopic investment—*See* investment.

I

immediate denture—*See* denture.

implant denture—*See* denture.

impression—A negative likeness of an object.

final impression—The impression that is used to form the master cast.

functional impression—An impression that captures the supporting structures in the form that they will assume during mastication, deglutition, and other normal functions.

pickup impression—An impression in which an object such as a framework or a crown is lifted off the teeth by the impression material. When the cast is poured the object will be in its proper place on the cast.

primary (preliminary) impression—An impression taken for the purpose of constructing a customized tray in which the final impression will be registered.

sectional impression—An impression that is taken in sections. It is removed from the mouth in sections and assembled prior to forming the cast.

snap impression—Same as preliminary impression.

two piece impression—An impression taken in two separate steps with (usually) two different types of impression material. Example: the edentulous area of a mouth might be registered in zinc oxide-eugenol paste in an acrylic resin tray and the remaining natural teeth registered in another impression tray with alginate or rubber. The two impression trays are indexed to preclude movement or distortion, between them as the cast is poured.

impression compound—A material made up of synthetic resins that may be employed in various impression techniques.

incisal guidance—The contacting surfaces of the anterior teeth (labial of the mandibular and lingual of the maxillary) which influence condylar movement.

incisal guidance (of the articulator)—The metal plane upon which the incisal pin rests and upon which it moves when the upper member of the articulator is moved about to simulate mandibular movement.

incisal rest—*See* rest.

index—A record made in compound or plaster of two or more parts, so that they can be taken apart and then reassembled in their original positions by means of the index.

indirect retainer—*See* retainer.

induction heating—A method of melting a metal or alloy by means of an electric current of extremely high frequency.

infrabulge—The part of the crown of a tooth located below the survey line.

infrabulge clasp—*See* clasp.

infraocclusion—A term to describe a tooth which has failed to erupt into its normal position, with the result that it is below the occlusal plane.

injection molding—A process used to introduce, under pressure, the denture plastic into the mold through sprue holes.

interarch space—The vertical space between the residual ridges at a given degree of jaw opening.

interceptive occlusal contact—An interfering, premature contact between opposing teeth, which prevents proper closure into centric occlusion.

intercuspate—To interlock or fit together the cusps, grooves, fossae, and embrasures of opposing teeth.

interfacial tension—The attraction of two substances separated by a thin moisture film.

interim denture—*See* denture.

internal attachment—Same as precision attachment.

interocclusal record—A record, made in wax, compound, zinc oxide-eugenol paste, or plaster, of the teeth with the jaws in a desired positional relationship.

interocclusal space (gap) (freeway space)—The distance between the occlusal surfaces of the upper and lower teeth when the mandible is in rest position.

interproximal space—The space above and below the contact points between adjoining teeth.

intraoral—Within the mouth.

investing—The act of investing an object.

investment—A gypsum material used to envelope an object so as to form a mold into which a plastic material can be packed or a molten metal can be cast to form a dental restoration. Investment is also used to hold two metal objects in apposition so that they can be joined by solder.

high heat investment—A gypsum material compounded so that it can withstand the high heat of the burnout oven and of the molten metal.

hydroscopic investment—An investment compounded to expand a controlled amount when the mixed (but not set) investment is brought into contact with water.

investment cast—*See* cast.

ipsilateral—Situated on the same side of the dental arch.

irreversible hydrocolloid—*See* hydrocolloid.

K

Kennedy bar—Same as double lingual bar or continuous lingual clasp.

key/keyway device—A frictional type of direct retainer comprised of a slot or channel (keyway) that is fitted into the crown of an abutment tooth and a protuberant part (key) that is attached to the metal framework that closely fits into the slot.

kinematic facebow—A facebow designed so that the location of the hinge axis can be established and recorded on the skin of the face.

knife edge ridge—A residual ridge which, as a result of atrophy, has become abnormally thin and sharp.

Knoop hardness number—*See* hardness.

L

L clasp—*See* clasp.

labial—Pertaining to the lip.

labial bar—A mandibular major connector which has been positioned on the labial aspect of the mandible, rather than in the usual location for the major connector, lingual to the anterior teeth.

labial frenum—The cordlike fold of epithelium that attaches to the lips and to the alveolar ridge at or near the midline.

labial vestibule—*See* vestibule.

lamine dura—The inner bony wall of the tooth socket.

laminagraphy—A method of sectional radiography.

lamina propria mucosae—The sublayer of the oral mucosa. The oral mucous membrane is composed of two layers: the layer lining the mouth is the surface epithelium, and the underlayer is the lamina propria.

land—The area of plaster, stone, or investment which extends from the periphery of the lower half flasked denture to the edge of the denture flask.

lateral (incisor)—The anterior tooth located just distal to the central incisor.

lateral checkbite—An interocclusal record in wax or plaster of the occluded teeth with the mandible in a left or right working position.

ledging—1. The process of forming a ledge in the blockout wax on an abutment tooth of the master cast, as the area to be occupied by the retentive terminal of the clasp. 2. The technique of creating a ledge in the lingual surface of the wax pattern of a crown, to create a place to be occupied by the lingual (reciprocal) arm of a circumferential type clasp.

leverage—A mechanical principle in which the magnitude of a force is multiplied by extending the lifting force farther from a fulcrum and on the opposite side of the fulcrum from the object to be moved.

line angle—The angle formed by the union of two surfaces of a tooth. *Example:* The junction of the labial surface of an incisor with the mesial surface forms the mesiolabial line angle.

lingual—Pertaining to the tongue.

lingual apron—Same as lingual plate or lingual strap.

lingual frenum—The band of tissue that attaches the under surface of the tongue to the floor of the mouth.

lingual notch—The indentation in the lingual flange of a denture made by or created for the lingual frenum.

lingual plate—The solid metal portion of the framework which is a continuous extension of the lingual bar superiorly, to cover the cingula of the lower anterior teeth.

lingual rest—*See* rest.

lingual strap—*See* strap.

linguoversion—A tooth in a position which is lingual to its normal or customary position in the arch.

long axis—An imaginary line that might be drawn through the center of an object (a tooth) in a vertical plane.

low fusing alloy—One of the alloys that melts at extremely low temperature, such as Melotte's metal which melts at approximately 200° F.

lug—The occlusal rest is sometimes referred to as an occlusal lug.

luting—The process of attaching one object to another with melted wax.

M

magnetic stabilizer—Magnetized metal inserts which are manufactured to be incorporated into upper and lower complete dentures to aid in the retention. Inserts with the same magnetic charge are placed in each denture. The dentures thus repel one another which tends, theoretically at least, to stabilize both dentures.

major connector—A plate or bar which unites the two sides of a removable partial denture.

malar process—The zygomatic or cheek bone.

male attachment—The projecting part of a precision attachment made to fit the female part of the attachment.

malleability—The property of a metal or alloy which permits it to be extended in all directions without breaking.

malocclusion—An abnormal occlusion.

mandibular axis—Same as hinge axis.

mandibular protraction—A facial anomaly in which the gnathion lies anterior to the orbital plane.

mandibular retraction—A type of facial anomaly in which the gnathion lies posterior to the orbital plane.

masking—The process of camouflaging the metal parts of a prosthesis to prevent the metal from showing through a veneering material such as porcelain.

masseter muscle—One of the pairs of muscles of mastication which extend from the external surface of the angle of the mandible to the zygomatic process.

master cast—*See* cast.

mastication—The process of comminuting the food—chewing it up for swallowing.

Masticators—Trade name for a metal, mechanical type of posterior tooth.

maxillary protraction—A type of facial anomaly in which the subnasion lies anterior to the orbital plane.

mechanical tooth—An artificial tooth that conforms to a mechanical concept rather than to the anatomy of the natural teeth.

median palatine raphe—The fibrous band that extends along the midline of the hard palate.

Melotte's metal—A low fusing metal composed of bismuth, lead, and zinc.

melting point—The point at which a metal melts. Actually, melting of a metal takes place within a range of temperatures rather than at a fixed point of temperature.

melting range—The interval between the temperature at which the alloy begins to melt (the *solidus*) and the temperature at which it is completely molten (the *liquidus*).

meniscus—The disc of fibrocartilage that lies between the head of the condyle and its articulating surface in the temporal fossa.

menton—A reference point on the anterior aspect of the mandible at the midline. Closely related to, but not the same as, pogonion and gnathion.

mesial—Toward the middle of the arch; toward the midline of the mouth.

mesiodistal clasp—*See* clasp.

methyl-methacrylate—A synthetic resin widely used as a denture base material.

mill in—The final refinement of the occlusion done by placing abrasive paste on the occlusal and incisal surfaces of the teeth and moving the upper member of the articulator against the lower to simulate functional movements. It is sometimes accomplished intraorally with the dentures in place.

milled rest—A semiprecision type of direct retainer. A key/keyway type of attachment made in the laboratory, as distinguished from the manufactured type of attachment.

minor connector—The part of a removable partial denture framework which unites rests and clasps with the major connector.

modeling compound—Same as modeling plastic.

modeling plastic—An impression material widely used in prosthetic practice. Same as modeling compound.

modiolus—An area at the corner of the mouth which marks the fusion of several facial muscles with the buccinator.

modulus of elasticity—A measure of the stiffness of a metal or alloy. A high modulus of elasticity indicates stiffness.

monomer—The methyl-methacrylate liquid.

Monson curve—A curve of occlusion in which the biting surfaces of all the teeth conform to a segment of an 8-inch sphere the center of which is at or near the glabella. The plane of occlusion is thus concave upward.

mounting (noun)—The plaster or stone which attaches the casts to the articulator.

mounting (verb)—The act of attaching the casts to the upper and lower members of the articulator with plaster or stone.

mucobuccal fold—The approximate junction of the cheeks and lips with the alveolar process in the buccal vestibule. Same as vestibular fornix.

mucositis—Inflammation of the mucous membrane.

mucostatic—An impression philosophy which holds that the tissues should be registered in an impression while they are in a state of complete rest.

muscle trimming—A misnomer for border molding.

mushbite—An intraocclusal record of centric relation made by introducing a mass of soft wax between the edentulous jaws and guiding the mandible into closure. Same as biscuit bite.

mylohyoid ridge—A bony prominence located in the posterior region of the lingual surface of the mandible, to which the mylohyoid muscle attaches. It is an important landmark in obtaining the impression and in the fitting of a mandibular prosthesis.

N

nasion—A bony landmark, the junction of the nasal and frontal bones.

needle point tracer—Same as Gothic arch tracer.

Nesbett—A unilateral type of partial denture, usually replacing one tooth. Named after the dentist who introduced it to the profession.

Ney-Chayes attachment—A type of precision attachment named for the company that manufactures it and the dentist who introduced it to the profession.

NIC (noninterfering cusp) tooth—A type of nonanatomic tooth. Commonly referred to as "nicks."

noble metal—A metal not readily oxidized at room temperature. Gold is a noble metal.

nonanatomic teeth—Artificial teeth which do not conform in occlusal configuration to natural teeth.

O

oblique ridge—The transverse ridge of enamel which crosses the occlusal surface of the upper molars between the mesiolingual and the distobuccal cusps.

obturator—A prosthesis used to close an abnormal opening between the oral and nasal cavities.

occlude—To bring together, hence to bring the upper and lower teeth into contact.

occlusal equilibration—The process of refining and perfecting the intercuspating surfaces of the teeth.

occlusal plane—A theoretical plane which in an ideal occlusion would be touched by the incisal edges and occlusal surfaces of all the teeth except the maxillary lateral incisors.

occlusal rest—*See* rest.

occlusal stop—Same as occlusal rest.

occlusal vertical dimension—*See* vertical dimension.

occlusion—Intercuspation of the upper and lower teeth.

    balanced occlusion—An occlusion in which opposing anterior and posterior teeth of both right and left sides contact each other in function, so that tipping and dislodging stresses on the dentures are neutralized.

    centric occlusion—The relation of opposing tooth surfaces which provides maximum planned contact and/or intercuspation.

    functional occlusion—The intercuspation of the teeth during function.

    protrusive occlusion—The relationship of opposing teeth when the mandible is thrust forward so that the incisors are edge to edge.

    traumatic occlusion—An occlusion in which interceptive and deflective contacts have the potential of causing injury to the teeth and the periodontal apparatus.

    traumatogenic occlusion—Same as traumatic occlusion.

occlusion rim—Wax or compound platforms attached to the baseplates and used to establish intraoral records, principally vertical dimension and centric relation.

orthognathic—A normal relationship of the maxilla and mandible; neither prognathic nor retrognathic.

osteoporosis—A diminution of bone formation coupled with a withdrawal of minerals to produce a more porous bone. Bone so affected is translucent in the radiograph. It is usually of systemic origin and may be exacerbated by malnutrition, menopause, senescence, or disuse.

osteosclerosis—Increased bone formation which results in smaller trabecular spaces and increased radiopacity.

overbite—Vertical overlap of the maxillary over the mandibular teeth.

overjet—Horizontal overlap of the maxillary over the mandibular teeth.

ovoid arch form—A dental arch which is roughly oval in outline.

P

palatal bar—A type of major connector which unites the two sides of a maxillary removable partial denture. In common parlance, the bar is distinguished from the palatal strap by being narrower in width.

palatal strap—*See* strap.

Passavant's cushion (also pad)—A small bulge of soft tissue found on the posterior and lateral walls of the nasopharynx at the level of the soft palate. It aids in closing the opening between the nasal and oral cavities during the act of swallowing.

passivity—Refers to the state of inactivity of the partial denture clasp when the partial denture is in place but not in function.

path of insertion—The route traversed by a removable partial denture as it is inserted and removed from the mouth.

pathosis—A diseased condition.

pennyweight—One-twentieth of a troy ounce (abbreviated DWT).

periodontal apparatus—The enveloping structures of the teeth. Collectively, the lamina dura, the periodontal membrane, the gingival attachment, and the cementum.

peripheral roll—The border of an impression formed by the lips, cheeks, and floor of the mouth. Also, the same border of the denture.

perleche—Fissuring of the skin at the corners of the mouth accompanied by inflammation. May be a symptom of riboflavin deficiency and may be aggravated by a diminished vertical dimension of occlusion. The terms perleche and cheilosis are customarily used interchangeably.

philtrum—The depression on the surface of the upper lip in the midline just below the nasal septum.

physiological rest position—The position of the mandible when the muscles of mastication, the postcervical, the infrahyoid, and suprahyoid muscles are all in a state of balanced tonic contraction.

pickling—The removal of oxides from the surface of a gold alloy by the action of heat and acid or other pickling agent.

pickup impression—*See* impression.

pier—An intermediate or middle abutment in a bridge of three abutments.

Pilkington-Turner tooth—An anatomical type of artificial posterior tooth with a cusp angulation of 30°.

plane—A straight line drawn between two landmarks.

planigraphy—A method of sectional radiography.

planning cast—*See* cast.

Pleasure curve—A plane of occlusion in which the occlusal surfaces of the molars curve downward distally instead of upward. Same as anti-Monson or reverse curve.

pogonion—The most anterior point on the symphysis of the mandible.

polymer—Methyl-methacrylate powder.

polymerization—The chemical reaction which takes place between the powder and liquid as methyl-methacrylate cures.

pontic—The artificial tooth affixed between the abutments of a fixed partial denture.

post dam (noun)—The special provision incorporated into the posterior border of the upper denture for the purpose of sealing the denture against the resilient soft tissue at approximately the junction of the hard and soft palates.

post dam (verb)—The act of creating the post dam seal either in the impression or in the cast.

post dam bead—the narrow, elevated ridge of base material which is incorporated onto the tissue surface of the posterior border of the denture for the purpose of excluding air, thereby providing a seal.

precision attachment—A specially machined direct retainer for a removable partial denture. Consists of male and female parts, one of which is attached to the denture and the other to the abutment tooth.

precision rest—*See* rest.

primary impression—*See* impression.

primary stress bearing area—An area of the mouth which is especially suited to withstand heavy stress from a denture, for example, the buccal shelf of the mandible.

processing cast—*See* cast.

prognathic—A forward position of the mandible in relation to the maxilla.

proportional limit—The amount of stress that a metal will withstand before it is permanently stretched or bent. It is a measure of the strength or toughness of an alloy.

prosthesis—The artificial replacement of a lost body part.

prosthetics—The art and science of replacing lost body parts.

prosthetist—A person who engages in the construction of lost body parts.

prosthodontics—That branch of dentistry which is primarily concerned with the replacement of lost dental tissues and parts.

prosthodontist—A dentist who specializes in the practice of dental prosthetics.

protrusive checkbite—A registration, made with wax or similar material of the occlusion with the mandible in a forward position as in "biting a thread."

protrusive occlusion—*See* occlusion.

protrusive relation—The forward position of the mandible.

provisional denture—*See* denture.

pterygomaxillary notch (hamular notch)—The fissure formed by the junction of the maxilla and the pterygoid process of the sphenoid bone.

ptyalism—Hypersecretion of saliva. Normal flow of saliva in 24 hours is between 2 and 3 pints. In ptyalism the flow can reach up to 10 quarts in 24 hours.

Q

quadrant—One-fourth of the mouth or one-half of the dental arch from the midline back to the terminus of either arch.

quench—To plunge a hot casting into water or alcohol to cool it.

quick-cure resin—Same as autopolymerizing resin. A methyl-methacrylate that polymerizes without heat.

R

radiograph—An x-ray.

radiolucent—Bone which has large marrow spaces is easily penetrated by the x-rays. This produces an image on the radiograph which is gray or even black. Such an image is said to be radiolucent.

radiopaque—The x-ray cannot readily penetrate bone that has few and small marrow spaces, and the resulting radiograph is white or whitish gray or radiopaque.

Rational posterior—A type of artificial posterior tooth.

rebase—A method of refitting the denture in which the base material is completely replaced with new material without changing the position of the teeth.

reciprocal clasp arm—The arm of the clasp which opposes and counteracts the force exerted by the retentive arm.

reciprocate—To counteract a force with an equal and opposite force.

record base—The baseplate and occlusion rim employed to obtain interocclusal records.

refractory cast—*See* cast.

relief—The special provision made to reduce pressure in a given area. The most common example is the "relief" provided in the hard palate area of a maxillary denture.

relief chamber—A recessed area provided in the palate of a maxillary complete denture to eliminate or minimize pressure in the area covered by the relief.

reline—To resurface the tissue side of a denture to make it fit more accurately.

removable partial denture—*See* denture.

recess—The special preparation made in the surface of the abutment tooth or in a restoration, to house the occlusal (incisal, lingual, cingulum) rest.

residual ridge—The remnant of the alveolar ridge following extraction of the teeth.

resin—A term frequently used to refer to methyl-methacrylate.

    autopolymerizing resin—One which cures or polymerizes without the application of heat.

resorption—The reduction in size of an organ or tissue as a result of physiological or pathological processes.

rest—A projection of the clasp which lies in a prepared recess of the abutment tooth and acts to support and stabilize the removable partial denture.

    cingulum rest—The rest which engages a prepared recess in the cingulum of an anterior tooth.

    incisal rest—A projection of the clasp which lies in a prepared recess on the incisal edge of an anterior tooth. An incisal rest may also be designed independently of a clasp and employed as an indirect retainer.

    lingual rest—A rest which engages the lingual surface of (usually) an anterior tooth. Much less commonly, a lingual rest may lie in the lingual groove of a molar.

    occlusal rest—A projection of the clasp which lies in a prepared recess on the occlusal surface of a posterior tooth. Sometimes referred to as occlusal lug.

    precision rest—A key/keyway type of attachment for supporting, stabilizing, and retaining a denture.

rest position—The position of the mandible when the postcervical muscles, the muscles of mastication, and the infrahyoid and suprahyoid groups of muscles are all in tonic equilibrium.

rest seat—The prepared recess in a tooth created to receive the occlusal, incisal, or lingual rest.

rest vertical dimension—*See* vertical dimension.

restoration—A generic term sometimes used to designate an inlay, crown, bridge, partial denture, or even a complete denture.

retainer—A device used to secure the removable partial denture to the tooth.

    direct retainer—A clasp or precision attachment which acts directly on the abutment tooth to secure the removable partial denture in place.

    indirect retainer—A part of the removable partial denture that provides retention by resisting dislodging stress exerted against the denture on the opposite side of the fulcrum line.

retentive undercut—*See* undercut.

retrognathic—A relationship of the jaws in which the mandible is recessive and the maxilla is forward.

retromolar pad—A pear-shaped mass of soft tissue located just posterior to the last tooth. When the teeth are not present, it lies on the crest at the distal terminus of the residual ridge.

retromylohyoid area—The area in the alveolingual sulcus, just lingual to the retromolar pad, which extends lingually down to the floor of the mouth and posteriorly to the retromylohyoid curtain.

retrusion—Backward movement.

reverse approach circlet clasp—*See* clasp.

reverse curve—Same as anti-Monson or Pleasure curve.

reverse loop clasp—*See* clasp.

reversible hydrocolloid—*See* hydrocolloid.

ridge lap—The part of an artificial tooth that is abutted to the residual ridge when no flange is employed.

rima oris—The line formed by the junction of the lips.

ring clasp—*See* clasp.

Roach clasp—*See* clasp.

Rockwell hardness number—*See* hardness.

rugae—The elevated folds of mucosa which are situated just posterior to the anterior maxillary teeth in the anterior third of the plate.

S

saddle—The base of a removable partial denture.

sagittal plane—The plane that divides the body at the midline into two equal halves.

sanitary pontic—A conical shaped pontic contoured to allow a space between it and the residual ridge so that the saliva can wash beneath it and thus maintain cleanliness.

scribe—To make a mark with a scriber.

secondary stress bearing area—An area of the mouth not suited to bear the principal load of a denture, but which does contribute some measure of support. *Example:* the median palatine raphe.

sectional impression—*See* impression.

semianatomic tooth—A posterior tooth form that bears a resemblance to the natural bicuspids and molars but has been modified by reducing cusp height.

semirigid bridge—Same as broken stress bridge. A fixed partial denture in which one of the connections between the units is composed of a male and female joint which allows some movement, instead of the usual soldered joint.

serpentine tooth—*See* Hardy tooth.

setting expansion—The increase in size of a gypsum product which occurs as it sets or hardens.

setting time—The time necessary for a substance to harden or solidify.

setup (noun)—The arrangement of artificial teeth in the wax of the record base.

setup (verb)—The act of arranging the teeth in the record base for try-in.

shellac baseplate—A baseplate fabricated of shellac resin.

Shore durometer—An instrument for measuring the surface hardness of a relatively soft substance such as a dental plastic.

simple circlet clasp—*See* clasp.

slotted attachment—A precision attachment with a key/keyway arrangement.

sluiceways—Grooves which permit the escape of food from between occluding tooth surfaces during mastication. Same as spillways.

slurry—A fluid mixture of a partially dissolved solid in a liquid.

slurry concentrate—A concentrated solution of calcium sulfate used to accelerate the set of plaster when taking intraocclusal checkbites. It is made by grinding up discarded stone casts and collecting the slurry as it comes from the cast trimmer. The solution is permitted to set for 90 minutes, after which the liquid which accumulates at the top of the solution is poured off. It is then allowed to set overnight and the next day all but 1 to 1½ inches of the accumulated liquid is again poured off. Each time that the solution is used it must be shaken vigorously.

slurry water—A saturated solution of gypsum made by dissolving discarded stone casts in water. A dental cast can be wetted or soaked in such a solution without danger of being etched or partially dissolved.

smile line—The approximate vertical level of the patient's upper lip when he smiles. It is customarily indicated with a mark on the labial surface of the wax occlusion rim.

snap impression—*See* impression.

solder—To attach two metals or alloys together by means of a lower fusing metal and heat.

span—The distance between two abutment teeth.

specific gravity—The weight of a substance as compared with the weight of an equal volume of water.

spillways—The grooves and fissures in teeth which permit the crushed food to make an exit as the occluding surfaces are brought together. Same as sluiceways.

spindle—The perpendicular part of the cast surveyor containing a chuck which has been designed to hold the various tools, e.g., analyzing rod, undercut gauge.

spit plate—A one- or two-tooth temporary, or interim type, of claspless partial denture. A better term is interim partial denture.

splint (noun)—A device which unites two or more objects together. *Example:* two teeth. May be fixed or removable, rigid or flexible.

splint (verb)—The act of uniting two or more teeth with a restoration or restorations. Most commonly used to denote the uniting of two teeth with metallic crowns.

splint bar—The truss arm which lies on the residual ridge connecting two teeth on opposite sides of the arch. The bar is usually attached to crowns on the teeth by means of solder. Also called gingival bar.

split cast mounting—A method of cast mounting on the articulator. The sides or the base of the cast are grooved so that it can be removed from the articulator and then returned to its original position by means of these index grooves.

split cast mounting technique—A method of testing the accuracy of interocclusal records by means of index grooves which have been placed in the sides or the base of the cast prior to mounting it on the articulator.

split remounting plate—A manufactured device consisting of two machined metal plates which are held together by an interlocking key. One part is embedded in the base of the cast, the other part in the articulator mounting. By means of this device the cast can be easily removed and accurately replaced on the articulator at will.

spoon plate—A claspless type of interim partial denture usually replacing only one or two anterior teeth, so called because of its resemblance in contour to a spoon. It is retained altogether by interfacial tension and tongue control.

spot grinding—The process of perfecting the occlusion by marking premature occlusal contacts with carbon paper (or similar substance) and then removing the interferences with stones.

sprue—The wax or metal that is used to create the entranceway by which the melted metal is enabled to enter the mold. Also the metal which later fills these entranceways.

sprue former—The base to which the sprue is attached while the wax pattern is being invested in a refractory material.

stabilized baseplate—A baseplate which has been "lined" with a corrective impression material, such as zinc oxide-eugenol paste, to make it fit the mouth more accurately.

standard—The minor connector which connects the body of the clasp with the major connector. Same as strut.

stay plate—A one- or two-tooth claspless temporary denture.

Steel's backing—The base metal backing made to fit the Steel's facing.

Steel's facing—An interchangeable facing manufactured by the Columbus Dental Co.

stellite metal (alloy)—Refers to a group of extremely hard, corrosion-resistant alloys made up principally of chromium, cobalt, and tungsten.

stock impression tray—A manufactured impression tray.

strap—A connector, usually made of metal, used in fabrication of the removable partial denture.

   lingual strap—Same as lingual plate or lingual apron.

   palatal strap—A major connector which crosses the palate to unite the two sides of a maxillary removable partial denture. The strap is distinguished from the palatal bar by being considerably wider and thinner.

stressbreaker—A device placed between the clasp and the denture base of a removable partial denture which permits the base to move in function independently of the clasp.

stress checker—Same as stressbreaker.

strut—A minor connector.

study cast—*See* cast.

stylus—The tracer of a Gothic arch tracing device.

stylus tracing—The tracing made on a waxed (or smoked) surface by a tracer as the mandible moves about.

sublingual crescent—The crescent-shaped area in the floor of the mouth formed by the lingual wall of the mandible and the adjacent part of the floor of the mouth.

sublingual fold—The crescent-shaped area on the floor of the mouth following the inner wall of the mandible and tapering toward the molar regions. It is formed by the sublingual gland and the submaxillary duct.

subnasion—The point of the angle formed between the nasal septum and the upper lip.

substructure—The portion of an implant denture that lies between the oral mucosa and the bone.

suction chamber—Same as relief chamber.

superstructure—The part of an implant denture that lies above the mucosa and is supported by the substructure.

support—The resistance of a partial denture to a force which is primarily vertical in direction.

suprabulge—The portion of the crown of a tooth that is above the survey line.

surgical template—A translucent acrylic resin denture form made to fit the mouth as it will be when the teeth have been extracted. It is used as a guide for preparing the extraction site to receive the immediate denture.

survey line—The line marked on the abutment tooth of the cast which indicates the greatest circumference of that tooth in that horizontal plane.

surveying—The process of analyzing the planning cast for the purpose of establishing the structural details of the removable partial denture.

surveyor—The cast surveyor. The parallelometer used to analyze the planning cast in the design of the prosthesis.

swage—To shape a piece of metal or alloy by hammering or by exposing it to pressure between a die and a counterdie.

T

tail (of a clasp)—The minor connector which connects the body of the clasp with the major connector.

T bar clasp—*See* clasp.

tang—Synonym for tail of a clasp. A minor connector uniting clasp and bar.

tapered blockout tool—A tool for the surveyor which is shaped to produce a fixed degree of taper in the blockout wax on the master cast prior to duplication.

technique—A method of accomplishing an end; hence, a method of fabricating a prosthesis or a part of a prosthesis or of carrying out a clinical procedure.

temporary denture—*See* denture.

tensile strength—A measure of the resistance of a metal to breakage from a stretching or pulling force.

therapy—Remedial treatment of a bodily condition.

thermal expansion—The increase in size that takes place in a gypsum mold when it is brought up to a high heat in the burnout and casting process.

thermoplastic—A material which can be softened by heat and which hardens upon being cooled.

thermoset—A material, such as plaster, that hardens by a chemical reaction.

thirty-degree tooth—An anatomical type of posterior tooth. The cusp inclines form an angle of approximately 30° with the horizontal.

thirty-three degree tooth—An anatomical type of artificial posterior tooth.

three-quarter veneer—A crown which covers all but the labial surface of an anterior tooth. A three-quarter crown on a posterior tooth may cover all but the buccal surface of a maxillary tooth and all but the lingual surface of a mandibular tooth.

tilt—The position of a cast on the surveyor table relative to the horizontal plane.

tissue borne—Supported by the soft tissue instead of by a tooth.

tomography—A method of sectional radiography. The purpose is to show detail in a desired plane of an object by blurring the structures in other planes.

torus mandibularis—A bony eminence often found on the lingual surface of the body of the mandible, most commonly in the cuspid-bicuspid region.

torus palatinus—A bony prominence found in the midline of the palate.

tooth borne—Supported by abutment teeth.

torque—A rotational or torsional force.

tracer—A device used to scribe mandibular movements on a marking plate.

tracing device—Refers to a contrivance used to record the excursive movements of the mandible on a flat surface. Consists of a scriber which is attached to one arch and a recording table that is attached to the other arch. A Gothic arch tracer is a tracing device.

transfer fork—Same as bitefork.

transitional denture—*See* denture.

translatory movement—Uniform motion of a body in a straight line.

transverse ridge—The ridge of enamel found at the junction of the buccal and lingual ridges on the occlusal surface of a bicuspid or molar.

traumatic occlusion—*See* occlusion.

traumatogenic occlusion—*See* occlusion.

tray (impression tray)—A device designed

to carry the impression material into the mouth so as to register the impression.

tray compound—High fusing modeling composition especially suited for use as an impression tray.

treatment partial denture—*See* denture.

treatment plan—The detailed plan of clinical procedures listed in the sequence in which each one will be carried out.

triangular ridge—The ridge of enamel which extends from the tip of the cusp down into the central groove of bicuspids and molars.

troy weight—The system of weight used in weighing gold alloy. The basic unit is the grain, 24 of which equal 1 pennyweight.

truss bar—The metal structure that is laid across an edentulous space between two fixed partial denture abutments upon which is constructed a pontic.

tube tooth—An artificial tooth that has been fabricated with a vertical cylindrical channel in its center so that it can be fitted over a post in the metal framework.

tubercle (genial)—The small bony eminences found on either side of the midline on the lingual aspect of the mandible which provide for insertion of the geniohyoid muscles.

Twenty-degree Tooth—A trade name denoting a nonanatomical type of posterior tooth, sometimes described as a semianatomical tooth. The cusps form a 20° angle with the horizontal.

two piece impression—*See* impression.

U

ultimate strength—The greatest stress to which a metal or alloy can be exposed without rupture.

undercut—The contour of an object when a part of greater cross sectional diameter overlies a part of lesser cross sectional diameter.

    retentive undercut—An area of the abutment tooth below the height of contour into which the clasp tip can be placed to aid in the retention of the prosthesis.

    undesirable undercut—An undercut area on the abutment tooth which cannot be used to retain the clasp. The undercut may also be composed of bone or soft tissue and would be undesirable if it had the potential of interfering with a desired design of the prosthesis.

undercut gauge—A tool for the surveyor which is shaped so that it can be used to measure the amount of undercut on the abutment tooth in thousandths of an inch.

undesirable undercut—*See* undercut.

unilateral partial denture—*See* denture.

upright—The minor connector that unites the body of the clasp with the major connector.

utility wax—A soft wax usually provided in rope form which has a variety of uses in prosthetic work, both in the clinic and in the laboratory. One major use is to rim the impression tray.

V

Vacuatrol—Trade name for a mechanical device that employs a bell jar to exclude the air from a mix of a gypsum material.

vacuum fired—Refers to the fusing of porcelain in a furnace that excludes air.

vacuum mixing—A process of mixing a gypsum material in a vacuum for the purpose of eliminating air bubbles.

vault—The palate or roof of the mouth.

velum rubber—A gum rubber to which sulfur has been added. It becomes tough and elastic but never hardens. At one time it found extensive use in the fabrication of maxillofacial prostheses, but it has largely been replaced by the silicone and polyvinyl chloride materials for this purpose.

veneer—A thin layer.

veneer crown—A type of crown in which a minimum amount of tooth structure has been removed in the tooth preparation. Also used to designate a full cast crown in one surface of which a window has been prepared to receive a thin layer of porcelain or plastic.

vermillion border (of the lips)—The bright red portion of the lips. The mucous membrane which extends outside the mouth.

vertical dimension—A vertical measurement of the face between two arbitrarily selected points which are located for convenience in measuring, one above and one below the mouth, usually in the midline.

    occlusal vertical dimension—The vertical dimension of the face when the teeth or the occlusion rims are in contact in centric occlusion.

    rest vertical dimension—The vertical dimension of the face with the jaws in rest position.

vertical overlap—Extension of the maxillary teeth over the mandibular teeth.

vertical projection clasp—*See* clasp

vestibule—The pouch formed by the cheeks or lips and the alveolar ridge.

> **buccal vestibule**—The pouch formed by the cheeks and the buccal alveolar ridge. Same as buccal corridor.
>
> **labial vestibule**—The pouch formed by the lips and the labial alveolar ridge.

vibrating line—The imaginary line situated in resilient tissue at the posterior part of the palate which marks the border between moving and nonmoving tissue.

Vickers hardness test—*See* hardness.

vitrification—A stage in the firing of dental porcelain represented by complete fusion of the material.

V. O. Vitallium occlusal posteriors—Artificial teeth made of plastic into which has been incorporated a thin metal strip for the purpose of reducing wear of the plastic and making the teeth more efficient masticators. Same as Hardy tooth.

W

wash—The corrective impression material.

wax pattern—A structure formed in wax which will be invested to form the mold into which the metal is poured.

web type lingual bar—Same as lingual plate.

wing bridge—Same as cantilever bridge.

working bite (occlusion)—The contact relation of the upper and lower bicuspids and molars when the mandible is moved laterally and the buccal cusps are in an edge-to-edge relationship.

working cast—The cast of the mouth or section of the mouth upon which the laboratory work is accomplished.

X

x-ray—Used colloquially as both a verb and a noun indicating the act of making a radiograph and the radiograph itself.

xerostomia—Dry mouth. Lack of normal salivary flow caused by some abnormal bodily condition.

Y

"Y" clasp—*See* clasp.

yield strength—The amount of stress that a metal or alloy will withstand before it is permanently deformed.

Z

Zero Mould—A trade name for a nonanatomic type of denture tooth.

zero tilt—Refers to the position of the cast on the surveyor when it is parallel with the horizontal plane.

Index